PSYCHIATRY - THEORY, APPLICATIONS AND TREATMENTS

# BIPOLAR DISORDER

## SYMPTOMS, MANAGEMENT AND RISK FACTORS

# Psychiatry - Theory, Applications and Treatments

Additional books in this series can be found on Nova's website under the Series tab.

Additional e-books in this series can be found on Nova's website under the e-book tab.

# Health Psychology Research Focus

Additional books in this series can be found on Nova's website under the Series tab.

Additional e-books in this series can be found on Nova's website under the e-book tab.

PSYCHIATRY - THEORY, APPLICATIONS AND TREATMENTS

# BIPOLAR DISORDER

# SYMPTOMS, MANAGEMENT AND RISK FACTORS

NICKOLAS B. MOORE
EDITOR

New York

**Library of Congress Cataloging-in-Publication Data**

Bipolar disorder : symptoms, management and risk factors / editors, Nickolas B. Moore.
pages cm
Includes index.
ISBN 978-1-62618-666-8 (hardcover)
1. Manic-depressive illness. I. Moore, Nickolas B.
RC516.B5265 2013
616.89'5--dc23

2013013158

*Published by Nova Science Publishers, Inc. † New York*

# Contents

# Preface

Bipolar disorder is a psychiatric disease that involves profound changes in mood accompanied by severe changes in feelings, thoughts and behaviors wherein emotions can move quickly from a deep depression to excessive excitement without apparent reason. In this book, the authors present current research in the study of the symptoms, management and risk factors of bipolar disorder. Topics include face emotion processing deficits in pediatric bipolar disorder; understanding bipolar disorder from clinical expression to therapeutic strategies; brain-derived neurotrophic factors and neurocognitive profiles in the psychosis spectrum; understanding lived experience and personal recovery in people with bipolar disorder; computerized self-management in bipolar disorder; prescription drug Memantine in the long-term prophylaxis of treatment-resistant bipolar mood disorders; P11 expression and PET as potential biomarkers for bipolar disorder; and neurocognitive impairment in bipolar disorder.

Chapter I – Bipolar disorder is a psychiatric disease that involves profound changes in mood accompanied by severe changes in feelings, thoughts and behaviors: emotions can move quickly from a deep depression to excessive excitement, without some apparent reason. BD is usually a chronic condition and may last for life with recurring episodes that often occur during adolescence or early adulthood, sometimes during childhood and usually requires treatment for life. In the manic phase the disorder typically occurs in forms of exasperated disinhibition and manic symptoms may include: an euphoric or irritable mood, angry and reactive state of mind; increased activity and feelings of strength and energy; ambitious and grandiose aspirations; poor self-criticism; greater interest in sexual activity and reduction in hours of sleep and need for sleep. On the other hand, depressive phases may be so serious that can also lead to episodes of self-harm. Depressive symptomatology may include: depressed or apathetic mood; reduced strength in activities, thinking and talking; feeling of being hopeless and helpless; pessimistic approach to reality, sometimes, with suicidal thoughts; alteration in the rhythm of appetite and in sleep patterns. Although it is not known a definitive cure, BD is a very treatable disease that can be kept under control. Drugs play a key role in the care of persons affected by BD, in particular medications commonly used to treat the manic episodes of BD are mood stabilizers. During depressive episodes, people with BD can be treated with antidepressants by evaluating administration and dosage with extreme caution because of the risk to switch to a manic phase. In addition to medications, psychotherapy and psychoeducational approaches are essential for individuals suffering from BD. At present BD is considered a multifactorial etiology condition in which many physiopathogenetic factors are involved, thus researchers have identified several causes such as biological differences, imbalance of neurotransmitters and hormones, genetic predisposition, traumatic life events, stress and environmental factors.

Chapter II – Pediatric bipolar disorder (PBD) is a severe and often debilitating psychiatric illnesses. Prevalence estimates find a forty-fold increase in the diagnosis of PBD in outpatient settings over a recent 10-year span. Of the many impairments of PBD, social deficits may most impact daily functioning. Prominent psychosocial deficits include impaired peer relationships marked by few friends and difficulty keeping friends, and problems with regulating emotions. Understanding human facial emotions is critical for emotional and social understanding, especially successful social interactions and the building of social relationships. Recent empirical evidence suggests that PBD youth exhibit profound difficulties in labeling facial expressions and this deficient processing of facial expressions contributes to social impairments among PBD youth. Further, neurological data find that dysfunction within a distributed fronto-striatal-limbic network characterizes these face emotion processing deficits. This chapter reviews empirical evidence for face emotion processing deficits and associated neurocognitive impairments in PBD youth. In addition, the authors review evidence of face misperception in other childhood psychopathologies, including major depressive disorder (MDD), anxiety (specifically social phobia), and autism spectrum disorders (ASD). In doing so, they attempt to distinguish face emotion processing deficits in PBD from other childhood mental disorders, and discuss how this might inform differential diagnosis and perhaps serve as a target for psychotherapeutic intervention.

Chapter III – Background: There has been recent interest in the role of brain-derived neurotrophic factor (BDNF) in the pathophysiology and treatment of bipolar disorder and schizophrenia. BDNF plays a role in neuroplasticity by promoting neuronal growth, survival, differentiation, neurostructure, and neurofunction in several brain areas. Its specific neuroplasticity-related role in affective and non-affective psychoses has shown several commonalities that cast doubts on traditional Kraepelinian distinctions between bipolar disorder and schizophrenia. Method: The authors review relevant studies of BDNF gene polymorphisms and expression in people with bipolar disorder and schizophrenia compared to healthy controls that suggest its putative role in etiology, mechanism, and phenotypic expression in both disorders. Results: Studies suggest that peripheral BDNF is low in people with bipolar disorder and schizophrenia and BDNF concentrations are inversely correlated with symptom severity. At the DNA level, studies of the Val66Met single nucleotide polymorphisms (SNP) of the BDNF gene suggests that the Met allele is associated with neurocognitive deficits present in both disorders. In contrast, several studies suggest that the Val allele may be associated with symptom severity and the incidence of both bipolar disorder and schizophrenia. Conclusions: BDNF appears to be a shared biomarker of bipolar disorder and schizophrenia with demonstrable associations with incidence, clinical symptoms, and neurocognitive phenotypes. This state of affairs supports a latent dimension or spectrum model of affective and non-affective psychoses rather than the traditional categorical distinctions. Despite growing evidence of BDNF's role in the psychosis spectrum, questions remain about its reliability and validity as a clinical biomarker and predictor of bipolar disorder and schizophrenia.

Chapter IV – Objective: The concept of personal recovery (PR) as defined by those who live with mental illness has gained significant momentum and has been adopted as a key principle in mental health services internationally. The philosophy of PR views living with mental illness as a dynamic journey with an emphasis on hope, self-determination, and quality of life despite the presence of symptoms. This differs from the clinical definition of recovery (CR), which focuses on improvements in functional outcomes and may view mental illness as chronic and refractory. Research on PR has largely focused on people living with schizophrenia or mixed diagnostic samples. Over the past decade, however, there has been increasing interest in understanding PR in those who live with bipolar disorder (BD). A review of qualitative literature that captures the lived experience of those with BD and their views on PR will consolidate the knowledge to date in order to inform clinical practice, the direction of future research, and the self-management strategies of those affected by BD. Methods: A systematic review of qualitative studies focusing on the topic of PR in people with BD was conducted. Data compilation consisted of two parallel searches of identified databases by two independent researchers. Approximately 1000 original studies were identified, of which 24 met the following inclusion criteria for review: peer reviewed qualitative studies involving samples of people living with BD (mixed diagnosis samples were not eligible for inclusion), studies employing a psychosocial perspective, and studies published in English. A thematic analysis of the studies under review was completed, resulting in a descriptive narrative which identifies and interprets the main concepts and conclusions in the qualitative findings. Results: Four overarching themes were identified: the negative impact of BD; ambivalence in relation to living with BD, personal transformation as a result of lived experience, and wellness strategies that highlighted behaviours or practices that contribute to recovery in BD. The authors' literature review found that the lived experience of BD encompasses both positive and negative aspects. Coping and symptom management may present challenges, there may be ambivalence about the diagnosis of BD and its treatment, and self-esteem may be impaired. However, purpose, hope, and wellness seemed more achievable when the traditional definition of CR was broadened to include a PR perspective, which allowed people to transcend the otherwise seemingly contradictory experiences associated with BD.

Chapter V – Bipolar Disorder (BD) is a highly recurrent affective disorder characterised by periods of extreme mood, including depression and mania or hypomania. It has been identified in 2% of the population and is estimated to cost the UK £5.2 billion per year. There is increasing evidence that people with BD respond well to psychological interventions, evidenced by fewer relapses, improvements in social functioning and reduced hospital admissions. Despite this, few service users receive psychological intervention within routine clinical services. Computerised interventions are an innovative way of addressing the accessibility problem by providing highly accessible, around the clock, self-directed support. Despite numerous interventions being developed for 'mild to moderate' depression and the majority studies demonstrating clinical effectiveness, the development of this approach in BD is in its infancy. This is somewhat surprising considering there is evidence that self-management is effective in BD, the effective components of self-help and face-to-face psychological therapy can be translated into computerised therapy with a similar treatment effect and the treatment effect in depression has also been observed in 'severely' depressed sample subgroups. Results have recently been published from a pilot trial failing to find a statistically significant treatment effect, and three other trials have not yet published on effectiveness outcome. However, positive findings have been reported, demostrating the strongest improvement in psychological and physical domains of quality life, wellbeing and recovery outcomes. Recovery and quality of life outcomes despite being service user priorities, and recovery focussed approaches being halied as one of the key prorities for modernising mental health care, have not until now been the primary focus of interventions in this area. Interventions have tended to focus on relapse prevention, symptom management and medication compliance. The content, structure and support provided in these interventions may be an important predictor of outcome and may be related to acceptability. Statistically powered, hypothesis testing trials are urgently needed to tease these differences apart. Future research needs to focus on the cost effectiveness of such interventions, explore the mechanisms of change and consider the impact of individual components on outcome. The relevance of this approach for people not routinely accessing the internet for self-help would support translation of interventions into practice. This budding research field is starting to demonstrate the promise computerised treatment approaches have to feasibly deliver evidence based psychological intervention to a large number of people with BD. Such approaches are a current government priority to improve access to psychological interventions for people with 'severe' mental health problems.

Chapter VI – Memantine is a non-competitve NMDA receptor antagonist with a low affinity for the receptor and a voltage/use dependent action. Interestingly, it has been recently demonstrated that the drug by selectively blocking the extrasynaptic (excitotoxic) receptor but preserving the normal synaptic function has a neuroprotective action. It is currently used in the treatment of moderate to severe Alzheimer's Disease (AD). Although its efficacy on the AD patient's quality of life has proven to be moderate, several studies have demonstrated the excellent safety and tolerability profile of the drug. Moreover, Memantine has been used off-label in a number of neurological and psychiatric conditions, including depression, with conflicting and inconclusive results. The authors have recently suggested the use of memantine as an antimanic and mood-stabilizing agent in treatment-resistant bipolar disorder. This use is absolutely at variance with the prevalent hypotheses which take NMDA receptor antagonists to be potential antidepressant drugs (mainly on the basis of their effect on the forced swimming test). In keeping with the authors' hypothesis, based on experimental pharmacological evidence obtained in an animal model of bipolar disorder, the authors have observed a clinically relevant antimanic and sustained mood-stabilizing effect of memantine, as augmenting agent, in treatment-resistant bipolar disorders.

Chapter VII – Bipolar disorder (BD) is a complex, chronic psychiatric condition characterized by recurring episodes of depression and mania or hypomania. It is subdivided into BD-I and BD-II, based on the nature and severity of the mood episodes experienced. Substantial evidence demonstratesthat p11 (S100A10) and positron emission tomography (PET) are potential biomarkers for BD. For example, peripheral blood mononuclear cell (PBMC) p11 mRNA was over-expressed in BD compared with non-BD controls. Comparing BD patients to healthy controls (HCs), normalized glucose metabolism (NGM) was higher in the hippocampus, parahippocampus, and amygdala, but lower in the anterior cingulate cortex (aCC), medial prefrontal cortex (mPFC), dorsolateral prefrontal cortex (dlPFC), insula and thalamus. Compared to BD-II, BD-I had hypometabolism of glucose in the aCC, bilateral middle and inferior temporal gyrus, insula and striatum, and hypermetabolism of glucose in the left parahippocampus. In addition, PBMC p11 mRNA levels were significantly positively correlated with NGM in the mPFC, aCC, left insula, bilateral orbitofrontal cortex (OFC), and left middle, inferior and superior temporal gyri, and withthe number of depressive episodes in BD patients, especially in BD-I patients. These data demonstrate that PBMC p11 mRNA expression is associated with neural activation in the brain of BD patients and warrants a larger translational study to determine its clinical utility. In this chapter, the authors will discuss the background information of p11 as a potential biomarker for BD. In addition, the authors develop the concept of combining blood p11 levels with PET as biomarkers for BD diagnosis. The authors will also discuss the current status of this research, including methods, such as blood sample collection, mRNA purification, real time PCR and PET data analysis for BD biomarker identification. Specifically, they will discuss the strategies for developing a blood test and PET for BD diagnosis from bench to bedside and/or from bedside to bench, a two-way approach.

Chapter VIII – Bipolar disorder was once thought to be an episodic affective disease with complete inter-episodic remission. However research in the area of neurocognition has demonstrated varying degree of impairment even in the period of remission. Cognitive deficits within bipolar disorders have been studied and overall pattern of impairment in tests of attention, executive function, and verbal memory has become evident. Increased cognitive dysfunction often is associated with greater symptom severity as well as greater likelihood of poor social and vocational outcomes. The further effect of psychotropic medication on cognitive slowing remains a challenging issue. Consensus is lacking with respect to the use of mood stabilizers and antipsychotics towards their effect on cognitive impairment or therapeutic effects on neurocognition. Use of non-pharmacological options such as social skills training, cognitive-behavioral therapy and cognitive remediation needs to be further studied. Neuroimaging techniques have identified endophenotypic markers whose identification would help to identify at-risk individuals and facilitate early intervention.

In: Bipolar Disorder
Editor: Nickolas B. Moore
ISBN: 978-1-62618-666-8


*Chapter I*

# Better Understanding of Bipolar Disorder from Clinical Expression to Therapeutic Strategies

***Giuseppe Marano, Gianandrea Traversi, Carola Nannarelli, Salvatore Mazza and Marianna Mazza****
Department of Neurosciences,
Catholic University of Sacred Heart of Rome, Italy

## Abstract

Bipolar disorder is a psychiatric disease that involves profound changes in mood accompanied by severe changes in feelings, thoughts and behaviors: emotions can move quickly from a deep depression to excessive excitement, without some apparent reason. BD is usually a chronic condition and may last for life with recurring episodes that often occur during adolescence or early adulthood, sometimes during childhood and usually requires treatment for life.

In the manic phase the disorder typically occurs in forms of exasperated disinhibition and manic symptoms may include: an euphoric or irritable mood, angry and reactive state of mind; increased activity and feelings of strength and energy; ambitious and grandiose aspirations; poor self-criticism; greater interest in sexual activity and reduction in hours of sleep and need for sleep.

On the other hand, depressive phases may be so serious that can also lead to episodes of self-harm. Depressive symptomatology may include: depressed or apathetic mood; reduced strength in activities, thinking and talking; feeling of being hopeless and helpless; pessimistic approach to reality, sometimes, with suicidal thoughts; alteration in the rhythm of appetite and in sleep patterns.

* Corresponding author: Marianna Mazza, MD, PhD Department of Neurosciences, Institute of Psychiatry and Clinical Psychology UniversitàCattolica del SacroCuore di Roma Via Ugo De Carolis, 48 00136 Roma (Italy). Tel: +39 06 35348285. Fax: +39 06 35501909. E-mail: mariannamazza@hotmail.com, marianna.mazza@rm.unicatt.it.

Although it is not known a definitive cure, BD is a very treatable disease that can be kept under control. Drugs play a key role in the care of persons affected by BD, in particular medications commonly used to treat the manic episodes of BD are mood stabilizers. During depressive episodes, people with BD can be treated with antidepressants by evaluating administration and dosage with extreme caution because of the risk to switch to a manic phase. In addition to medications, psychotherapy and psychoeducational approaches are essential for individuals suffering from BD.

At present BD is considered a multifactorial etiology condition in which many physiopathogenetic factors are involved, thus researchers have identified several causes such as biological differences, imbalance of neurotransmitters and hormones, genetic predisposition, traumatic life events, stress and environmental factors.

**Keywords**: Bipolar disorder, depressive symptomatology, genetics, mania, psychotropic drugs, therapeutic management

## Abbreviations

BD: Bipolar Disorder
DSM-IV: Diagnostic and Statistical Manual of Mental Disorders fourth edition
TCAs: Tricyclic Antidepressants
SSRIs: Selective Serotonin Reuptake Inhibitors
SNRIs: Serotonin-Norepinephrine Reuptake Inhibitors
BDNF: Brain Derived Neurotrophic Factor
COMT: Catechol O-methyltransferase
NAS: Bipolar disorder not otherwise specified

## Introduction

Bipolar Disorder (BD) or manic-depressive disorder is a serious disease with complex origins. Hippocrates (Marneros A 2002) seems to be the first to discover BD linking to the black bile of melancholia with the yellow bile of mania. The idea of a relationship between mania and melancholia has been attributed to Aretaeus of Cappadocia (Marneros A 2002), who recognized that these two states had the same etiology, namely a dysfunction of the brain and other organs, and the possibility of switching between these two states in the same person at different times.

A first systematic and rigorous description of BD was made by the German psychiatrist Emil Kraepelin(Kraepelin 1921, Akiskal HS 2002), who introduced the term manic-depressive illness distinguishing it from dementia praecox otherwise schizophrenia (Sedler 1983). In addition, Kraepelin led to the manic-depressive illness not only the traditional forms of mania and melancholia, but also some recurrent depressive conditions that arose alternating with maniac episodes of reduced intensity, known as hypomania. He also described the temperamental dispositions such as hyperthymic, cyclothymic or irritable type, and understood the role of family history in the manic-depressive illness (Goodwin 2007).

Kraepelin's reflections helped to develop a concept of bipolarity that embraces clinical syndromes and identifies a bipolar spectrum also including persons who are potentially predisposed to develop bipolar illness and generally have a dysthymic, cyclothymic, hyperthymic or mixed temperament but should not be considered to have a form of overt disease.

Finally, BD may occur with multiple shades assuming an episodic character or expressing a constant character if it is a syndrome, but in any case it represents an alteration of well-being state with mood fluctuations. This results in an state of mental alteration entailing, on the one hand, psychological sufferance and, on the other hand, a failure in personal, relational, social and professional functioning.

For a long time elevated mood was related to creativity (Jamison 2011). Jamison (Jamison 1989) was interested in understanding the overlapping between hypomania and intense creative states in writers and artists such as Vincent Van Gogh, Virginia Woolf and Ernest Hemingway. Then other authors (Janka 2004, Hankir 2011) have analyzed the link between bipolarity and creativity supposing that artistic creativity was related to hypomanic states characterized by euphoria, increased self-esteem and little need for sleep. The link might exist, but it has not already been demonstrated conclusively (Johnson, Murray et al. 2012), because it has emerged mainly from studies of individual cases rather than from large epidemiological studies with a scientific solidity. In addition, the link does not seem to be linear, because creativity does not appear to be expressed in people suffering from severe mania but only in those who are affected by the milder forms. According to Johnson, the attitude of openness to new ideas and new experiences would be essential to the development of creativity as well as the extrovert attitude is characteristic of artists such as actors or musicians who express themselves through contacts with the public. From a neurobiological point of view, it seems that creativity can be supported by the neurotransmitter dopamine, a substance of mesolimbic area, whose alteration causes mood disorders responsible for the genesis of positive moods but also for phenomena related to maniacality.

## Bipolar Disorders: Symptoms and Diagnosis

Pathology occurs when the normal balance that links temperament, character, mood and personality changes for a specific period of time and pervasively involves the entire life of the person in such a way as to affect global functioning with physical, cognitive and behavioral alterations and changes in the ability to deal with the events and to relate with others.

According to the Diagnostic and Statistical Manual of Mental Disorders (DSM-IV-TR) (American Psychiatric Association 2000), BD is the fluctuation of mood between the depressive pole and the euphoric pole. BD is so called because causes pathological changes between two poles, one that involves an increase in mood, mania, and another that leads to a lowering of mood, depression. This differentiates BD from unipolar depressive disorder where mood changes tend to mood decline.

There are different types of BD. Bipolar I disorder is characterized by the presence of at least one episode of mania or a mixed episode with the co-occurrence of both manic and depressive symptoms, with or without psychotic features. Mania is defined as a distinct period of abnormally and persistently elevated, expansive or irritable mood, lasting at least one week, or if it is necessary hospitalization, of any duration. Bipolar II disorder is characterized by the presence of one or more major depressive episodes alternating with at least one spontaneous hypomanic episode. Hypomania looks exactly like mania but has a shorter duration of four days. The cyclothymic disorder is defined by alternating episodes of very rapid hypomanic and depressive episodes less severe than major depressive episodes. Bipolar disorder not otherwise specified (NAS) includes disorders with bipolar features that do not meet the criteria for any specific BD such as recurrent hypomanic episodes without intercurrent depressive symptoms, manic or mixed episode overlapping to delusions.

The cardinal symptoms of the depressive phase are depressed mood and an emotional state characterized by sadness, pessimism, hopelessness, apathy and anhedonia. Cognitive function may be compromised and the content of thought is focused on issues of worthlessness and guilt. The deep sadness and pessimistic view of the future can lead to suicidal thoughts or acts. The manic phase has an onset generally faster than the depression phase: it may occur within a few hours, but more often is preceded by several days of unusual expansiveness, talkativeness, hyperactivity or irritability. Mania is characterized by euphoria, grandiosity, decreased need for sleep, increased talkativeness, distractibility, greater interest in sexual activity and psychomotor agitation. Manic speech is typically accelerated, the content of thoughts is represented by ideas of magnitude with hypervaluation, and cognitive functions are impaired by distractibility, difficulty of synthesis and lack of judgment.

The exact cause of BD is not completely understood, but many authors are now convinced that it is a multifactorial disorder that occur when many factors act together to cause disease. The study of pedigrees of patients showed that BD is a familial disease, and this suggests that there is a genetic predisposition, although a specific gene has not been identified (Mick, Kim et al. 2008, Craddock and Sklar 2009). The latest research also corroborate the hypothesis that there is not a single gene responsible for the disease, but rather that many genes act together creating a predisposition that interacts with environmental factors and even some types of stress such as physical, sexual or emotional abuse, breaking of a sentimental relationship, events of loss and separation from significant figures (Mick and Faraone 2009).

Another described risk factor for affective disorders is temperament, it is assumed that specific profiles or temperamental traits may predispose to BD (Hedelin, Lof et al. 2010, Nilsson, Straarup et al. 2012), also through a progressive exposure to stressful life events. BD would represent the evolution of the structural characteristics of the subject, intended as specific affective predispositions as well as dysthymic, irritable, hyperthymic or cyclothymic temperaments. The cyclothymic temperament seem to be more closely related to the subsequent development of a BD (Kesebir, Vahip et al. 2005, Hedelin, Lof et al. 2010, Nilsson, Straarup et al. 2012).

At present both functional and morphological neuroimaging studies indicate the existence of alterations in the brains of bipolar patients, although clinical significance of these changes has not been fully elucidated (Kurnianingsih, Kuswanto et al. 2011). Neurotransmitters modifications play a relevant role in BD.

It has been established that the emotions lost in depression and hyperintense in mania are under the control of the mesolimbic dopamine system. Dopamine plays a crucial role in the control of desire, motivation to act and pleasure, it is involved as a mediator in the areas of mental functioning related to the individual's relationship with the environment and the subjective emotional resonance of that relationship. This does not exclude, of course, the possibility of an interaction between dopamine and other neurotransmitters (Blumberg, Kaufman et al. 2004).

Currently, in fact, there is a consensus in considering at the origin of the manic state activation, a multifactorial pathogenesis, in which various neurotransmitter systems act in functional interdependence. Probably, different neurotransmitters have a role in the pathogenesis of the various components of clinical depression and mania.

Both the functional dopaminergic and noradrenergic hypertone would be at the basis of raising mood, whereas the noradrenergic system would be primarily responsible for the cognitive impairment and surveillance, the dopaminergic system would be related to hyperactivity and particular ways of relating to the environment, the serotonergic hypotone would induce sleep disturbance, eating disorders and increase in libido (Blumberg, Kaufman et al. 2004, Eley, Liang et al. 2004).

Psychopharmacological research indicate, furthermore, the efficacy of antiepileptic drugs in the therapy of BD. This leads to the assumption of a mechanism of kindling at the basis of behavioral and affective alterations of bipolar patients.

Kindling is an animal model of epilepsy produced by focal electrical stimulation of the brain (McNamara 1986). It has been neurophysiologically defined (Cullen and Goddard 1975) as an high-frequency but subthreshold short electrical pulses that would sensitize to the stimulus neurons in limbic and cortical areas inducing the onset of epileptiform discharge. Recently this hypothesis has been imported into the psychiatric context and applied to BD, because the cyclical alternation of altered mood episodes can facilitate the development of further episodes (Mazza, Di Nicola et al. 2007, Post 2007, Bender and Alloy 2011).

## Global Distribution of Prevalence for BipolarDisorders

Epidemiological studies have highlighted that BD is widespread in all cultures and ethnicities with invariant features and immutable characteristics. BD may begin at any age, the average age of onset is around 21 years (Angst 1998), with a lifetime prevalence of 0.6% for bipolar I disorder, 0.4% for bipolar II disorder in the general population, where the USA showed the higher prevalence rate of 4.4% and India had the lowest rate 0.1% (Merikangas, Jin et al. 2011). Furthermore, a spectrum of bipolar conditions, including subthreshold bipolar manifestations, have a prevalence of 2.4%. In a recent prospective study on adolescents, Merikangas and Lamers (Merikangas and Lamers 2012) estimate bipolar II prevalence rates at 3–4%. The World Health Organization recognized BD as the sixth leading cause of disability among people ages from 15 to 44 years (Woods 2000). The estimate can decrease when misdiagnosis may occur: for example depressive episodes in BD may be very difficult to distinguish from those occurring in major depressive disorder. On the other hand, BD is frequently in comorbidity with other mental conditions and can be associated with greater rates of disability, impairment and suicide (Mazza and Marano 2009, Gonda, Pompili et al. 2012).

BD is a chronic affective disorder that causes significant economic burden to patients, families and society. Bipolar patients need attention from health care services and mental health specialists, and may have contact with the social welfare and legal systems. In addition, BD result in poor occupational impairment and, sometimes, in morbidity and premature mortality through suicide. Cost-of-illness studies measuring economic burden of BD estimate a total costs of $ 255,072 billion, where bipolar I patients cost $ 160,671 and bipolar II patients $ 94,401 against $ 95,584 for unipolar patients (Parker, McCraw et al. 2012). In this context should be mentioned, however, intangible costs such as family burden, quality of life and social functioning that are difficult to quantify monetarily.

Shippee and colleagues (Shippee, Shah et al. 2011) have found that BD is more costly than depressive disorder because from their subgroup analysis arise that BDpopulation are not married and the rates of work loss, unemployment and social, cognitive, work and household limitations associated with BD are higher than subjects affected by major depressive disorder, more likely it may be due to the more severe and persistent characteristics of BD and the stronger effects of mania/hypomania than depression.

Some authors have studied gender differences in symptom expression and course of illness in bipolar patients to determine whether gender is important in influencing illness variables such as course, symptom expression and likelihood of comorbidity. Women, however, may be more likely than men to be hospitalized for manic episodes. Regarding gender differences women show high rates of comorbidity with anxiety disorders, whereas substance abuse, which worsens the course and prognosis of the disease, is more common in males (Diflorio and Jones 2010). Nivoli et al. (Nivoli, Pacchiarotti et al. 2011) have noticed that polarity seem to differ across genders: men may be more likely than women to have manic predominant polarity, whereas women showed a predominant depressive polarity. Forty and colleagues (Forty, Jones et al. 2009) examining the pattern and distribution of manic and depressive episodes in bipolar illness assessed their diagnostic, prognostic and therapeutic importance. Colom and coworkers (Colom, Vieta et al. 2006) were particularly interested in the analysis of episode polarity in BD and observed that bipolar I patients seemed to be predisposed to a predominant manic course whilst patients with depressive onset present a prevalent depressive polarity. As concerning maniac symptomatology status across gender, Bhattacharya et al. (Bhattacharya, Khess et al. 2011) provided data that are important for clinical management: they found that depressive episodes and anxiety symptoms predominated in the course of illness of female bipolar patients, whereas increased psychomotor activity was more frequent in male subjects.

The effect of marriage in men and women with BD may be different. Lieberman and colleagues (Lieberman, Massey et al. 2010) conducted a study to assess whether marital status may influence illness course. They found that bipolar I disorder was associated with a lower likelihood of being married for men, but not for women; married women presented lower rate of depressive symptoms than unmarried women, conversely married men were likely to have no differences in illness course.

## Bipolar Disorders: The Comorbid Factor

There is a complex interplay between BD and its commonly occurring comorbid psychiatric disorders that can be framed, on one hand, in Axis I such as anxiety disorder, substance abuse, eating disorders and, on the other hand, in Axis II such as histrionic, narcissistic, borderline and antisocial personality disorders. Comorbidity greatly influences presentation, diagnosis and prognosis, complicates treatment, significantly increases the morbidity and disease burden. McElroy et al.(McElroy, Altshuler et al. 2001) found that 65% of bipolar patients present at least one psychiatric comorbidity, 42% two or more, and 24% three or more comorbid conditions. As regards sex differences, in women with BD there seems to be a greater prevalence of anxiety and eating disorders, whereas in men there is a strong association with alcohol and substance abuse (Tohen, Greenfield et al. 1998).

The presence of comorbidities should be taken into account not only for diagnostic purposes of classification but also for prognosis and therapy, in fact it is associated with a lower response to treatment, a higher rate of chronicity and more severe social and work dysfunction (Mazza and Marano, 2009).

Comorbid disorders may occur simultaneously or alternately. Comorbidities may also be represented by a subthreshold symptomatology that even if do not comply with the diagnostic criteria for a disorder, contribute to a significant proportion of morbidity.

In the clinical practice dual diagnosis is very common and represents the concurrence of a psychiatric disorder and addictive condition. It has been estimated that the prevalence rate of substance abuse in bipolar population range from 35% to 60% (Lagerberg, Andreassen et al. 2010). The simultaneous presence of BD and substance abuse is a predictor for poor adherence to treatment and often affects the outcome. Poor adherence to medicaltreatment can have side effects undermining the necessary therapeutic alliance, and also creates distrust and skepticism both in patients and in therapist, induces resistance and aggravates sufferance and prognosis increasing economic burden of health. Lagerberg and colleagues (Lagerberg, Andreassen et al. 2010) conducted a studyin the Oslo University Hospitals noticing that bipolar patients with comorbid substance abuse had substantial psychosocial impairment. Several other studies, as the recent Systematic Treatment Enhancement Program for Bipolar Disorder (Ostacher, Perlis et al. 2010), emphasized the association between bipolar illness and comorbid substance use disorders that may contribute to greater risk of switch into manic or mixed states. Comorbid substance use disorders have been also widely reported among youth and adolescents affected by BD (Wilens, Biederman et al. 2007, Goldstein and Bukstein 2010, Duffy, Horrocks et al. 2012) with potentially serious effects on the disease, because often substance abuse masks the illness and aggravate consequences causing difficulties in management and in therapy adherence. Phenomena such as low self-esteem, feelings of inadequacy, inability to express emotions and feelings, difficulty in tolerating frustration would promote the use of substances as a therapeutic tool to quell anxiety, overcome depression, increase euphoria or cancel stages confusion. In the diverse range of comorbid psychiatric disorders it has also been reported a comorbidity with alcohol abuse in bipolar population (Nery, Stanley et al. 2010, Oquendo, Currier et al. 2010, Bouzyk-Szutkiewicz, Waszkiewicz et al. 2012, Moreno, Hasin et al. 2013). Acute or chronic excessive drinking can cause a cascade of behavioral symptoms such as hyperactivity and mood frailty that sometimes can be misdiagnosed as BD. On the other hand, there is the opposite risk, that mood disorders are considered as side effects of alcohol. The co-occurrence of alcohol abuse in BD is associated with a lower level of global functioning, negative predictors of outcomes, poorer responsiveness to treatment with the higher possibility of chronic alcohol abuse.

Di Nicola et al. (Di Nicola, Tedeschi et al. 2010) examined the association between behavioral addictions and BD, suggesting a significant association between these two psychiatric conditions. Their co-occurrence could be due to higher impulsivity traits and character immaturity in BD and could mean worse prognosis of these patients. Impulsivity in mixed episodes has been examined in a study conducted by Fleck and colleagues (Fleck, Kotwal et al. 2011) that found a frontosubcortical activation. Mixed states are associated with a high risk of suicide, in fact 43% of suicide attempts occurs during a mixed state and the increased risk is closely related to people with high impulsivity character (Hantouche, Angst et al. 2003, Marneros, Rottig et al. 2004).

BD has been closely linked to cigarette smoking in a number of epidemiological studies (Heffner, Strawn et al. 2011, Heffner, DelBello et al. 2012, Williams, Gandhi et al. 2012, Dickerson, Stallings et al. 2013): bipolar patients seem to be at high risk for early smoking, increased smoking amount and dependence on nicotine, because they attempt to reduce psychiatric symptoms through smoking. It is important to note that, even among smokers without comorbid BD, it is very difficult quitting smoking and relapse rates are very high, so the clinician should continue to treat BD in comorbidity encouraging the patient's motivation.

Individuals suffering from BD frequently present a comorbid anxiety disorder (Mazza 2011, Cazard and Ferreri 2012, Sala, Goldstein et al. 2012, Young, Pfaff et al. 2012). In the Systematic Treatment Enhancement Program for Bipolar Disorder, Simon and coworkers (Simon, Otto et al. 2004)indicated that 52.8% of patients experienced at least one lifetime anxiety disorder and 34.2% showed a comorbid anxiety disorders. The comorbidity had effects on the illness course, because it is associated with fewer periods of well-being, more frequent risk of relapse, poor quality of life, increased risk of suicide and substance use. Fagiolini et al.(Fagiolini, Frank et al. 2007) suggested the possible identification of three different specific subtypes of bipolarity in relation to the anxious-depressive symptomatology: 1) a subtype characterized by the presence of depressive, maniac, obsessive-compulsive, panic-agoraphobic spectrum; 2) a subtype distinguished by symptoms of manic and depressive spectrum, in the absence of symptoms of anxious spectrum; 3) a subtype marked by a limited number of symptoms of both anxious and depressive spectrum.

A significant number of epidemiological studies have reported the existence of an increased prevalence of eating disorders in bipolar patients. In a community study conducted on more than 4500 subjects, Angst (Angst 1998) found a significant association between BD and eating disorder with a frequency of bulimia nervosa of 22% during hypomanic episodes, 14% in the manic phase, 11% during depressive phase against the 5% found among healthy controls. In another population study, Wittchen and colleagues (Wittchen, Mhlig et al. 2003) have pointed out that in 2548 subjects recruited the comorbidity with hypomanic and manic patients was 9% and 8%, respectively. In a more recent study, Castrogiovanni et al.(Castrogiovanni, Soreca et al. 2009) observed increased binge eating behaviors in bipolar population significantly correlated with risk for obesity, morbidity, mortality and poor quality of life (Murray and Michalak 2012). The association between BD and weight increase can be explained by three main factors: the use of psychopharmacological therapies that determine weight gain, the habit of bipolar patients with lifestyle risk of weight gain and the hypothesis of pathophysiological elements common to BD and obesity (Rosmond and Bjorntorp 1998, Rybakowski and Twardowska 1999, Cervantes, Gelber et al. 2001).

The signs of bipolar illness can be traced even in sexual behavior: Mazza and colleagues (Mazza, Harnic et al. 2011) conducted a study to examine the sexual sphere of female bipolar patients and ascertained that female bipolar I patients showed an increased level of interest in sex in comparison with female bipolar II patients.

BD is often associated with other psychiatric illnesses, but it also occurs with a variety of other medical conditions such as obesity (Keck and McElroy 2003, Bond, Kauer-Sant'Anna et al. 2010), diabetes mellitus (Cassidy, Ahearn et al. 1999, Regenold, Thapar et al. 2002), migraine (McIntyre, Konarski et al. 2006), metabolic syndrome (Babic, Maslov et al. 2010), hypothyroidism (Valle, Ayuso-Gutierrez et al. 1999) and cardiovascular disease (Marano, Harnic et al. 2009, Marano, Traversi et al. 2011, Weiner, Warren et al. 2011). In fact, persons suffering from BD experience twice the cardiovascular mortality (Murray, Weiner et al. 2009). Vemuriet al.(Vemuri, Kenna et al. 2011) evaluated the gender-associated differences in lipid profile in a bipolar cohort and found that women had lower means triglycerides and LDL cholesterol, but a correspondingly higher mean HDL cholesterol ratio than men. Bipolar patients affected by dyslipidemia should be carefully evaluated using adequate measures to prevent atherosclerosis and cardiovascular risk. A fairly large body of literature extols a bidirectional relation between affective disorders and epilepsy (Mazza, Orsucci et al. 2004, Schmitz 2005, Mazza, Di Nicola et al. 2007) with complex etiology including epileptogenic dysregulation within limbic circuits and psychotropic adverse effects of antiepileptic agents. Mazza et al .(Mazza, Di Nicola et al. 2007) analyzed common biological mechanism at the level of ion channels to determine whether and how this bidirectional influence occurs. These findings provide an important basis for clinicians that should take in account that treatment for one condition should involve assessment and possible concomitant treatment for comorbid conditions.

## Genetic-Molecular Characterization of Bipolar Disorder

BD is a complex disease resulting from the interaction of genetic susceptibility with biological, psychological and social factors. Neurochemical and genetic mechanisms that underlie psychopathological symptoms are complicated and not well understood, and several factors work together through a hierarchy of predispositions.

The first hypotheses on the etiopathological mechanism at the basis of this disorder have been made on purely pharmacological observations. After identifying the molecules that had beneficial effects on bipolar patients, it could be argued that there were altered biochemical pathways. Currently, the precise molecular mechanisms by which originate BD are not known, however it is commonly accepted that developmental abnormalities resulting in neuronal impairment of proper synaptic connectivity can determine psychiatric disorders such as BD. To confirm this, all the candidate genes identified to date appear to be attributable, directly or indirectly, to alterations of the activity of neuronal transmission (Owen, Craddock et al. 2007, Linke, Witt et al. 2012).

There are many evidences to support the important role of genetic factors in the etiology of affective disorders and in particular of BD. The genes involved are different and the interaction between these and many environmental factors seem important in conferring susceptibility to developing the disease. Modern techniques of molecular biology have allowed us to evaluate the associations between specific genes and BD.

Studies of families, twins and adoptive children provide consistent evidence of a strong genetic contribution to BD. It has been calculated that the risk of developing the disease during life is closely related to the sharing ratio of the genetic material from a subject suffering from BD and one unaffected. The identical twin of a subject affected by BD has a risk of onset of 40-70%, whereas a first-degree relative has a risk of 5-10% and an unrelated subject of 0,5-1,5% (Craddock and Jones 2001, Hayden and Nurnberger 2006, Squassina, Manchia et al. 2008). In addition, studies of twins have found a higher concordance rate for monozygotic twins than in heterozygotes ranging from 40 to 60% versus 19%, this correlation is maintained even if the twins are separately bred (Jones, Tai et al. 2006).

In the identification and localization of a component that contributes to genetic susceptibility to a disease it is important to assess the presence of linkage between pathology and a genetic marker. The linkage studies appraise the cosegregation of the marker and the disease within families and give an indication of the possible association between the marker locus and the disease locus. There is large number of linkage studies that have identified the presence of linkage between BD and various chromosomal areas and recent studies of genome-wide scans that have identified new susceptibility loci or confirmed data previously reported (Alsabban, Rivera et al. 2011, Mandelli L 2011, Smith, Koller et al. 2011, Yosifova, Mushiroda et al. 2011, Hare, Contreras et al. 2012, Price and Morris 2013).

Backlund et al. (Backlund, Nikamo et al. 2011) have identified in the chromosome 12 the gene P2RX7 as a susceptibility gene to BD and in particular responsible for cognitive manic symptoms of this disease. Dagdan and coworkers (Dagdan, Morris et al. 2011) suggested that rs3788266 as a functional promoter variant in the S100B gene is associated with a risk for BD. Gella et al.(Gella, Segura et al. 2011) and Leussis et al.(Leussis, Madison et al. 2012) supported that ANK3 is a susceptibility gene specific to BD. Ovadiaet al.(Ovadia and Shifman 2011) evaluated RELN gene related to a susceptibility to BD. Greenwood and coworkers (Greenwood, Nievergelt et al. 2012) provided additional evidence for at least one locus for BP disorder in chromosomes 6 and 17. Jackson and colleagues (Jackson, Fanous et al. 2013) indicated compelling evidence of an association between the 15q25 gene cluster and BD.

Association studies with candidate genes is usually a next step and genes are selected on the basis of both the results of linkage studies and considering the biological function of the factors for which they code. A large number of studies have investigated the association between markers located in the sequence of candidate genes and BD reporting often conflicting results. The majority of scientific studies has so far been devoted to the analysis of genes coding for components of the serotonergic and dopaminergic systems. The gene coding for the D3 receptor, located on chromosome region 3q13.3, is of particular interest because it is almost exclusively expressed in limbic areas, regions that are involved in the emotions processing. Although it has been reported a positive association for this gene, Elvidge and colleagues (Elvidge, Jones et al. 2001) do not confirm this finding. Similarly the gene encoding the tyrosine hydroxylase has been studied by several authors and firstly it has been reported to be associated with BD (Leboyer, Malafosse et al. 1990), but then the result was not confirmed (Turecki, Rouleau et al. 1997). The gene encoding for Catechol O-methyltransferase (COMT) has been analyzed in several studies that report a significant association with BD (Lee, Chen et al. 2013) and especially this candidate gene seems to affect related cognitive domains (Soeiro-de-Souza, Machado-Vieira et al. 2012) and modulate facial emotion recognition (Soeiro-de-Souza, Bio et al. 2012).

The gene coding for the serotonin transporter, place of selective action of many antidepressants located on chromosome regions 17q11.1-12, has been the subject of numerous studies of association. Several polymorphisms were evaluated in positive association with BD (Cho, Meira-Lima et al. 2005, Kenna, Roder-Hanna et al. 2012, Tharoor, Kotambail et al. 2012). The serotonin transporter seems associated with certain personality traits such as anxiety, irritability and aggression (Chou, Lin et al. 2012). Mazzaet al.(Mazza, Mandelli et al. 2010) studied gene 5HTR2C and its polymorphisms assessing that it is implicated in BD. Lee and colleagues (Lee, Chen et al. 2012) provide initial evidence that the ALDH2 and 5-HT2A genes interact only in bipolar I disorder, and that bipolar I disorder and bipolar II disorder are genetically distinct. In this context, Huang and coworkers (Huang, Chang et al. 2012) found association between brain derived neurotrophic factor (BDNF) and DRD2 in bipolar II disorder, but not in bipolar I disorder.

The BDNF gene, a member of the family of neurotrophins, plays an important role in promoting neuronal growth and it is involved in neuronal plasticity. Growing evidence suggests that BDNF and its polymorphisms are involved in the pathophysiology of mood disorders and in particular affecting the risk for BD (Fan and Sklar 2008, Mandelli, Mazza et al. 2010, Kenna, Roder-Hanna et al. 2012, Teh, Lee et al. 2012).

The association between the clock genes of the circadian system and the BD has been tested in several studies (Mansour, Monk et al. 2005, McClung 2007, Dallaspezia and Benedetti 2009, Milhiet, Etain et al. 2011). Soria and colleagues (Mansour, Monk et al. 2005) have hypothesized that circadian dysfunction could underlie, at least partially, the liability for mood disorder and have examined polymorphisms of 19 circadian genes. Associations of unipolar major depression with CRY1 and NPAS2 were detected, evidence for association of BD with CLOCK and VIP was found elucidating genetic mechanisms specific to each mood disorder. McGrath et al. (McGrath, Glatt et al. 2009) reported that clock genes are involved in the molecular basis of BD. In addition, PERIOD3 and ARNTL (Nievergelt, Kripke et al. 2006), CLOCK 3111T/C (Lee, Song et al. 2010) showed suggestive evidence of association with several circadian phenotypes identified in bipolar patients.

The genetic constitution of an individual appears somehow to create a personality more susceptible to overreact to external stress. Genetics then plays a predisposing role, whereas the environment exerts a triggering role.

## Neural Correlates in Bipolar Disorders

Several neuroimaging studies have suggested structural changes in association with BD, but the findings are heterogeneous and have not identified the exact brain areas responsible for the pathogenesis of the condition. Some studies (Vita, De Peri et al. 2009, De Peri, Crescini et al. 2012) were conducted using meta-analytic techniques to investigate the specificity of brain structural abnormalities in bipolar patients, although no clear relation has already emerged.

Womer et al. (Womer, Wang et al. 2009) performed a quantitative analysis of the cerebellar vermis volumes and found increased cerebellar vermis volumes in male BD patients. Whereas Monkul and colleagues (Monkul, Hatch et al. 2008) showed an inverse correlation between affective episodes and vermis area among male BD subjects. On the other hand, Baldaçara and colleagues (Baldacara, Nery-Fernandes et al. 2011) investigated the structural volumes of the cerebellum of patients with euthymic BD type I in comparison with healthy subjects. The results demonstrated smaller cerebellar volumes in patients with euthymic BD type I supporting that this specific aspect of regional anatomy might be associated with the characteristics of the illness considering that the cerebellum is an important brain area in emotional and cognitive development. In a more recent study, Schutter et al.(Schutter, Koolschijn et al. 2012) provide evidence that cerebellar volumes are associated with brain reactivity to emotional stimuli and may contribute to a predisposition for psychiatric disorders.

A study spearheaded by Chang (Chang, Karchemskiy et al. 2005) followed the trend according to which BD is associated with volume abnormalities in brain regions known to support affect regulation and investigated amygdalar volume in children and adolescents with early-onset BD that showed volume reductions in the left and right amygdale. More recently, they (Karchemskiy, Garrett et al. 2011) evaluated amygdalar volumes in offspring of parents BD offspring to identify possible structural abnormalities that may be associated with risk for BD. Bipolar offspring do not seem to have decreased cerebral amygdalar volume, possibly because these alterations might be later sequelae of BD rather than as a preexisting risk factor. Taken together, these results suggest that BD is associated with decreased volumes in the amygdala that play a critical role in the rapid, automatic and non-conscious processing of emotional and social stimuli.

A number of neuroimaging studies have focused on abnormalities of brain structure in BD, but there is a paucity of research examining sex differences at a neurobiological and mechanistic level in bipolar patients (Jogia, Dima et al. 2012). Mackay et al. (Mackay, Roddick et al. 2010) sustained that BD reflect an interaction between brain growth and sex along the anteriorposterior axis of the brain highlighting that male subjects with BD had larger and more symmetric brains in comparison with healthy male controls, whereas female patients showed smaller and more symmetric brains than healthy controls. These results suggest that brain morphology and gender differences in patients suffering from BD may play an important role in onset of the illness.

Overall, cerebral structural abnormalities may occur in different brain areas and the pattern of structural change may differ but these findings have important implications for future neurobiological studies and functional brain imaging methods offer a promising approach for investigate the biological mechanisms involved in emotion processing (Marano, Traversi et al. 2012).

Further studies are clearly warranted emphasizing the importance of longitudinal studies examining patients before and after the onset of a psychiatric disorders and evaluating whether structural changes over time may be associated with vulnerability for developing subsequent BD. Prospective research should deepen the relationship between brain changes and subsequent development of BD to elucidate the role of specific brain area in either conferring risk for or protecting against the development of BD.

## Bipolar Disorders: Therapeutic Treatment

The pharmacological treatment of BD represent a complex part of psychiatric practice. In fact there are different classes of psychotropic agents proposed for the acute and long-term treatment of this disorder tending to chronicity and characterized by significant levels of social disability. The choice of the most appropriate drug treatment, the optimal dose and planning of treatment duration constitute the basis of an adequate pharmacological approach to bipolar patients.

The treatment of affective disorders contemplates various stages of intervention, aimed both at the resolution of the acute episode, and the prevention of new episodes of mood designing a maintenance therapy. In the acute treatment it is essential to make an accurate diagnosis and to take account of the characteristics and symptoms severity. During preparation of maintenance therapy, which should be prolonged in time, it is important to consider the characteristics of the course of the disease and the possible presence of concomitant medical conditions.

The main goal of treatment of the depressive episode, when it occurs as part of BD, is the remission of the depressive symptoms and the return to normal operating levels. However, it requires the adoption of precautionary strategies, because of the high possibility that the treatment of depression triggers a manic or hypomanic episode in a bipolar patient. The risk of pharmacological induction of mania in bipolar patients would be around 20-40% (Goldberg and Truman 2003), whereas the risk of mood elevations after antidepressant therapy in bipolar II patients is intermediate between that found for the bipolar I disorder and major depression disorder (Bond, Noronha et al. 2008).

Current guidelines (American Psychiatric Association, 2000) consider contraindications to the use of antidepressant monotherapy in the depressive phase of BD. The choice of treatment depends on the severity of the current episode: for mild to moderate severity episodes it is suggested the use of a mood stabilizer drug and the possible association of antidepressant is reserved for cases of non-response or to more severe forms of depression and should be limited to the acute phase. The use of antidepressants in BD should not be understood as the first tool to treat depressive or anxious symptoms. Antidepressants can promote excitatory episodes, and happens because the excitatory symptoms are not always observable, sometimes they can be intermittent, and are not often reported by the patient as such and the past manic episodes are often omitted or minimized by the patient's spontaneous narrative.

Some authors have devoted their scientific researches whether or not to use antidepressants in patients suffering from BD. Amit and Weizman(Amit and Weizman 2012) concluded that although the risk of antidepressant-induced manic switch appears to be strongly reduced when antidepressants are given in combination with a mood stabilizer, the randomized controlled trials do not show significant benefits of antidepressants in the treatment of acute bipolar depression. In a review article, Bauer and colleagues (Bauer, Ritter et al. 2012) identified two common possibilities in the management of bipolar depression. The first case would be representative of a patient not optimally treated and without mood stabilizers in the pharmacological treatment, then in order to deal with a depressive episode the choice of treatment should be between quetiapine or olanzapine, or alternatively, carbamazepine and lamotrigine.

The antidepressant is a medication that should not be used for a long-term therapy in bipolar patients, and there are still conflicting opinions whether it has to be prescribed in monotherapy or in combination with a mood stabilizer. Instead, the second case would be that of a patient already treated adequately with a mood stabilizer, therefore lamotrigine may be an alternative because there is evidence that antidepressants provide benefits when a patient is being treated with a mood stabilizer (Bauer, Ritter et al. 2012). But psychotherapy remains an important part of the treatment and should span all phases of the illness. On the other hand, Mazza et al. (Mazza, Squillacioti et al. 2008) have reported the effectiveness of aripiprazole in the treatment of bipolar depression both as additional agent and as monotherapy in bipolar patients unresponsive to mood stabilizers: aripiprazole maintained a good safety and tolerability profile with very small changes in mean body weight. In a subsequent study, Mazza and coworkers (Mazza, Squillacioti et al. 2009) observed the specificity of anti-anhedonic and anti-depressant properties of aripiprazole in bipolar patients: anhedonia was present in 52% of the sample and was significantly reduced during treatment with aripiprazole. Furthermore, Mazza and colleagues (Mazza, Mandelli et al. 2011, Mazza, Mandelli et al. 2012) have analyzed factors associated with the course of symptoms comparing depression to mixed states and they found that mixed features may persist relatively stable throughout a depressive episode, having a negative impact over clinical and functional outcome, but not on social adjustment. In a recent review, Sidor et al. (Sidor and MacQueen 2012) analyzed the use of antidepressants in the treatment of BD. New-generation antidepressants are preferred over old tricyclic antidepressants (TCAs) that are more likely to induce a switch of the patient in a manic phase. Within the new generation antidepressants, venlafaxine seems to be related to the higher risk of mania induction, whereas bupropion expresses the lowest rate of the same risk.

Since recent studies have argued against the efficacy of antidepressants in the treatment of bipolar depression and scientific evidence is discordant and conflicting, it is important to be cautious and evaluate their use because of the unclear risk-to-benefit ratio; further well-designed studies are needed.

The manic and mixed episodes may represent a medical emergency and may require hospitalization, which must sometimes be made against the will of the patient due to lack of awareness of the disease. The goal of treatment is the rapid resolution of symptoms with a return to previous levels of functioning. Treatment of a manic episode must consider the characteristics of symptoms, their severity and the presence or absence of psychotic symptoms. In clinical practice combination therapy is frequently used to improve response and remission rates. The primary role of mood stabilizers in the treatment of acute mania has long been well-documented in the literature, and a first-line approach traditionally involves the combination of a an atypical antipsychotic with lithium or valproate (Geoffroy, Etain et al. 2012). For serious manic or mixed episodes the use of lithium or valproate is preferred in association with an antipsychotic, for less serious cases it may be sufficient a monotherapy with lithium or valproate (American Psychiatric Association 2000). Atypical antipsychotics have a greater effectiveness on psychomotor agitation and on any psychotic symptoms, whereas typical antipsychotics present a less favorable tolerability profile and can cause disturbing adverse effects such as induction of depressive symptoms and tardive dyskinesia after treatment discontinuation. In turn lithium or valproate would seem be more effective on mood disorders exerting important antimanic effects. Several agents with mood-stabilizing properties such as carbamazepine, lamotrigine, gabapentin and topiramate are frequently used in clinical practice, however the most consistent evidence concerns the use of lithium and valproate.

Lithium has long been used as the first agent to treat acute mania in subjects affected by BD, it is effective for preventing the occurrence of mania and to treat maniac episodes. Lithium has a latency of therapeutic effect of a few weeks, but its action can be maximized by rapid titration of plasma concentrations, up to reach values within the therapeutic range of

0,8-1,2 mEq/l. Due to this low therapeutic index it has poor manageability and at values equal to or greater of 1.5 mEq/l it becomes toxic (McKnight, Adida et al. 2012).

Valproate is an anti-convulsant agent that has been used to treat epilepsy since 1983, but it has been approved as a treatment for manic episodes in bipolar patients in 1995. Valproate has shown an antimanic efficacy comparable to that of lithium and has a wide therapeutic index, so it is generally well tolerated (Chiu, Wang et al. 2013). The antimanic properties seem to be correlated to plasma values between 50 and 125 μg/ml.

A new option for the treatment of BD is asenapine, a second-generation antipsychotic agent with sublingual administration. The use of asenapine as adjunctive treatment in patients suffering from bipolar I disorder in the manic phase resulted in a significant improvement in symptoms (McIntyre, Cohen et al. 2010) and it has been used as adjunctive therapy to reduce the rate of mania (Szegedi, Calabrese et al. 2012). Weight gain associated with asenapine is relatively modest so it can be used in bipolar patients with comorbid metabolic diseases (Chwieduk and Scott 2011). Baruch et al. (Baruch, Tadger et al. 2013) reported the effectiveness of asenapine in the treatment of acute manic episodes for elderly bipolar manic patients and its good tolerability profile.

BD is a chronic disease tending to a relapsing course. The primary goal of a long-term pharmacological treatment is therefore to reduce the risk of manic and depressive recurrence and improve psychopathological conditions during stabilized phases. Due to the high risk of recurrence and morbidity that is associated with BD, generally the maintenance pharmacological therapy is aimed at preventing new episodes of mood and controlling subsyndromal symptoms. The decision to establish a maintenance therapy is rather complex and linked to numerous factors such as patient's age, age of onset of the disease, frequency, duration and severity of past episodes, response to previous pharmacological treatments and consequences of a new episode for the patient. Recent guidelines recommend a preventive intervention even after a single manic episode and the use of an antipsychotic as an adjunctive treatment has been suggested in stabilized patients that continue to manifest subthreshold symptoms or breakthrough episodes of mood disturbance (American Psychiatric Association, 2000).

In the long term, the combination of psychological interventions with pharmacotherapy is beneficial as it ensures adherence and monitoring of tolerability (Fountoulakis, Kasper et al. 2012).

Vieta et al. (Vieta, Gunther et al. 2011) conducted a review of studies and data available in the literature with particular attention to studies with a double-blind, placebo-controlled trials that evaluated the efficacy of mood stabilizers and antipsychotics medications in the maintenance phase of BD. The results confirmed that lithium (Licht 2012) and valproate remain the gold standard in maintenance therapy of BD together with some atypical antipsychotics, such as aripiprazole, olanzapine, quetiapine and risperidone, that seem to prevent manic phases or hypomanic relapses. The authors conclude that sometimes the monotherapy in maintenance treatment does not seem to be sufficient for the management of bipolar patients. In case of combined therapy for the prophylactic treatment of BD they suggested ziprasidone and lithium or divalproex, risperidone and lithium or divalproex to reduce the risk of manic relapses, but only quetiapine and lithium or valproate to decrease risk for relapse at both the manic/mixed and depressed poles of BD (Vieta, Gunther et al. 2011).

Oxcarbazepine may represent a useful alternative to lithium and valproate. Mazza and coworkers (Mazza, Bria et al. 2007, Mazza, Di Nicola et al. 2007) reported that oxcarbazepine has efficacy in the maintenance treatment of BD and can be particularly useful as add-on treatment in bipolar patients if previous treatments have failed or in patients who have difficulty tolerating adequate dosages of standard approved treatments.

Oxidative stress, that occurs during the physiological cellular activity and antioxidant defense mechanisms of the body, is believed to be involved in the pathogenesis of various neuropsychiatric disorders, because these diseases share some characteristics that predispose to oxidative stress and enhance it by triggering cascade mechanisms. There are numerous studies showing that the levels of markers of oxidative stress increase in tissues during disease progression and immunocytochemistry evidence exists of oxidative damage to biomacromolecules in brain areas affected by the disease (Gergerlioglu, Savas et al. 2007, Andreazza, Kauer-Sant'anna et al. 2008, Pandya, Howell et al. 2012). Since the oxidative stress exists at or before the onset of the illness, the use of antioxidants as adjuvant therapy may reduce the oxidative injury and improve the outcome of illness (Mazza, Pomponi et al. 2007, Pomponi, Janiri et al. 2013). In this perspective, oxidative stress leads to an increase of senescent cells that have a characteristic shortening in the length of telomeres, terminal regions of chromosome consist of a sequence repeated in tandem, composed of six nucleotides TTAGGG and rich in guanine and cytosine. Telomere length is mainly determined by the relationship between oxidative stress and antioxidant defense capacity of the individual. If the antioxidant capacity is reduced, the telomeres under the influence of the production of free radicals will shorten and induce an altered cell proliferation bringing the cell to senescence. Thus, telomere shortening may contribute to a general decline of many homeostatic mechanisms, including brain function. Elvsåshagen et al. (Elvsashagen, Vera et al. 2011) valued leukocyte telomere length, they found that average telomere length in bipolar II patients was 552 base pairs shorter than that in controls, corresponding to approximately thirteen years of accelerated cell aging. Veryrecently, Marazziti et al.(Marazziti, Baroni et al. 2012) and Nierenberg et al.(Nierenberg, Kansky et al. 2013) have focused their scientific interest on mitochondrial metabolism achieving data converging towards the hypothesis that mitochondrial dysfunction contributes to metabolic errors and apoptosis playing an important role in the pathophysiology of BD as well as other neuropsychiatric disorders. In such perspective, the development of new pharmacological agents should have mitochondrial function as a target obtaining consequently a protective effect from oxidative stress.

The issue of compliance to the treatment regimen is central to help the patient to maintain or improve health. Poor adherence to therapy is now considered one of the most delicate barriers to the achievement of successful treatment. It is essential to the continuity of care in chronic pathologies, such as BD, to ensure an optimum adhesion, but it is not simple because sometimes bipolar patients might be burdened of comorbidities and subjected to polytherapy schemes, making the adhesion to treatment even more complex. The main barriers to adherence may depend by forgetfulness, other priorities, decision to skip a dose, lack of adequate information and emotional factors. The clinician has to favorite therapeutic adherence providing the patient with clear and simple information and involving patient's relatives because patients who are more adherent to therapy are those with better health outcomes (Sajatovic, Levin et al. 2011). Enhancement of treatment adherence in bipolar patients is a necessary and promising management component as an adjunct to pharmacotherapy. Kriegshauseret al.(Kriegshauser, Sajatovic et al. 2010) investigated factors associated with medication adherence in bipolar patients across gender differences and found that men engaged in less significant social relations whereas women exhibited more meaningful interpersonal relationships and, consequently, more robust social support that showed a positive correlation with treatment adherence. Sajatovic and colleagues (Sajatovic, Micula-Gondek et al. 2011) evaluated medication adherence in bipolar patients and found that being male or female was not associated with adherence status, whereas men with high self-perceived masculinity demonstrate poor medication adherence. Jonsdottir et al. (Jonsdottir, Opjordsmoen et al. 2013) investigated clinical predictors of functional outcome in patients affected by BD and found that neurocognitive impairment is not a predictor index of the risk of non-adherence to medical therapies, whereas the presence of substance abuse may be indicative of a partial or total risk of non-adherence to treatment. Mazza and coworkers (Mazza, Mandelli et al. 2009) conducted a study on a sample of bipolar patients with comorbid substance use disorder and demonstrated that substance use disorder comorbidity did not represent a risk factor for treatment drop-out, while in their sample young age, low treatment dosage and bipolar I diagnosis were significantly associated with drop-out. On the other hand, Moon et al.(Moon, Chang et al. 2012) and Lerner et al.(Lerner and Levinson 2012) examining drop-out rates outlined that psychoeducation interventions had a clear impact on treatment adherence and might be promising target for the treatment of BD.

## Non-Pharmacological Methods in the Management of Bipolar Disorders

Other possible treatments for BD are represented by psychological and psychoeducational interventions, electroconvulsive therapy (Dierckx, Heijnen et al. 2012), light therapy (Pail, Huf et al. 2011, Araki, Terao et al. 2012), good sleep hygiene (Soreca, Wallace et al. 2012), regular exercise (Dakwar, Blanco et al. 2012, Vancampfort, Correll et al. 2013) and dietary advice (Elmslie, Mann et al. 2001).

Electroconvulsive therapy may be used in cases with particularly serious manic or depressive episodes, manic episodes with simultaneous presence of relevant psychotic symptoms, severe depressive symptoms that constitute a serious threat for life or in cases of medical contraindications to pharmacological therapy. A significant body of evidence indicates the efficacy of electroconvulsive therapy for the treatment of both unipolar and bipolar depressive patients resistant to pharmacological treatment (Bailine, Fink et al. 2010, Dierckx, Heijnen et al. 2012). There is little evidence for differences in response to electroconvulsive therapy between patients with bipolar or unipolar major depression. Bailine and coworkers (Bailine, Fink et al. 2010) suggested that electroconvulsive therapy has antidepressive efficacy both in unipolar and bipolar depression. Medda and colleagues (Medda, Perugi et al. 2009) has observed that unipolar patients obtained more benefits from this therapy while bipolar patients tended to exhibit residual manic and psychotic symptomatology. Dierckx et al. (Dierckx, Heijnen et al. 2012) estimated electroconvulsive therapy as an equally useful tool for depression showing more promising remission rates for bipolar patients.

With regard to non-pharmacological treatment of BD psychological intervention deserves a particular attention. Psychotherapy, together with psychopharmacological therapy, should be considered in case of inadequate response to drug treatment and discomfort in facing problems and distress. The combined treatment of psychotherapy and psychopharmacotherapy showed better efficacy compared to only psychopharmacological treatment. Psychotherapy appears to be effective in the prevention of depressive recurrences since it tries to understand and prevent psychosocial stressors to which the patient is subjected (Schottle, Huber et al. 2011).

Psychopharmacotherapy would be most active on vegetative symptoms, anhedonia, ideomotor apraxia, whereas psychotherapy has different target symptoms and act on feelings of inadequacy and guilt, interpersonal problems, lack of motivation. Furthermore, psychotherapy can be of great utility in the critical phases in order to provide an adequate psychoeducational intervention on the disorder and improve compliance to psychopharmacological treatment.

Beyond any theoretical model psychotherapic intervention is very important because it aims to help patients to find meaning in illness, identify strategies to deal with stress, improve quality of life, work functioning and interpersonal relationships.

Psychoeducation is an educational intervention involving exposing and interactive methods but, above all, practical use to prevent and appropriately deal with discomforts and mental illness. It has been reported that psychoeducational interventions helped bipolar patients and their families to recognize early signs and enhance communication within family, aimed at reducing the number of relapses and improving adherence to pharmacological treatment (Vieta 2005, Colom, Vieta et al. 2009, Reinares, Colom et al. 2010).

The approach to treatment of BD more than a single strategy should be an integrated treatment aimed to increase compliance and ameliorate global functioning. In the analysis of the variables involved in the favorable prognosis of bipolar patients, psychoeducation treatment can sometimes give controversial results: Barros Pellegrinelli and coworkers (de Barros Pellegrinelli, de et al. 2013) did not report a reduction in the rating depression in bipolar patients after sixteen sessions of psychoeducation, while Gonzalez and colleagues (Gonzalez Isasi, Echeburua et al. 2012) demonstrated that psychoeducation treatment is effective for long term treatment of refractory bipolar patients.

Some non-pharmacological treatments such as transcranial magnetic stimulation and vagus nerve stimulation have shown promising results and may represent a viable strategy in treatment-resistant depression, with some limitations because there are data referable to a small number of patients and inadequate controls or randomization (Poon, Sim et al. 2012). Bersani et al. (Bersani, Minichino et al. 2013) performed a review to assess the effectiveness of transcranial magnetic stimulation: it is a non-invasive method to stimulate nerve cells that is generally considered tolerable and safe, but shows some minor side effects. It is used for severe refractory depression, as an add-on treatment to drug therapy or in monotherapy. Factors associated with successful treatment are patient's age of 48–65 and stimulation intensity higher than 64.6 (Bersani, Minichino et al. 2013).

Light therapy, commonly used to treat skin diseases, has also become a widely used remedy for mental illnesses such as BD. Exposure to light with high intensity produces antidepressant effects, and benefits have been also found in patients that show sensitivity to seasonal change (Dauphinais, Rosenthal et al. 2012). It is important to remember that the use of this method cannot be separated from psychopharmacological therapy.

Finally, some studies suggest sleep deprivation as short-term treatment and as an adjunct to psychotropic agents. Sleep deprivation during one night determines, however, only a transient improvement in symptomatology (Poon, Sim et al. 2012).

## Conclusion

BD is chronic and recurrent disease, meaning that lasts a lifetime, although not with the same severity, and the episodes tend to recur over time. BD is a complex and heterogeneous illness that strongly impact on subjects life also because it may occur with other comorbid medical conditions. The quality of life is compromised in bipolar patients even during periods of euthymia determining greater impairment in all domains because of the psychosocial impact of chronic condition.

The objectives of treatment are to reduce symptoms of acute episodes, to make the episodes less frequent and severe, to avoid switching from one phase to another, to decrease the need for hospital admissions, to improve the functioning of the patient during inter-episodic phase, to prevent self-harm actions and suicide risk.

Psychotropic agents play a key role in the care of bipolar population. Maintenance treatment with a mood stabilizer sharply reduces the frequency, severity and duration of manic and depressive episodes, although manic episodes and depression that require specific treatment may occur. During the evolution of the disorder, changes in dose or type of medication may become necessary as well as changes in the method of treatment. Together with pharmacologic treatment psychological interventions are essential, in form of psychotherapy, psychoeducation training and family implementation resources, in order to help the patient to recognize the disease and to develop the capacity to face the causes that can trigger acute episodes.

The origin of BD is not well understood and can be recognized in a combination of causes such as predisposing genetic factors and specific alterations in brain circuits that control mood, emotions, impulses and some basic biological functions as appetite, sleepand sexuality. Other factors that may contribute to the onset of BD include defects in the mechanisms of stress response and significant changes in hormone levels, but also the environment plays a key role, being able to facilitate the elicitation of symptoms.

Although different hypotheses have been formulated to explain the mechanisms that contribute to trigger bipolar illness, much remains to be done to fully understand the specific set and sequence of events that produce the disease and its cardinal features. Further neuropathologic and neuroimaging investigations may elucidate pathobiological mechanisms hiding under the ontogeny, magnitude and progression of the disease. In addition, understanding the pathophysiologic underpinnings of this medical condition would provide insight into the molecular biology of the nervous system and a gateway toward developing novel treatment strategies.

## References

Akiskal HS, P. O. (2002). The soft bipolar spectrum: footnotes to Kraepelin on the interface of hypomania, temperament and depression. Bipolar Disorders. 100 years after manic-depressive insanity. A. J. Marneros A. NewYork, Boston, Dordrecht, London, Moscow, Kluwer Academic Publishers: pp. 37-62.

Alsabban, S., M. Rivera and P. McGuffin (2011). Genome-wide searches for bipolar disorder genes. *Curr. Psychiatry Rep.* 13(6): 522-527.

Amit, B. H. and A. Weizman (2012). Antidepressant treatment for acute bipolar depression: an update. *Depress Res. Treat.* 2012: 684725.

Andreazza, A. C., M. Kauer-Sant'anna, B. N. Frey, D. J. Bond, F. Kapczinski, L. T. Young and L. N. Yatham (2008). Oxidative stress markers in bipolar disorder: a meta-analysis. *J. Affect Disord.* 111(2-3): 135-144.

Angst, J. (1998). The emerging epidemiology of hypomania and bipolar II disorder. *J. Affect Disord.* 50(2-3): 143-151.

Araki, Y., T. Terao, N. Hoaki, Y. Wang and S. Goto (2012). Bipolar temperaments and light. *J. Affect Disord.* 136(3): 740-742.

American Psychiatric Association (2000). Diagnostic and Statistical Manual of Mental Disorders. Washington, DC.

Babic, D., B. Maslov, M. Martinac, K. Nikolic, S. Uzun and O. Kozumplik (2010). Bipolar disorder and metabolic syndrome: comorbidity or side effects of treatment of bipolar disorder. *Psychiatr. Danub* 22(1): 75-78.

Backlund, L., P. Nikamo, D. S. Hukic, I. R. Ek, L. Traskman-Bendz, M. Landen, G. Edman, M. Schalling, L. Frisen and U. Osby (2011). Cognitive manic symptoms associated with the P2RX7 gene in bipolar disorder. *Bipolar Disord.* 13(5-6): 500-508.

Bailine, S., M. Fink, R. Knapp, G. Petrides, M. M. Husain, K. Rasmussen, S. Sampson, M. Mueller, S. M. McClintock, K. G. Tobias and C. H. Kellner (2010). Electroconvulsive therapy is equally effective in unipolar and bipolar depression. *Acta Psychiatr Scand.* 121(6): 431-436.

Baldacara, L., F. Nery-Fernandes, M. Rocha, L. C. Quarantini, G. G. Rocha, J. L. Guimaraes, C. Araujo, I. Oliveira, A. Miranda-Scippa and A. Jackowski (2011). Is cerebellar volume related to bipolar disorder? *J. Affect Disord.* 135(1-3): 305-309.

Baruch, Y., S. Tadger, I. Plopski and Y. Barak (2013). Asenapine for elderly bipolar manic patients. *J. Affect Disord.* 145(1): 130-132.

Bauer, M., P. Ritter, H. Grunze and A. Pfennig (2012). Treatment options for acute depression in bipolar disorder. *Bipolar Disord* 14 Suppl 2: 37-50.

Bender, R. E. and L. B. Alloy (2011). Life stress and kindling in bipolar disorder: review of the evidence and integration with emerging biopsychosocial theories. *Clin. Psychol. Rev.* 31(3): 383-398.

Bersani, F. S., A. Minichino, P. G. Enticott, L. Mazzarini, N. Khan, G. Antonacci, R. N. Raccah, M. Salviati, R. Delle Chiaie, G. Bersani, P. B. Fitzgerald and M. Biondi (2013). Deep transcranial magnetic stimulation as a treatment for psychiatric disorders: A comprehensive review. *Eur. Psychiatry* 28(1): 30-39.

Bhattacharya, A., C. R. Khess, S. K. Munda, A. K. Bakhla, S. K. Praharaj and M. Kumar (2011). Sex difference in symptomatology of manic episode. *Compr. Psychiatry* 52(3): 288-292.

Blumberg, H. P., J. Kaufman, A. Martin, D. S. Charney, J. H. Krystal and B. S. Peterson (2004). Significance of adolescent neurodevelopment for the neural circuitry of bipolar disorder. *Ann. N. Y. Acad. Sci.* 1021: 376-383.

Bond, D. J., M. Kauer-Sant'Anna, R. W. Lam and L. N. Yatham (2010). Weight gain, obesity, and metabolic indices following a first manic episode: prospective 12-month data from the Systematic Treatment Optimization Program for Early Mania (STOP-EM). *J. Affect Disord.* 124(1-2): 108-117.

Bond, D. J., M. M. Noronha, M. Kauer-Sant'Anna, R. W. Lam and L. N. Yatham (2008). Antidepressant-associated mood elevations in bipolar II disorder compared with bipolar I disorder and major depressive disorder: a systematic review and meta-analysis. *J. Clin. Psychiatry* 69(10): 1589-1601.

Bouzyk-Szutkiewicz, J., N. Waszkiewicz and A. Szulc (2012). Alcohol and psychiatric disorders. *Pol. Merkur. Lekarski* 33(195): 176-181.

Cassidy, F., E. Ahearn and B. J. Carroll (1999). Elevated frequency of diabetes mellitus in hospitalized manic-depressive patients. *Am. J. Psychiatry* 156(9): 1417-1420.

Castrogiovanni, S., I. Soreca, D. Troiani and M. Mauri (2009). Binge eating, weight gain and psychosocial adjustment in patients with bipolar disorder. *Psychiatry Res.* 169(1): 88-90.

Cazard, F. and F. Ferreri (2012). Bipolar disorders and comorbid anxiety: Prognostic impact and therapeutic challenges. Encephale.

Cervantes, P., S. Gelber, F. N. Kin, V. N. Nair and G. Schwartz (2001). Circadian secretion of cortisol in bipolar disorder. *J. Psychiatry Neurosci.* 26(5): 411-416.

Chang, K., A. Karchemskiy, N. Barnea-Goraly, A. Garrett, D. I. Simeonova and A. Reiss (2005). Reduced amygdalar gray matter volume in familial pediatric bipolar disorder. *J. Am. Acad. Child Adolesc. Psychiatry* 44(6): 565-573.

Chiu, C. T., Z. Wang, J. G. Hunsberger and D. M. Chuang (2013). Therapeutic potential of mood stabilizers lithium and valproic acid: beyond bipolar disorder. *Pharmacol. Rev.* 65(1): 105-142.

Cho, H. J., I. Meira-Lima, Q. Cordeiro, L. Michelon, P. Sham, H. Vallada and D. A. Collier (2005). Population-based and family-based studies on the serotonin transporter gene polymorphisms and bipolar disorder: a systematic review and meta-analysis. *Mol. Psychiatry* 10(8): 771-781.

Chou, Y. H., C. L. Lin, S. J. Wang, J. F. Lirng, K. C. Yang, A. Chien Chang and M. H. Liao (2012). Aggression in bipolar II disorder and its relation to the serotonin transporter. *J. Affect Disord.*

Chwieduk, C. M. and L. J. Scott (2011). Asenapine: a review of its use in the management of mania in adults with bipolar I disorder. *CNS Drugs* 25(3): 251-267.

Colom, F., E. Vieta, C. Daban, I. Pacchiarotti and J. Sanchez-Moreno (2006). Clinical and therapeutic implications of predominant polarity in bipolar disorder. *J. Affect Disord.* 93(1-3): 13-17.

Colom, F., E. Vieta, J. Sanchez-Moreno, R. Palomino-Otiniano, M. Reinares, J. M. Goikolea, A. Benabarre and A. Martinez-Aran (2009). Group psychoeducation for stabilised bipolar disorders: 5-year outcome of a randomised clinical trial. *Br. J. Psychiatry* 194(3): 260-265.

Craddock, N. and I. Jones (2001). Molecular genetics of bipolar disorder. *Br. J. Psychiatry* 178 (Suppl 41): S128-133.

Craddock, N. and P. Sklar (2009). Genetics of bipolar disorder: successful start to a long journey. *Trends Genet* 25(2): 99-105.

Cullen, N. and G. V. Goddard (1975). Kindling in the hypothalamus and transfer to the ipsilateral amygdala. *Behav. Biol.* 15(2): 119-131.

Dagdan, E., D. W. Morris, M. Campbell, M. Hill, M. Rothermundt, F. Kastner, C. Hohoff, C. von Eiff, P. Krakowitzky, M. Gill, P. McKeon and S. Roche (2011). Functional assessment of a promoter polymorphism in S100B, a putative risk variant for bipolar disorder. *Am. J. Med. Genet. B. Neuropsychiatr. Genet.* 156B(6): 691-699.

Dakwar, E., C. Blanco, K. H. Lin, S. M. Liu, D. Warden, M. Trivedi and E. V. Nunes (2012). Exercise and mental illness: results from the National Epidemiologic Survey on Alcohol and Related Conditions (NESARC). *J. Clin. Psychiatry* 73(7): 960-966.

Dallaspezia, S. and F. Benedetti (2009). Melatonin, circadian rhythms, and the clock genes in bipolar disorder. *Curr. Psychiatry Rep.* 11(6): 488-493.

Dauphinais, D. R., J. Z. Rosenthal, M. Terman, H. M. DiFebo, C. Tuggle and N. E. Rosenthal (2012). Controlled trial of safety and efficacy of bright light therapy vs. negative air ions in patients with bipolar depression. *Psychiatry Res.* 196(1): 57-61.

de Barros Pellegrinelli, K., O. C. L. F. de, K. I. Silval, V. V. Dias, M. C. Roso, M. Bandeira, F. Colom and R. A. Moreno (2013). Efficacy of psychoeducation on symptomatic and functional recovery in bipolar disorder. *Acta Psychiatr. Scand.* 127(2): 153-158.

De Peri, L., A. Crescini, G. Deste, P. Fusar-Poli, E. Sacchetti and A. Vita (2012). Brain structural abnormalities at the onset of schizophrenia and bipolar disorder: a meta-analysis of controlled magnetic resonance imaging studies. *Curr. Pharm. Des.* 18(4): 486-494.

Di Nicola, M., D. Tedeschi, M. Mazza, G. Martinotti, D. Harnic, V. Catalano, A. Bruschi, G. Pozzi, P. Bria and L. Janiri (2010). Behavioural addictions in bipolar disorder patients: role of impulsivity and personality dimensions. *J. Affect Disord.* 125(1-3): 82-88.

Dickerson, F., C. R. Stallings, A. E. Origoni, C. Vaughan, S. Khushalani, J. Schroeder and R. H. Yolken (2013). Cigarette smoking among persons with schizophrenia or bipolar disorder in routine clinical settings, 1999-2011. *Psychiatr. Serv.* 64(1): 44-50.

Dierckx, B., W. T. Heijnen, W. W. van den Broek and T. K. Birkenhager (2012). Efficacy of electroconvulsive therapy in bipolar versus unipolar major depression: a meta-analysis. *Bipolar. Disord.* 14(2): 146-150.

Diflorio, A. and I. Jones (2010). Is sex important? Gender differences in bipolar disorder. *Int. Rev. Psychiatry* 22(5): 437-452.

Duffy, A., J. Horrocks, R. Milin, S. Doucette, G. Persson and P. Grof (2012). Adolescent substance use disorder during the early stages of bipolar disorder: a prospective high-risk study. *J. Affect Disord.* 142(1-3): 57-64.

Eley, T. C., H. Liang, R. Plomin, P. Sham, A. Sterne, R. Williamson and S. Purcell (2004). Parental familial vulnerability, family environment, and their interactions as predictors of depressive symptoms in adolescents. J. *Am. Acad. Child Adolesc. Psychiatry* 43(3): 298-306.

Elmslie, J. L., J. I. Mann, J. T. Silverstone, S. M. Williams and S. E. Romans (2001). Determinants of overweight and obesity in patients with bipolar disorder. *J. Clin. Psychiatry* 62(6): 486-491; quiz 492-483.

Elvidge, G., I. Jones, F. McCandless, P. Asherson, M. J. Owen and N. Craddock (2001). Allelic variation of a BalI polymorphism in the DRD3 gene does not influence susceptibility to bipolar disorder: results of analysis and meta-analysis. *Am. J. Med. Genet.* 105(4): 307-311.

Elvsashagen, T., E. Vera, E. Boen, J. Bratlie, O. A. Andreassen, D. Josefsen, U. F. Malt, M. A. Blasco and B. Boye (2011). The load of short telomeres is increased and associated with lifetime number of depressive episodes in bipolar II disorder. *J. Affect Disord.* 135(1-3): 43-50.

Fagiolini, A., E. Frank, P. Rucci, G. B. Cassano, S. Turkin and D. J. Kupfer (2007). Mood and anxiety spectrum as a means to identify clinically relevant subtypes of bipolar I disorder. *Bipolar Disord.* 9(5): 462-467.

Fan, J. and P. Sklar (2008). Genetics of bipolar disorder: focus on BDNF Val66Met polymorphism. *Novartis Found Symp.* 289: 60-72; discussion 72-63, 87-93.

Fleck, D. E., R. Kotwal, J. C. Eliassen, M. Lamy, M. P. Delbello, C. M. Adler, M. Durling, M. A. Cerullo and S. M. Strakowski (2011). Preliminary evidence for increased frontosubcortical activation on a motor impulsivity task in mixed episode bipolar disorder. *J. Affect Disord.* 133(1-2): 333-339.

Forty, L., L. Jones, I. Jones, D. J. Smith, S. Caesar, C. Fraser, K. Gordon-Smith, S. Hyde and N. Craddock (2009). Polarity at illness onset in bipolar I disorder and clinical course of illness. *Bipolar Disord.* 11(1): 82-88.

Fountoulakis, K. N., S. Kasper, O. Andreassen, P. Blier, A. Okasha, E. Severus, M. Versiani, R. Tandon, H. J. Moller and E. Vieta (2012). Efficacy of pharmacotherapy in bipolar disorder: a report by the WPA section on pharmacopsychiatry. *Eur. Arch. Psychiatry Clin. Neurosci.* 262 Suppl 1: 1-48.

Gella, A., M. Segura, N. Durany, B. Pfuhlmann, G. Stober and M. Gawlik (2011). Is Ankyrin a genetic risk factor for psychiatric phenotypes? *BMC Psychiatry* 11: 103.

Geoffroy, P. A., B. Etain, C. Henry and F. Bellivier (2012). Combination therapy for manic phases: a critical review of a common practice. *CNS Neurosci. Ther.* 18(12): 957-964.

Gergerlioglu, H. S., H. A. Savas, F. Bulbul, S. Selek, E. Uz and M. Yumru (2007). Changes in nitric oxide level and superoxide dismutase activity during antimanic treatment. *Prog. Neuropsychopharmacol. Biol. Psychiatry* 31(3): 697-702.

Goldberg, J. F. and C. J. Truman (2003). Antidepressant-induced mania: an overview of current controversies. *Bipolar Disord.* 5(6): 407-420.

Goldstein, B. I. and O. G. Bukstein (2010). Comorbid substance use disorders among youth with bipolar disorder: opportunities for early identification and prevention. *J. Clin. Psychiatry* 71(3): 348-358.

Gonda, X., M. Pompili, G. Serafini, F. Montebovi, S. Campi, P. Dome, T. Duleba, P. Girardi and Z. Rihmer (2012). Suicidal behavior in bipolar disorder: epidemiology, characteristics and major risk factors. *J. Affect Disord.* 143(1-3): 16-26.

Gonzalez Isasi, A., E. Echeburua, J. M. Liminana and A. Gonzalez-Pinto (2012). Psychoeducation and cognitive-behavioral therapy for patients with refractory bipolar disorder: A 5-year controlled clinical trial. *Eur. Psychiatry.*

Goodwin FK, J. K. (2007). Manic-Depressive Illness: Bipolar Disorders and Recurrent Depression: Bipolar Disorders and Recurrent Depression., Oxford University Press.

Greenwood, T. A., C. M. Nievergelt, A. D. Sadovnick, R. A. Remick, P. E. Keck, Jr., S. L. McElroy, T. Shekhtman, R. McKinney and J. R. Kelsoe (2012). Further evidence for linkage of bipolar disorder to chromosomes 6 and 17 in a new independent pedigree series. *Bipolar Disord.* 14(1): 71-79.

Hankir, A. (2011). Review: bipolar disorder and poetic genius. *Psychiatr Danub.* 23 Suppl 1: S62-68.

Hantouche, E. G., J. Angst and H. S. Akiskal (2003). Factor structure of hypomania: interrelationships with cyclothymia and the soft bipolar spectrum. *J. Affect Disord.* 73(1-2): 39-47.

Hare, E., J. Contreras, H. Raventos, D. Flores, A. Jerez, H. Nicolini, A. Ontiveros, L. Almasy and M. Escamilla (2012). Genetic structure of personality factors and bipolar disorder in families segregating bipolar disorder. *J. Affect Disord.* 136(3): 1027-1033.

Hayden, E. P. and J. I. Nurnberger, Jr. (2006). Molecular genetics of bipolar disorder. *Genes Brain Behav.* 5(1): 85-95.

Hedelin, M., M. Lof, M. Olsson, T. Lewander, B. Nilsson, C. M. Hultman and E. Weiderpass (2010). Dietary intake of fish, omega-3, omega-6 polyunsaturated fatty acids and vitamin. *BMC Psychiatry* 10: 38.

Heffner, J. L., M. P. DelBello, R. M. Anthenelli, D. E. Fleck, C. M. Adler and S. M. Strakowski (2012). Cigarette smoking and its relationship to mood disorder symptoms and co-occurring alcohol and cannabis use disorders following first hospitalization for bipolar disorder. *Bipolar Disord.* 14(1): 99-108.

Heffner, J. L., J. R. Strawn, M. P. DelBello, S. M. Strakowski and R. M. Anthenelli (2011). The co-occurrence of cigarette smoking and bipolar disorder: phenomenology and treatment considerations. *Bipolar Disord.* 13(5-6): 439-453.

Huang, C. C., Y. H. Chang, S. Y. Lee, S. L. Chen, S. H. Chen, C. H. Chu, S. Y. Huang, N. S. Tzeng, I. H. Lee, T. L. Yeh, Y. K. Yang and R. B. Lu (2012). The interaction between BDNF and DRD2 in bipolar II disorder but not in bipolar I disorder. *Am. J. Med. Genet. B Neuropsychiatr. Genet.* 159B(5): 501-507.

Jackson, K. J., A. H. Fanous, J. Chen, K. S. Kendler and X. Chen (2013). Variants in the 15q25 gene cluster are associated with risk for schizophrenia and bipolar disorder. *Psychiatr. Genet.* 23(1): 20-28.

Jamison, K. R. (1989). Mood disorders and patterns of creativity in British writers and artists. *Psychiatry* 52(2): 125-134.

Jamison, K. R. (2011). Great wits and madness: more near allied? *Br. J. Psychiatry* 199(5): 351-352.

Janka, Z. (2004). [Artistic creativity and bipolar mood disorder]. *Orv. Hetil* 145(33): 1709-1718.

Jogia, J., D. Dima and S. Frangou (2012). Sex differences in bipolar disorder: a review of neuroimaging findings and new evidence. *Bipolar Disord.* 14(4): 461-471.

Johnson, S. L., G. Murray, B. Fredrickson, E. A. Youngstrom, S. Hinshaw, J. M. Bass, T. Deckersbach, J. Schooler and I. Salloum (2012). Creativity and bipolar disorder: touched by fire or burning with questions? *Clin. Psychol. Rev.* 32(1): 1-12.

Jones, S. H., S. Tai, K. Evershed, R. Knowles and R. Bentall (2006). Early detection of bipolar disorder: a pilot familial high-risk study of parents with bipolar disorder and their adolescent children. *Bipolar Disord.* 8(4): 362-372.

Jonsdottir, H., S. Opjordsmoen, A. B. Birkenaes, C. Simonsen, J. A. Engh, P. A. Ringen, A. Vaskinn, S. Friis, K. Sundet and O. A. Andreassen (2013). Predictors of medication adherence in patients with schizophrenia and bipolar disorder. *Acta Psychiatr. Scand.* 127(1): 23-33.

Karchemskiy, A., A. Garrett, M. Howe, N. Adleman, D. I. Simeonova, D. Alegria, A. Reiss and K. Chang (2011). Amygdalar, hippocampal, and thalamic volumes in youth at high risk for development of bipolar disorder. *Psychiatry Res.* 194(3): 319-325.

Keck, P. E. and S. L. McElroy (2003). Bipolar disorder, obesity, and pharmacotherapy-associated weight gain. *J. Clin. Psychiatry* 64(12): 1426-1435.

Kenna, G. A., N. Roder-Hanna, L. Leggio, W. H. Zywiak, J. Clifford, S. Edwards, J. A. Kenna, J. Shoaff and R. M. Swift (2012). Association of the 5-HTT gene-linked promoter region (5-HTTLPR) polymorphism with psychiatric disorders: review of psychopathology and pharmacotherapy. *Pharmgenomics Pers. Med.* 5: 19-35.

Kesebir, S., S. Vahip, F. Akdeniz, Z. Yuncu, M. Alkan and H. Akiskal (2005). Affective temperaments as measured by TEMPS-A in patients with bipolar I disorder and their first-degree relatives: a controlled study. *J. Affect Disord.* 85(1-2): 127-133.

Kraepelin (1921). Manic Depressive Insanity and Paranoia. Edinburgh, E and S Livingstone.

Kriegshauser, K., M. Sajatovic, J. H. Jenkins, K. A. Cassidy, D. Muzina, O. Fattal, D. Smith and B. Singer (2010). Gender differences in subjective experience and treatment of bipolar disorder. *J. Nerv. Ment Dis.* 198(5): 370-372.

Kurnianingsih, Y. A., C. N. Kuswanto, R. S. McIntyre, A. Qiu, B. C. Ho and K. Sim (2011). Neurocognitive-genetic and neuroimaging-genetic research paradigms in schizophrenia and bipolar disorder. *J. Neural Transm.* 118(11): 1621-1639.

Lagerberg, T. V., O. A. Andreassen, P. A. Ringen, A. O. Berg, S. Larsson, I. Agartz, K. Sundet and I. Melle (2010). Excessive substance use in bipolar disorder is associated with impaired functioning rather than clinical characteristics, a descriptive study. *BMC Psychiatry* 10: 9.

Leboyer, M., A. Malafosse, S. Boularand, D. Campion, F. Gheysen, D. Samolyk, B. Henriksson, E. Denise, A. des Lauriers and J. P. Lepine (1990). Tyrosine hydroxylase polymorphisms associated with manic-depressive illness. *Lancet* 335(8699): 1219.

Lee, K. Y., J. Y. Song, S. H. Kim, S. C. Kim, E. J. Joo, Y. M. Ahn and Y. S. Kim (2010). Association between CLOCK 3111T/C and preferred circadian phase in Korean patients with bipolar disorder. *Prog. Neuropsychopharmacol. Biol. Psychiatry* 34(7): 1196-1201.

Lee, S. Y., S. L. Chen, Y. H. Chang, C. H. Chu, S. Y. Huang, N. S. Tzeng, C. L. Wang, S. H. Lin, I. H. Lee, T. L. Yeh, Y. K. Yang and R. B. Lu (2012). The ALDH2 and 5-HT2A genes interacted in bipolar-I but not bipolar-II disorder. *Prog. Neuropsychopharmacol. Biol. Psychiatry* 38(2): 247-251.

Lee, S. Y., S. L. Chen, Y. S. Wang, Y. H. Chang, S. Y. Huang, N. S. Tzeng, I. H. Lee, T. L. Yeh, Y. K. Yang and R. B. Lu (2013). COMT and BDNF interacted in bipolar II disorder not comorbid with anxiety disorder. *Behav. Brain Res.* 237: 243-248.

Lerner, Y. and D. Levinson (2012). Dropout from outpatient mental health care: results from the Israel National Health Survey. *Soc. PsychiatryPsychiatr. Epidemiol.* 47(6): 949-955.

Leussis, M. P., J. M. Madison and T. L. Petryshen (2012). Ankyrin 3: genetic association with bipolar disorder and relevance to disease pathophysiology. *Biol. Mood Anxiety Disord.* 2(1): 18.

Licht, R. W. (2012). Lithium: still a major option in the management of bipolar disorder. *CNS Neurosci Ther.* 18(3): 219-226.

Lieberman, D. Z., S. H. Massey and F. K. Goodwin (2010). The role of gender in single vs married individuals with bipolar disorder. *Compr. Psychiatry* 51(4): 380-385.

Linke, J., S. H. Witt, A. V. King, V. Nieratschker, C. Poupon, A. Gass, M. G. Hennerici, M. Rietschel and M. Wessa (2012). Genome-wide supported risk variant for bipolar disorder alters anatomical connectivity in the human brain. *Neuroimage* 59(4): 3288-3296.

Mackay, C. E., E. Roddick, T. R. Barrick, A. J. Lloyd, N. Roberts, T. J. Crow, A. H. Young and I. N. Ferrier (2010). Sex dependence of brain size and shape in bipolar disorder: an exploratory study. *Bipolar Disord.* 12(3): 306-311.

Mandelli, L., M. Mazza, G. Martinotti, D. Tavian, E. Colombo, S. Missaglia, M. Di Nicola, D. De Ronchi, G. Negri, R. Colombo, L. Janiri and A. Serretti (2010). Further evidence supporting the influence of brain-derived neurotrophic factor on the outcome of bipolar depression: independent effect of brain-derived neurotrophic factor and harm avoidance. *J. Psychopharmacol.* 24(12): 1747-1754.

Mandelli L, P. S., Fabbri C, Serretti A (2011). The Genetic Basis of Bipolar Disorder. Bipolar Disorder: Causes, Diagnosis and Treatment. P. J. M, Nova Science Publishers: pp.1-74.

Mansour, H. A., T. H. Monk and V. L. Nimgaonkar (2005). Circadian genes and bipolar disorder. *Ann. Med.* 37(3): 196-205.

Marano, G., D. Harnic, M. Lotrionte, G. Biondi-Zoccai, A. Abbate, E. Romagnoli and M. Mazza (2009). Depression and the cardiovascular system: increasing evidence of a link and therapeutic implications. *ExpertRev. Cardiovasc. Ther.* 7(9): 1123-1147.

Marano, G., G. Traversi, C. Nannarelli, S. Pitrelli, S. Mazza and M. Mazza (2012). Functional neuroimaging: points of intersection between biology and psychotherapy. *Clin. Ter.* 163(6): e443-456.

Marano, G., G. Traversi, E. Romagnoli, V. Catalano, M. Lotrionte, A. Abbate, G. Biondi-Zoccai and M. Mazza (2011). Cardiologic side effects of psychotropic drugs. *J. Geriatr. Cardiol.* 8(4): 243-253.

Marazziti, D., S. Baroni, M. Picchetti, P. Landi, S. Silvestri, E. Vatteroni and M. Catena Dell'Osso (2012). Psychiatric disorders and mitochondrial dysfunctions. *Eur. Rev. Med. Pharmacol. Sci.* 16(2): 270-275.

Mazza, M. and Marano G. (2009). Are Bipolar Disorder Patients with Co-morbid Substance Use Disorder More Compromised in Social Functioning? *European Psychiatric. Review* 2(2): 30-33.

Marneros A, A. J. (2002). Bipolar disorders: roots and evolution. Bipolar Disorders. 100 years after manic-depressive insanity. A. J. Marneros A. NewYork, Boston, Dordrecht, London, Moscow, Kluwer Academic Publishers: pp. 1-36.

Marneros, A., S. Rottig, A. Wenzel, R. Bloink and P. Brieger (2004). Affective and schizoaffective mixed states. *Eur. Arch. Psychiatry Clin. Neurosci.* 254(2): 76-81.

Mazza, M., P. Bria and S. Mazza (2007). Efficacy and safety of oxcarbazepine in bipolar disorder. *Can. J. Psychiatry* 52(4): 272; author reply 272-273.

Mazza, M., M. Di Nicola, G. Della Marca, L. Janiri, P. Bria and S. Mazza (2007). Bipolar disorder and epilepsy: a bidirectional relation? Neurobiological underpinnings, current hypotheses, and future research directions. *Neuroscientist* 13(4): 392-404.

Mazza, M., M. Di Nicola, G. Martinotti, C. Taranto, G. Pozzi, G. Conte, L. Janiri, P. Bria and S. Mazza (2007). Oxcarbazepine in bipolar disorder: a critical review of the literature. *Expert Opin. Pharmacother* 8(5): 649-656.

Mazza, M., D. Harnic, V. Catalano, M. Di Nicola, A. Bruschi, P. Bria, A. Daniele and S. Mazza (2011). Sexual behavior in women with bipolar disorder. *J. Affect Disord.* 131(1-3): 364-367.

Mazza, M., L. Mandelli, M. Di Nicola, D. Harnic, V. Catalano, D. Tedeschi, G. Martinotti, R. Colombo, P. Bria, A. Serretti and L. Janiri (2009). Clinical features, response to treatment and functional outcome of bipolar disorder patients with and without co-occurring substance use disorder: 1-year follow-up. *J. Affect Disord.* 115(1-2): 27-35.

Mazza, M., L. Mandelli, G. Martinotti, M. Di Nicola, D. Tavian, G. Negri, E. Colombo, S. Missaglia, D. De Ronchi, R. Colombo, L. Janiri and A. Serretti (2010). Further evidence supporting the association between 5HTR2C gene and bipolar disorder. *Psychiatry Res.* 180(2-3): 151-152.

Mazza, M., L. Mandelli, L. Zaninotto, M. D. Nicola, G. Martinotti, D. Harnic, A. Bruschi, V. Catalano, D. Tedeschi, R. Colombo, P. Bria, A. Serretti and L. Janiri (2011). Factors associated with the course of symptoms in bipolar disorder during a 1-year follow-up: depression vs. sub-threshold mixed state. *Nord J. Psychiatry* 65(6): 419-426.

Mazza, M., L. Mandelli, L. Zaninotto, M. D. Nicola, G. Martinotti, D. Harnic, A. Bruschi, V. Catalano, D. Tedeschi, R. Colombo, P. Bria, A. Serretti and L. Janiri (2012). Bipolar disorder: pure versus mixed depression over a 1-year follow-up. *Int. J. Psychiatry Clin. Pract.* 16(2): 113-120.

Mazza M, M. G., Traversi G (2011). The Comorbid Factor: Evidence for a Positive Association between Bipolar Disorders and Anxiety Disorders. Bipolar Disorder: Causes, Diagnosis and Treatment. J. M. Plunkett. Nova Publishers: pp.265-280.

Mazza, M., F. Orsucci, S. De Risio, P. Bria and S. Mazza (2004). Epilepsy and depression: risk factors for suicide? *Clin. Ter.* 155(10): 425-427.

Mazza, M., M. Pomponi, L. Janiri, P. Bria and S. Mazza (2007). Omega-3 fatty acids and antioxidants in neurological and psychiatric diseases: an overview. *Prog Neuropsychopharmacol Biol Psychiatry* 31(1): 12-26.

Mazza, M., M. R. Squillacioti, R. D. Pecora, L. Janiri and P. Bria (2008). Beneficial acute antidepressant effects of aripiprazole as an adjunctive treatment or monotherapy in bipolar patients unresponsive to mood stabilizers: results from a 16-week open-label trial. *Expert Opin. Pharmacother* 9(18): 3145-3149.

Mazza, M., M. R. Squillacioti, R. D. Pecora, L. Janiri and P. Bria (2009). Effect of aripiprazole on self-reported anhedonia in bipolar depressed patients. *Psychiatry Res.* 165(1-2): 193-196.

McClung, C. A. (2007). Circadian genes, rhythms and the biology of mood disorders. *Pharmacol. Ther.* 114(2): 222-232.

McElroy, S. L., L. L. Altshuler, T. Suppes, P. E. Keck, Jr., M. A. Frye, K. D. Denicoff, W. A. Nolen, R. W. Kupka, G. S. Leverich, J. R. Rochussen, A. J. Rush and R. M. Post (2001). Axis I psychiatric comorbidity and its relationship to historical illness variables in 288 patients with bipolar disorder. *Am. J. Psychiatry* 158(3): 420-426.

McGrath, C. L., S. J. Glatt, P. Sklar, H. Le-Niculescu, R. Kuczenski, A. E. Doyle, J. Biederman, E. Mick, S. V. Faraone, A. B. Niculescu and M. T. Tsuang (2009). Evidence for genetic association of RORB with bipolar disorder. *BMC Psychiatry* 9: 70.

McKnight RF, Adida M, Budge K, Stockton S, Goodwin GM, Geddes JR (2012). Lithium toxicity profile: a systematic review and meta-analysis. *Lancet.* 25;379(9817):721-8.

McIntyre, R. S., M. Cohen, J. Zhao, L. Alphs, T. A. Macek and J. Panagides (2010). Asenapine in the treatment of acute mania in bipolar I disorder: a randomized, double-blind, placebo-controlled trial. *J. Affect Disord.* 122(1-2): 27-38.

McIntyre, R. S., J. Z. Konarski, K. Wilkins, B. Bouffard, J. K. Soczynska and S. H. Kennedy (2006). The prevalence and impact of migraine headache in bipolar disorder: results from the Canadian Community Health Survey. *Headache* 46(6): 973-982.

McNamara, J. O. (1986). Kindling model of epilepsy. *Adv. Neurol.*44: 303-318.

Medda, P., G. Perugi, S. Zanello, M. Ciuffa and G. B. Cassano (2009). Response to ECT in bipolar I, bipolar II and unipolar depression. *J. Affect Disord.* 118(1-3): 55-59.

Merikangas, K. R., R. Jin, J. P. He, R. C. Kessler, S. Lee, N. A. Sampson, M. C. Viana, L. H. Andrade, C. Hu, E. G. Karam, M. Ladea, M. E. Medina-Mora, Y. Ono, J. Posada-Villa, R. Sagar, J. E. Wells and Z. Zarkov (2011). Prevalence and correlates of bipolar spectrum disorder in the world mental health survey initiative. *Arch. Gen. Psychiatry* 68(3): 241-251.

Merikangas, K. R. and F. Lamers (2012). The 'true' prevalence of bipolar II disorder. *Curr. Opin. Psychiatry* 25(1): 19-23.

Mick, E. and S. V. Faraone (2009). Family and genetic association studies of bipolar disorder in children. *Child Adolesc. Psychiatr Clin. N. Am.* 18(2): 441-453, x.

Mick, E., J. W. Kim, J. Biederman, J. Wozniak, T. Wilens, T. Spencer, J. W. Smoller and S. V. Faraone (2008). Family based association study of pediatric bipolar disorder and the dopamine transporter gene (SLC6A3). *Am. J. Med. Genet. B Neuropsychiatr. Genet.* 147B(7): 1182-1185.

Milhiet, V., B. Etain, C. Boudebesse and F. Bellivier (2011). Circadian biomarkers, circadian genes and bipolar disorders. *J. Physiol. Paris* 105(4-6): 183-189.

Monkul, E. S., J. P. Hatch, R. B. Sassi, D. Axelson, P. Brambilla, M. A. Nicoletti, M. S. Keshavan, N. D. Ryan, B. Birmaher and J. C. Soares (2008). MRI study of the cerebellum in young bipolar patients. *Prog. Neuropsychopharmacol. Biol. Psychiatry* 32(3): 613-619.

Moon, E., J. S. Chang, M. Y. Kim, M. H. Seo, B. Cha, T. H. Ha, S. Choi, H. S. Cho, T. Park and K. Ha (2012). Dropout rate and associated factors in patients with bipolar disorders. *J. Affect Disord.* 141(1): 47-54.

Moreno, C., D. S. Hasin, C. Arango, M. A. Oquendo, E. Vieta, S. Liu, B. F. Grant and C. Blanco (2013). The bipolar-depressive continuum in the National Epidemiologic Survey on Alcohol and Related Conditions. *Bipolar Disord.* 15(1): 112-113.

Murray, D. P., M. Weiner, M. Prabhakar and J. G. Fiedorowicz (2009). Mania and mortality: why the excess cardiovascular risk in bipolar disorder? *Curr. Psychiatry Rep.* 11(6): 475-480.

Murray, G. and E. E. Michalak (2012). The quality of life construct in bipolar disorder research and practice: past, present, and possible futures. *Bipolar Disord.* 14(8): 793-796.

Nery, F. G., J. A. Stanley, H. H. Chen, J. P. Hatch, M. A. Nicoletti, E. S. Monkul, B. Lafer and J. C. Soares (2010). Bipolar disorder comorbid with alcoholism: a 1H magnetic resonance spectroscopy study. *J. Psychiatr. Res.* 44(5): 278-285.

Nierenberg, A. A., C. Kansky, B. P. Brennan, R. C. Shelton, R. Perlis and D. V. Iosifescu (2013). Mitochondrial modulators for bipolar disorder: A pathophysiologically informed paradigm for new drug development. *Aust. N. Z. J. Psychiatry* 47(1): 26-42.

Nievergelt, C. M., D. F. Kripke, T. B. Barrett, E. Burg, R. A. Remick, A. D. Sadovnick, S. L. McElroy, P. E. Keck, Jr., N. J. Schork and J. R. Kelsoe (2006). Suggestive evidence for association of the circadian genes PERIOD3 and ARNTL with bipolar disorder. *Am. J. Med. Genet. B. Neuropsychiatr. Genet.* 141B(3): 234-241.

Nilsson, K. K., K. N. Straarup, C. R. Jorgensen and R. W. Licht (2012). Affective temperaments' relation to functional impairment and affective recurrences in bipolar disorder patients. *J. Affect Disord.* 138(3): 332-336.

Nivoli, A. M., I. Pacchiarotti, A. R. Rosa, D. Popovic, A. Murru, M. Valenti, C. M. Bonnin, I. Grande, J. Sanchez-Moreno, E. Vieta and F. Colom (2011). Gender differences in a cohort study of 604 bipolar patients: the role of predominant polarity. *J. Affect Disord.* 133(3): 443-449.

Oquendo, M. A., D. Currier, S. M. Liu, D. S. Hasin, B. F. Grant and C. Blanco (2010). Increased risk for suicidal behavior in comorbid bipolar disorder and alcohol use disorders: results from the National Epidemiologic Survey on Alcohol and Related Conditions (NESARC). *J. Clin. Psychiatry* 71(7): 902-909.

Ostacher, M. J., R. H. Perlis, A. A. Nierenberg, J. Calabrese, J. P. Stange, I. Salloum, R. D. Weiss and G. S. Sachs (2010). Impact of substance use disorders on recovery from episodes of depression in bipolar disorder patients: prospective data from the Systematic Treatment Enhancement Program for Bipolar Disorder (STEP-BD). *Am. J. Psychiatry* 167(3): 289-297.

Ovadia, G. and S. Shifman (2011). The genetic variation of RELN expression in schizophrenia and bipolar disorder. *PLoS One* 6(5): e19955.

Owen, M. J., N. Craddock and A. Jablensky (2007). The genetic deconstruction of psychosis. *Schizophr. Bull.* 33(4): 905-911.

Pail, G., W. Huf, E. Pjrek, D. Winkler, M. Willeit, N. Praschak-Rieder and S. Kasper (2011). Bright-light therapy in the treatment of mood disorders. *Neuropsychobiology* 64(3): 152-162.

Pandya, C. D., K. R. Howell and A. Pillai (2012). Antioxidants as potential therapeutics for neuropsychiatric disorders. *Prog. Neuropsychopharmacol. Biol. Psychiatry.*

Parker, G., S. McCraw, D. Hadzi-Pavlovic and K. Fletcher (2012). Costs of the principal mood disorders: A study of comparative direct and indirect costs incurred by those with bipolar I, bipolar II and unipolar disorders. *J. Affect Disord.*

Pomponi, M., L. Janiri, G. La Torre, E. Di Stasio, M. Di Nicola, M. Mazza, G. Martinotti, P. Bria, S. Lippa, R. Natili and M. F. Pomponi (2013). Plasma levels of n-3 fatty acids in bipolar patients: Deficit restricted to DHA. *J. Psychiatr. Res.* 47(3): 337-342.

Poon, S. H., K. Sim, M. Y. Sum, C. N. Kuswanto and R. J. Baldessarini (2012). Evidence-based options for treatment-resistant adult bipolar disorder patients. *Bipolar Disord.* 14(6): 573-584.

Post, R. M. (2007). Kindling and sensitization as models for affective episode recurrence, cyclicity, and tolerance phenomena. *Neurosci. Biobehav. Rev.* 31(6): 858-873.

Price, F. S. and J. A. Morris (2013). The genetics of bipolar disorder. *BMJ* 346: f530.

Regenold, W. T., R. K. Thapar, C. Marano, S. Gavirneni and P. V. Kondapavuluru (2002). Increased prevalence of type 2 diabetes mellitus among psychiatric inpatients with bipolar I affective and schizoaffective disorders independent of psychotropic drug use. *J. Affect Disord.* 70(1): 19-26.

Reinares, M., F. Colom, A. R. Rosa, C. M. Bonnin, C. Franco, B. Sole, F. Kapczinski and E. Vieta (2010). The impact of staging bipolar disorder on treatment outcome of family psychoeducation. *J. Affect Disord.* 123(1-3): 81-86.

Rosmond, R. and P. Bjorntorp (1998). The interactions between hypothalamic-pituitary-adrenal axis activity, testosterone, insulin-like growth factor I and abdominal obesity with metabolism and blood pressure in men. *Int. J. Obes. Relat. Metab. Disord.* 22(12): 1184-1196.

Rybakowski, J. K. and K. Twardowska (1999). The dexamethasone/ corticotropin-releasing hormone test in depression in bipolar and unipolar affective illness. *J. Psychiatr. Res.* 33(5): 363-370.

Sajatovic, M., J. Levin, E. Fuentes-Casiano, K. A. Cassidy, C. Tatsuoka and J. H. Jenkins (2011). Illness experience and reasons for nonadherence among individuals with bipolar disorder who are poorly adherent with medication. *Compr. Psychiatry* 52(3): 280-287.

Sajatovic, M., W. Micula-Gondek, C. Tatsuoka and C. Bialko (2011). The relationship of gender and gender identity to treatment adherence among individuals with bipolar disorder. *Gend. Med.* 8(4): 261-268.

Sala, R., B. I. Goldstein, C. Morcillo, S. M. Liu, M. Castellanos and C. Blanco (2012). Course of comorbid anxiety disorders among adults with bipolar disorder in the U.S. population. *J. Psychiatr. Res.* 46(7): 865-872.

Schmitz, B. (2005). Depression and mania in patients with epilepsy. *Epilepsia* 46 Suppl 4: 45-49.

Schottle, D., C. G. Huber, T. Bock and T. D. Meyer (2011). Psychotherapy for bipolar disorder: a review of the most recent studies. *Curr. Opin. Psychiatry* 24(6): 549-555.

Schutter, D. J., P. C. Koolschijn, J. S. Peper and E. A. Crone (2012). The cerebellum link to neuroticism: a volumetric MRI association study in healthy volunteers. *PLoS One* 7(5): e37252.

Sedler, M. J. (1983). Falret's discovery: the origin of the concept of bipolar affective illness. Translated by M. J. Sedler and Eric C. Dessain. *Am. J. Psychiatry* 140(9): 1127-1133.

Shippee, N. D., N. D. Shah, M. D. Williams, J. P. Moriarty, M. A. Frye and J. Y. Ziegenfuss (2011). Differences in demographic composition and in work, social, and functional limitations among the populations with unipolar depression and bipolar disorder: results from a nationally representative sample. *Health Qual Life Outcomes* 9: 90.7.

Sidor, M. M. and G. M. MacQueen (2012). An update on antidepressant use in bipolar depression. *Curr. Psychiatry Rep.* 14(6): 696-704.

Simon, N. M., M. W. Otto, S. R. Wisniewski, M. Fossey, K. Sagduyu, E. Frank, G. S. Sachs, A. A. Nierenberg, M. E. Thase and M. H. Pollack (2004). Anxiety disorder comorbidity in bipolar disorder patients: data from the first 500 participants in the Systematic Treatment Enhancement Program for Bipolar Disorder (STEP-BD). *Am. J. Psychiatry* 161(12): 2222-2229.

Smith, E. N., D. L. Koller, C. Panganiban, S. Szelinger, P. Zhang, J. A. Badner, T. B. Barrett, W. H. Berrettini, C. S. Bloss, W. Byerley, W. Coryell, H. J. Edenberg, T. Foroud, E. S. Gershon, T. A. Greenwood, Y. Guo, M. Hipolito, B. J. Keating, W. B. Lawson, C. Liu, P. B. Mahon, M. G. McInnis, F. J. McMahon, R. McKinney, S. S. Murray, C. M. Nievergelt, J. I. Nurnberger, Jr., E. A. Nwulia, J. B. Potash, J. Rice, T. G. Schulze, W. A. Scheftner, P. D. Shilling, P. P. Zandi, S. Zollner, D. W. Craig, N. J. Schork and J. R. Kelsoe (2011). Genome-wide association of bipolar disorder suggests an enrichment of replicable associations in regions near genes. *PLoS Genet.* 7(6): e1002134.

Soeiro-de-Souza, M. G., D. S. Bio, D. P. David, D. Rodrigues dos Santos, Jr., D. S. Kerr, W. F. Gattaz, R. Machado-Vieira and R. A. Moreno (2012). COMT Met (158) modulates facial emotion recognition in bipolar I disorder mood episodes. *J. Affect Disord.* 136(3): 370-376.

Soeiro-de-Souza, M. G., R. Machado-Vieira, D. Soares Bio, C. M. Do Prado and R. A. Moreno (2012). COMT polymorphisms as predictors of cognitive dysfunction during manic and mixed episodes in bipolar I disorder. *Bipolar Disord.* 14(5): 554-564.

Soreca, I., M. L. Wallace, E. Frank, B. P. Hasler, J. C. Levenson and D. J. Kupfer (2012). Sleep duration is associated with dyslipidemia in patients with bipolar disorder in clinical remission. *J. Affect Disord.* 141(2-3): 484-487.

Squassina, A., M. Manchia, F. Manconi, M. Piccardi, R. Ardau, C. Chillotti, G. Severino and M. Del Zompo (2008). A case-control association study of the PDLIM5 gene and bipolar disorder in a Sardinian sample. *Psychiatr Genet.* 18(3): 128-132.

Szegedi, A., J. R. Calabrese, L. Stet, M. Mackle, J. Zhao and J. Panagides (2012). Asenapine as adjunctive treatment for acute mania associated with bipolar disorder: results of a 12-week core study and 40-week extension. *J. Clin. Psychopharmacol.* 32(1): 46-55.

Teh, C. A., T. S. Lee, M. Kuchibhatla, A. Ashley-Koch, J. Macfall, R. Krishnan and J. Beyer (2012). Bipolar disorder, brain-derived neurotrophic factor (BDNF) Val66Met polymorphism and brain morphology. *PLoS One* 7(7): e38469.

Tharoor, H., A. Kotambail, S. Jain, P. S. Sharma and K. Satyamoorthy (2012). Study of the association of serotonin transporter triallelic 5-HTTLPR and STin2 VNTR polymorphisms with lithium prophylaxis response in bipolar disorder. *Psychiatr Genet.*

Tohen, M., S. F. Greenfield, R. D. Weiss, C. A. Zarate, Jr. and L. M. Vagge (1998). The effect of comorbid substance use disorders on the course of bipolar disorder: a review. *Harv. Rev. Psychiatry* 6(3): 133-141.

Turecki, G., G. A. Rouleau, J. Mari, R. Joober and K. Morgan (1997). Lack of association between bipolar disorder and tyrosine hydroxylase: a meta-analysis. *Am. J. Med. Genet.* 74(4): 348-352.

Valle, J., J. L. Ayuso-Gutierrez, A. Abril and J. L. Ayuso-Mateos (1999). Evaluation of thyroid function in lithium-naive bipolar patients. *Eur. Psychiatry* 14(6): 341-345.

Vancampfort, D., C. U. Correll, M. Probst, P. Sienaert, S. Wyckaert, A. De Herdt, J. Knapen, D. De Wachter and M. De Hert (2013). A review of physical activity correlates in patients with bipolar disorder. *J. Affect Disord.* 145(3): 285-291.

Vemuri, M., H. A. Kenna, P. W. Wang, T. A. Ketter and N. L. Rasgon (2011). Gender-specific lipid profiles in patients with bipolar disorder. *J. Psychiatr. Res.* 45(8): 1036-1041.

Vieta, E. (2005). Improving treatment adherence in bipolar disorder through psychoeducation. *J. Clin. Psychiatry* 66 Suppl 1: 24-29.

Vieta, E., O. Gunther, J. Locklear, M. Ekman, C. Miltenburger, M. L. Chatterton, M. Astrom and B. Paulsson (2011). Effectiveness of psychotropic medications in the maintenance phase of bipolar disorder: a meta-analysis of randomized controlled trials. *Int. J. Neuropsychopharmacol.* 14(8): 1029-1049.

Vita, A., L. De Peri and E. Sacchetti (2009). Gray matter, white matter, brain, and intracranial volumes in first-episode bipolar disorder: a meta-analysis of magnetic resonance imaging studies. *Bipolar Disord.* 11(8): 807-814.

Weiner, M., L. Warren and J. G. Fiedorowicz (2011). Cardiovascular morbidity and mortality in bipolar disorder. *Ann. Clin. Psychiatry* 23(1): 40-47.

Wilens, T. E., J. Biederman, J. Adamson, M. Monuteaux, A. Henin, S. Sgambati, A. Santry and S. V. Faraone (2007). Association of bipolar and substance use disorders in parents of adolescents with bipolar disorder. *Biol. Psychiatry* 62(2): 129-134.

Williams, J. M., K. K. Gandhi, S. E. Lu, M. L. Steinberg and N. L. Benowitz (2012). Nicotine intake and smoking topography in smokers with bipolar disorder. *Bipolar Disord.* 14(6): 618-627.

Wittchen, H. U., S. Mhlig and L. Pezawas (2003). Natural course and burden of bipolar disorders. *Int. J. Neuropsychopharmacol.* 6(2): 145-154.

Womer, F. Y., F. Wang, L. G. Chepenik, J. H. Kalmar, L. Spencer, E. Edmiston, B. P. Pittman, R. T. Constable, X. Papademetris and H. P. Blumberg (2009). Sexually dimorphic features of vermis morphology in bipolar disorder. *Bipolar Disord.* 11(7): 753-758.

Woods, S. W. (2000). The economic burden of bipolar disease. *J. Clin. Psychiatry* 61 Supp 13: 38-41.

Yosifova, A., T. Mushiroda, M. Kubo, A. Takahashi, Y. Kamatani, N. Kamatani, D. Stoianov, R. Vazharova, S. Karachanak, I. Zaharieva, I. Dimova, S. Hadjidekova, V. Milanova, N. Madjirova, I. Gerdjikov, T. Tolev, N. Poryazova, M. C. O'Donovan, M. J. Owen, G. Kirov, D. Toncheva and Y. Nakamura (2011). Genome-wide association study on bipolar disorder in the Bulgarian population. *Genes. Brain Behav.* 10(7): 789-797.

Young, S., D. Pfaff, K. E. Lewandowski, C. Ravichandran, B. M. Cohen and D. Ongur (2012). Anxiety Disorder Comorbidity in Bipolar Disorder, Schizophrenia and Schizoaffective Disorder. *Psychopathology*.

In: Bipolar Disorder
Editor: Nickolas B. Moore

ISBN: 978-1-62618-666-8


Chapter II

# Face Emotion Processing Deficits in Pediatric Bipolar Disorder and Other Childhood Psychopathologies

***Brendan A. Rich*** ***and Heather R. Rosen***
Department of Psychology, Catholic University of America, Washington, DC, US

## Abstract

Pediatric bipolar disorder (PBD) is a severe and often debilitating psychiatric illnesses. Prevalence estimates find a forty-fold increase in the diagnosis of PBD in outpatient settings over a recent 10-year span (Moreno et al., 2007). Of the many impairments of PBD, social deficits may most impact daily functioning. Prominent psychosocial deficits include impaired peer relationships marked by few friends and difficulty keeping friends (Geller et al., 2000), and problems with regulating emotions (Goldstein, Miklowitz, and Mullen, 2006).

Understanding human facial emotions is critical for emotional and social understanding, especially successful social interactions and the building of social relationships (DeSonneville et al., 2002). Recent empirical evidence suggests that PBD youth exhibit profound difficulties in labeling facial expressions and this deficient processing of facial expressions contributes to social impairments among PBD youth (Rich et al., 2008). Further, neurological data find that dysfunction within a distributed fronto-striatal-limbic network characterizes these face emotion processing deficits (Rosen and Rich, 2010).

This chapter reviews empirical evidence for face emotion processing deficits and associated neurocognitive impairments in PBD youth. In addition, we review evidence of face misperception in other childhood psychopathologies, including major depressive disorder (MDD), anxiety (specifically social phobia), and autism spectrum disorders (ASD). In doing so, we attempt to distinguish face emotion processing deficits in PBD

* Contact Information: Brendan A. Rich, PhD - Assistant Professor, Department of Psychology, Catholic University of America, 620 Michigan Ave, NE, Washington, DC 20064. Ph: 202-319-5823. Fax: 202-319-6263. Email: richb@cua.edu.

from other childhood mental disorders, and discuss how this might inform differential diagnosis and perhaps serve as a target for psychotherapeutic intervention.

## Introduction

Bipolar disorder (BD) is one of the most severe and impairing psychiatric illnesses. Early-onset BD (i.e., onset of illness before late adolescence) may be a particularly insidious form of the illness. Youth who develop BD in childhood or early adolescence experience a more severe and longer course of illness than individuals who develop BD in adulthood (Geller and Luby, 1997). Bipolar youth have poorer response to treatment and greater rates of relapse in comparison to individuals with adult-onset BD (Geller et al., 2001), and have a 10-fold increased risk of suicide relative to the general population (Joshi and Wilens, 2009). The prevalence of BD in youth has increased dramatically in the past decade: a four-fold increase in the diagnosis of BD in youth discharged from U.S. community hospitals (Blader and Carlson, 2007; Case, Olfson, Marcus, and Siegel, 2007), and more alarming, a forty-fold increase in the diagnosis of BD in youth in outpatient settings (Moreno et al., 2007). Thus, due to the severity, complexity, and chronicity of symptoms, and the increasing rate of diagnosis, pediatric BD (PBD) is an important public health concern.

One particular area of research that has received a significant amount of scholarly attention in PBD is emotion processing. The human face is the key player in conveying emotional and social information. The ability to detect facial emotion is present at three years of age, and adult competency is reached by age ten (Knapp, 1992). Faces contain vital cues about social interaction and other people's mental states (Ekman et al., 1969) and thus play an integral role in social functioning. Perception of face emotions is particularly important for considering the mental representation of others, and deficits in processing these may impact how one responds in social interchanges (Herba and Phillips, 2004). In sum, the accurate identification and interpretation of facial expressions is imperative for successful social interactions, including the regulation of emotion, the building of social relationships, and the resolution of interpersonal problems (DeSonneville et al., 2002).

Empirical evidence finds that BD youth exhibit profound difficulties in labeling facial expressions (Guyer et al., 2007; Rich et al., 2006). Further, research indicates that deficient processing of facial expressions contributes to social impairments among BD youth (Rich et al., 2008). Such social deficits are highly debilitating and may have the greatest impact on BD youths' day-to-day functioning. Some of the most profound psychosocial deficits experienced by BD youth include poor parent-child relationships, impaired peer relationships marked by few friends and difficulty keeping friends (Geller et al., 2000), and problems with regulating emotions (Goldstein, Miklowitz, and Mullen, 2006). In addition, neurological data find that emotion processing deficits in PBD involve dysfunction within a distributed fronto-striatal-limbic network that regulates emotional and behavioral processes and responses (Rosen and Rich, 2010).

Interestingly, face misperception is evident in other childhood psychopathologies, including major depressive disorder (MDD), anxiety, and autism spectrum disorders (ASD). For example, youth with MDD are more likely to misclassify face emotions and rate facial expressions as more negative relative to healthy controls (Arsenio et al., 2004). Research indicates that youth with anxiety, particularly social anxiety, are less accurate than healthy comparisons in identifying facial emotions (Easter et al., 2005; Simonian et al., 2001). Finally, compared to healthy comparisons, youth with ASD are less likely to attend to facial features with high emotional salience (Klin et al., 2002) and have trouble recognizing and identifying facial emotions (Golan, Baron-Cohen, Hill, and Golan, 2006). There is evidence to suggest that face processing deficits may be greater in PBD youth than those with anxiety, MDD, and disruptive behavior disorders (Guyer et al., 2007).

This chapter reviews empirical evidence for face emotion processing deficits and associated neurocognitive impairments in PBD youth. Given that face processing deficits are ubiquitous to child psychopathology, we attempt to distinguish this deficit in PBD from three other childhood mental disorders (i.e., MDD, anxiety, and ASD), and discuss how this might inform differential diagnosis. We discuss the nature of face expression misperception, its role in the prominent psychosocial deficits in PBD, and its potential as a target for psychotherapeutic intervention.

## Face Emotion Processing Abnormalities in Bipolar Youth

### Behavioral Deficits

In one of the first studies to document face processing deficits in BD youth, McClure and colleagues (2005) used the Diagnostic Analysis of Nonverbal Accuracy [DANVA; (1994)], in which subjects classified the emotions of child and adult faces depicting happiness, sadness, anger, and fear. Findings indicated that euthymic BD patients performed significantly worse than controls in identifying the emotions of both child and adult faces, with particular deficits for happiness and anger in child faces, and sadness and anger in adult faces.

Rich and colleagues (2006) investigated cognitive and neurophysiological differences between BD youth and controls when rating the emotionality of facial expressions. Subjects viewed happy, angry, fearful, and neutral faces and rated the displayed face according to: (1) the level of perceived threat; (2) their subjective fearful response; and (3) a facial feature without emotion (i.e., nose width). This study also found significant face emotion processing deficits in BD youth, where compared to controls, youth with BD rated neutral faces as significantly more fear producing and angry. Thus, BD youth misperceived threat in otherwise calm and nonemotional facial expressions. Rich et al. also identified associated neurological abnormalities that will be reviewed later.

Schenkel and colleagues (2007) investigated facial emotion processing deficits in both medicated, euthymic and unmedicated, acutely ill BD youth relative to controls. Subjects completed the Emotional Acuity and the Emotional Differentiation subtests of the Penn Computerized Neuropsychological Battery (Erwin et al., 1992; Silver, Shlomo, Turner, and Gur, 2002), which assess one's ability to distinguish between happy and sad facial expressions. Results demonstrated that across both tasks, compared to healthy controls, acutely ill BD patients made significantly more errors classifying happy and sad facial expressions, whereas euthymic BD patients were impaired on happy and sad faces only on the Emotional Acuity subtest. Secondary analyses indicated that BD youth with comorbid ADHD made significantly more classification errors on sad faces than BD patients without ADHD. Further, earlier age of BD onset correlated with more face emotion classification errors.

Rich and colleagues (2008) compared youth with BD to controls on a task that presented gradations of facial emotions. Results indicated that even when BD youth correctly identified face emotions, they required more intense displays of emotions on happy, fearful, disgusted, and surprised faces than controls. These impairments were still apparent in BD youth even when taking into account comorbid diagnoses, medication status, and mood state. These findings suggest that face emotion-processing deficits in PBD may be trait-based. In addition, impaired face emotion labeling was associated with social deficits in youth with BD: the more impaired the face emotion understanding in BD youth, the greater their social deficits.

A final study provides preliminary evidence that face processing deficits may in fact be a biomarker for BD in youth. Brotman and colleagues (2008) compared youth who are at-risk for BD illness (i.e., had a parent or sibling with BD) to those already diagnosed with BD, and to healthy controls between the ages of 4 and 18 using the DANVA. Both BD patients and at-risk youth misidentified a greater number of emotions on child and adult faces than controls. Thus, these types of facial affect misclassification may be evident in youth with a genetic predisposition for BD but who have not been diagnosed with the disorder.

In sum, studies consistently find BD youth to be deficient when processing a variety of facial emotional displays. Importantly, these deficits are seen across different BD samples and using diverse tasks of face processing. Although comorbid ADHD may exacerbate poor performance on face emotion recognition tasks, such deficits are apparent independent of mood state and medication status. These deficits are associated with social impairments typically seen in PBD and may serve as potential vulnerability markers for BD illness.

## Neurocognitive Deficits

A series of fMRI studies confirm the behavioral face processing deficits reviewed above and begin to clarify the neural mechanisms underlying these deficits in BD youth. In general, results from PBD studies are mostly consistent with those found in fMRI studies of adult patients with BD. In particular, fMRI studies suggest that adults with BD exhibit prefrontal cortex (PFC) abnormalities while processing facial expressions, including regions of the dorsolateral prefrontal cortex (DLPFC; Hassel et al., 2008), the ventrolateral prefrontal cortex (VLPFC; Foland-Ross et al., 2012), and the orbitofrontal cortex (OFC; Chen et al., 2010); however, the direction of activation for these regions remains inconsistent across studies. The presence of amygdala hyperactivation while viewing emotional faces is also inconsistent across the literature among BD adults (Altshuler et al., 2005; Hassel et al., 2009; Malhi et al., 2007; Robinson et al., 2008). Meta-analyses of fMRI studies with BD adults highlight similar deficits, where reduced VLPFC and greater limbic (i.e., parahippocampal, hippocampal, amygdala, and basal ganglia) activation are observed in response to emotional stimuli (Chen, Suckling, Lennox, Ooi, and Bullmore, 2011) and during tasks involving the processing of facial emotion (Delvecchio et al., 2012).

Findings from fMRI studies with BD youth show similar deficits, where amygdala activation in response to emotional faces is poorly inhibited by prefrontal regions. For example, Pavuluri and colleagues (2007) compared neural activity during passive viewing of emotional faces (i.e., angry, happy, neutral) between euthymic, unmedicated BD youth and controls. Subjects were instructed to press a button each time a new face was presented on the screen. Behavioral results indicated no significant between-group differences in reaction time (RT). In terms of functional data, Pavuluri et al. found that BD youth displayed reduced activation of the OFC and the DLPFC when passively viewing angry faces versus neutral faces compared to controls. Additionally, when viewing happy faces versus neutral faces, BD patients showed decreased activation of the OFC, medial PFC, and DLPFC, and increased activation of the right posterior parietal cortex, right amygdala, and bilateral pregenual ACC relative to healthy controls.

In another study, Pavuluri (2009) examined neural differences between directed/explicit emotion processing (i.e., classifying a facial expression as either positive/happy or negative/angry) and incidental/implicit emotion processing (i.e., indicating whether the face of the person was older or younger than 35 years). There were no significant group differences in response time accuracy between unmedicated, euthymic BD adolescents and controls. Analysis of fMRI data revealed that in comparison to controls, in the incidental emotion processing condition, BD youth exhibited greater activity of the right amygdala, left DLPFC, left posterior cingulate cortex, and right cuneus.

Results from fMRI implicated functional abnormalities in an amygdala-striatal-VLPFC circuit. Specifically, Rich et al. (2006) showed that on trials where BD youth misperceived threat in neutral faces, BD patients exhibited greater activation of the left amygdala, accumbens, putamen, and VLPFC than controls. Further, increased ratings of hostility were significantly associated with heightened amygdala activity. Thus, there was a direct relation between amygdala perturbations and facial affect misperceptions.

Extending this work, Rich and colleagues (2008) investigated the functional connectivity between brain regions implicated in aberrant face emotion processing among individuals with BD. Neural functional connectivity measures the extent to which activation in one brain region is temporally associated with neural activity in another brain region. Using the same face-processing task discussed above (2006), Rich and colleagues compared neural functional connectivity between BD youth and controls aged 7 to 18 years. Results demonstrated that in comparison to controls, BD youth displayed significantly decreased functional connectivity between the left amygdala and two other regions: 1) right posterior cingulate/precuneus and 2) right fusiform gyrus/parahippocampal gyrus. These brain regions are critical for the processing of facial expressions (Haxby, Hoffman, and Gobbini, 2002; Kanwisher, McDermott, and Chun, 1997) and comprehension of social situations (Amaral, Price, Pitaken, and Carmichael, 1992; Critchley et al., 2000; Haxby, Hoffman, and Gobbini, 2002), and are associated with emotional learning and memory (Fanselow and LeDoux, 1999; Yaniv, Schafer, LeDoux, and Richter-Levin, 2000). Interestingly, weaker neural connectivity in BD youth was unrelated to comorbid diagnoses (i.e., ADHD, ODD, anxiety), mood state, or medication use. Thus, deficient connectivity between the amygdala and temporal cortical regions may reflect a trait marker for BD itself. These findings further elucidate a possible neural network underlying the pathophysiology of BD and the neural mechanisms associated with the emotional processing and social deficits found in BD patients.

It is interesting to note that across these three face processing studies, BD youth consistently displayed amygdala hyperactivity as compared to controls. In an effort to connect functional amygdala abnormalities to structural amygdala abnormalities, Kalmar and colleagues (2009) found that compared to controls, BD adolescents had significantly decreased amygdala volume and significantly increased amygdala activation during a gender discrimination task with happy, fearful, and neutral facial expressions. In particular, BD adolescents with the smallest amygdala volume exhibited the greatest amygdala activation during the processing of facial emotion. Therefore, a possible link may exist between structural and functional amygdala abnormalities in BD youth.

Dickstein and colleagues (Dickstein et al., 2007) evaluated differences in functional activity when encoding emotional facial stimuli between BD adolescents and controls. Subjects viewed four types of emotional faces (i.e., angry, fearful, happy, neutral) followed by an unexpected recognition memory test 30 minutes after scanning. Behavioral results showed that compared to controls, adolescents with BD displayed reduced memory for emotional faces, especially fearful faces. Comparative fMRI revealed that, relative to controls, BD youth displayed increased activation of the OFC for angry faces later recalled, and greater activation of the caudate, putamen, ACC, and OFC for happy faces later recalled. Thus, these results suggest hyperactivation of the fronto-striatal region among BD youth during encoding of affective facial stimuli.

In a recent fMRI study exploring the temporal characteristics of abnormal amygdala and prefrontal (i.e., DLPFC) activation, Garrett and colleagues (2012) examined decreases (habituation) and increases (sensitization) in the magnitude of activation over time among euthymic BD youth while viewing a display of emotional faces. In healthy adults, fMRI studies suggest that reduced amygdala activation is associated with repeated exposure to displays of fearful and neutral facial expressions (habituation), demonstrating that after the stimulus has been processed, attentional resources can be properly redistributed (Breiter et al., 1996; Wright et al., 2001). Conversely, healthy adults display greater activation in response to non-repeated angry facial stimuli (sensitization) over time, indicating that additional time and resources are necessary to interpret and process novel and/or threatening stimuli. Irregular habituation of amygdala activity and an absence of sensitization in prefrontal activity may indicate an inability for prefrontal regions to properly modulate and regulate amygdala activity (or appropriately process and respond to emotional stimuli) and thus, result in poor emotion regulation, a core feature of BD.

Garrett et al. (2012) found that BD youth demonstrated increased activation in the superior temporal sulcus (STS)/insula (associated with perception of faces and social aspects of face processing) and visual cortex/poster cingulate (possibly indicating greater attention to facial emotion) from the early (first half) to late phase (second half) of each testing block viewing emotional faces (i.e., happy, sad, and neutral). Activation in these regions from the early to late phase of the block decreased slightly in healthy controls. These findings are consistent with previous literature demonstrating poor prefrontal cortex regulation of increased amygdala activation to emotional stimuli in PBD (Rosen and Rich, 2010). These results suggest that while healthy controls effectively process the faces and then allocate fewer neural resources, BD youth increase their attentional resources to the faces and have difficulty disengaging away from the emotional faces. This also potentially indicates problems with processing facial expressions, which is consistent with behavioral research demonstrating that BD youth misidentify facial emotions, as discussed earlier.

While the most consistent neurological finding across adult and pediatric BD patients is amygdala hyperactivity during implicit emotion processing (e.g., presentation of a facial stimulus with emotional valence and the task is to report on nonemotional features of the face, such as gender or width of the nose), only one study to date has directly compared amygdala function in pediatric versus adult BD patients. In a cross-sectional fMRI study, Kim and colleagues (2012), compared amygdala activity in youth (ages 7-18 years) and adults (ages 19-60 years) with BD and in healthy controls during implicit processing of angry, fearful, and neutral facial expressions from the Pictures of Facial Affect series (gray-scale images depicting men and women displaying a variety of facial expressions) (Ekman and Frieson, 1976). Fearful faces were used since research has consistently shown that fearful faces elicit amygdala hyperactivity in both adults and youth with BD. Angry faces served as a negative comparison condition and neutral faces served as a control condition. Participants were instructed to respond whether the face presented was male or female. Results indicated that relative to healthy controls, both adults and youth with BD displayed heightened right amygdala activity in response to fearful expressions, which is consistent with previous research consisting of only BD adult or BD child samples (Kalmar et al., 2009; Lawrence et al., 2004; Yurgelun-Todd et al., 2002). Interestingly, however, BD youth showed greater right amygdala activation when responses to all three facial expressions were combined compared to both BD adults and healthy youth. These findings could suggest that facial stimuli themselves vary in their degree of valence to adults versus youth with BD, particularly when it comes to deciphering neutral faces. Thus, these results could speak to the developmental differences between adults and youth with BD in terms of the salience and interpretation of different facial expressions. In this vein, meta-analyses have noted that decreased amygdala volume is more prominent and reliably seen in BD youth than in adults with BD (Pfeifer, Welge, Strakowski, Adler, and DelBello, 2008; Usher, Leucht, Falkai, and Scherk, 2010). Further, behavioral research indicates that although face emotion labeling (explicit processing) deficits are observed in both adults and youth with BD, such deficits are more consistently displayed by BD youth (Kohler et al., 2011). In addition, research overwhelmingly suggests that PBD is a more severe form of adult-onset BD (e.g., Axelson et al., 2006; Birmaher et al., 2009; Carlson, Bromet, Driessens, Mojtabai, and Schwartz, 2002; Dickstein et al., 2007; Geller and Luby, 1997; Lewinsohn, Klein, and Seeley, 1995; Lewinsohn, Klein, and Seeley, 2000; McWhirter and Walters, 2008). Therefore, such pervasive cognitive and neurological deficits would be expected to be more pronounced in child-onset BD than adult BD.

Finally, as discussed earlier, behavioral data suggest that youth with a first-degree BD relative exhibit difficulties with face emotion identification (Brotman et al., 2008a; Brotman et al., 2008b); however, research on the neural substrates of these behavioral deficits in youth at-risk for BD is extremely limited. To date, only one study has investigated the neural correlates of face emotion processing deficits in unaffected and unmedicated youth at-risk for BD. Olsavsky and colleagues (2012) examined amygdala activity in response to emotional (i.e., "How hostile is the face?"; "How afraid are you of this face?") and nonemotional aspects (i.e., "How wide is the nose?") of happy and fearful faces among a sample of BD, unaffected first-degree relatives (i.e., siblings or offspring) of BD patients, and healthy control youths.

Results showed that both BD and unaffected at-risk subjects displayed greater right amygdala activation while rating their fear of fearful faces compared to healthy controls, with no differences in amygdala activation between BD and at-risk youth, even after controlling for at-risk familial status (i.e., sibling versus offspring of BD proband). Amygdala hyperactivation to fearful faces was still apparent in BD youth even when taking into account comorbid diagnoses and mood state. In addition, there were no differences in amygdala activity between groups in response to happy faces. Identifying neurobiological aberrations in unaffected first-degree relatives of patients with BD may help to elucidate potential endophenotypes of the illness, and examining unaffected at-risk youth in particular may clarify if neurobiological abnormalities can be used ultimately to predict full manifestation of BD.

Face emotions may hold particular promise for clarifying the pathophysiology of BD in youth and identifying behavioral and cognitive deficits that characterize the disorder. As discussed, research has consistently shown that BD youth misidentify face emotions across patient samples and face-processing tasks. Additionally, findings from fMRI implicate a fronto-striatal-limbic circuit in the processing of face emotion, with amygdala hyperactivation as a consistent neural correlate of face emotion processing deficits in BD youth.

## Face Emotion Processing Deficits in Depressed Youth

Major depressive disorder (MDD) typically starts in childhood or adolescence and is often continuous with and predicts affective disorders in adulthood (Pine et al., 1998). Depressed youth, particularly adolescents, are at heightened risk of suicide, other psychiatric disorders, and substance abuse, and are more likely to experience recurrent lifelong depressive episodes than individuals with onset later in life (Birmaher, Arbelaez, and Brent, 2002). Depression is relatively rare in preschool-aged children, with a 3 to 6 month prevalence of 1 to 2% (Egger et al., 2006), and has low prevalence rates of 1 to 3% in school-aged children (Garber and Horowitz, 2002). However, the prevalence of MDD dramatically rises in adolescence, with an estimated point prevalence of 5 to 6% and a cumulative lifetime rate in the 15 to 20% range (Costello et al., 2003). Depressed youth suffer significant impairment across several domains of functioning, including school, family, and peers (Garber and Horowitz, 2002).

### Behavioral Deficits

Individuals with MDD display a number of negative emotional biases involving attention, appraisal, and memory that are thought to contribute to both the development and maintenance of the depressed state (Beck et al., 1979). One of the most consistent findings in MDD is a tendency to selectively recall negative information (i.e., emotional memory bias) (Bradley, Mogg, and Williams, 2005; Zakzanis, Leach, and Kaplan, 1998), a deficit that is rather specific to MDD (McNally, 1997). While there has been a growth in research addressing patterns of face emotion processing in recent years, there is a paucity of behavioral research on this topic with depressed youth.

Amongst the research that is available are data indicating that pediatric MDD is associated with a deficit in memory for face emotions. Pine and colleagues (2004) investigated the relationship between MDD and biases in facial memory in offspring (ages 9-19) of parents with MDD, anxiety disorders (panic disorder or social phobia), and healthy comparisons. Offspring were assessed for a history of MDD. The behavioral task consisted of an encoding paradigm where subjects viewed emotional faces, and the recall paradigm assessed subjects' ability to recall an individual displaying a neutral expression whereas he/she was seen previously expressing a high-valence emotion.

Pine et al. (2004) found that compared to non-MDD subjects, youth with a history of MDD displayed a deficit in selective memory for fearful faces (but not happy or angry faces), and found no relationship between face-memory performance and parental history of MDD. Both age and gender separately predicted memory, where recall was better in older adolescents and female subjects, which is consistent with previous work (e.g., Nelson et al., 2002). These results suggest that youth with MDD have impaired encoding of fearful facial expressions, which has been observed in other work with adults with MDD (Sheline et al., 2001) and linked to neuroimaging research indicating perturbed amygdala functioning in youth with MDD (Monk et al., 2008).

Schepman and colleagues (2012) investigated face emotion recognition in depressed youth (ages 8-18) with and without comorbid conduct disorder (CD), a disorder where depression often co-occurs (Angold and Costello, 1993). Subjects were presented with printed photographs of blended/morphed expressions along four continua (happy-neutral; sad-neutral; fear-neutral; anger-neutral). After the presentation of each face, subjects rated the face as happy, sad, fearful, or angry. Results indicated that groups did not differ in their general ability to identify facial emotions. Youth with MDD displayed significant biases when processing low-intensity expressions. In particular, MDD youth recognized low-intensity sad and fearful faces better than controls, and non-MDD controls more frequently misclassified low-intensity negative emotions as happy than MDD youth. There were no significant group differences on performance and the intensity level for happy and angry faces. Additionally, there were no differences in performance between MDD youth with and without CD, or between youth with comorbid MDD/CD and controls.

Findings from this study suggest that instead of possessing a gross impairment in facial affect recognition, MDD youth appear to exhibit face emotion processing *biases* compared to youth without MDD, where they differ in the processing of ambiguous faces. In general, depressed youth display a reduced 'happy bias' and an increased 'sad bias' for low-intensity emotions, which are more likely to be important for everyday functioning and social interactions. Perceiving people as happier or sadder than they really are may have particular consequences in relationships with others.

## Neuroimaging Deficits

Given that the amygdala is engaged during the viewing of fearful faces (Monk et al., 2003; Nelson et al., 2003) and that the adult MDD literature suggests amygdala hyperactivation in response to fearful and sad faces compared to controls (Sheline et al., 2001; Surguladze et al., 2005), the majority of research on face emotion processing in depressed youth has stemmed from this research and has further explored perturbed amygdala functioning in response to facial affect. However, findings from fMRI studies are inconsistent in depressed youth. For example, one study found that a small sample of girls (aged 8-16 years) with MDD ($n = 5$) exhibited decreased left amygdala activation during passive viewing of fearful faces compared to both anxious and control girls (Thomas et al., 2001). Yet, Roberson-Nay and colleagues (2006) found contrary results. In their fMRI study, depressed, anxious, and healthy adolescents were compared on a face emotion encoding task (described earlier: Pine et al., 2004). Behavioral results indicated that MDD adolescents showed poorer memory for faces relative to healthy adolescents. Neuroimaging results demonstrated increased left amygdala activation in adolescents with MDD compared to healthy and anxious adolescents during successful (versus unsuccessful) encoding of emotional faces. There were no between-group differences in brain activation for specific facial emotions examined independently of memory performance. These findings are consistent with extensive research on amygdala function in adult MDD (Drevets, 2003; Drevets et al., 2002; Whalen et al., 2002), and specifically the finding of increased left amygdala activation during exposure to emotional faces among depressed adults (Sheline et al., 2001). Given these findings among adults with MDD, this study indicates that adolescent and adult MDD may involve similar underlying deficits in amygdala functioning.

Hyperactivation of the amygdala in response to fearful faces has also been observed in youth at risk for MDD. For example, Monk et al. (2008) compared activation of the amygdala and nucleus accumbens (responds to rewards such as money and happy facial displays; Ernst et al., 2005) in youth (aged 10-18 years) at high (offspring of parents with MDD) and low (offspring of parents without history of MDD, anxiety, or psychotic disorders) risk for MDD. Subjects viewed morphed faces that varied in intensity of happy or fearful expression and neutral faces. Monk and colleagues found that high-risk offspring displayed increased amygdala and nucleus accumbens activation to fearful faces compared to low risk offspring during passive viewing. In addition, high-risk offspring exhibited lower nucleus accumbens activation than low-risk offspring in response to happy faces during passive viewing. Group differences in both the amygdala and nucleus accumbens to emotional faces were observed only during passive viewing and not during the other two conditions, suggesting that the attention conditions may be activating other structures (e.g., the PFC) thought to regulate abnormal activation in the amygdala and nucleus accumbens. Indeed, results indicated that high-risk offspring exhibited heightened medial PFC activation to fearful faces in the two attention-constraining tasks (subjective fear and nose width rating) relative to low-risk subjects. Findings from this study indicate that amygdala and nucleus accumbens dysfunction in response to facial affect may reflect vulnerability markers for MDD.

Manni and colleagues (2011) also explored frontolimbic response to emotional faces in a sample of unaffected adolescents/young adult offspring (aged 16-21 years) of parents with MDD and healthy comparisons. During fMRI scanning, subjects performed a simple task of matching fearful and happy facial expressions. Manni et al. found that compared to controls, offspring subjects showed decreased activation in the left DLPFC to the presentation of fearful faces. Impaired activation of the DLPFC has been observed in depressed patients when performing cognitive or emotional tasks (Fales et al., 2008; Siegle et al., 2007). The PFC plays an integral role in the regulation of limbic areas, including the amygdala. In acutely depressed individuals, depressed mood is correlated with increased limbic activity and inversely related to reduced prefrontal activity (Drevets, 2003; Sheline et al., 2001). Interestingly, amygdala activation did not differ between groups when responding to fearful faces. This finding is contrary to those reported by Monk et al. (2008), where offspring of depressed parents exhibited increased amygdala in response to passively viewing fearful faces. However, when the fearful faces were presented within attentional constraints (i.e., Monk et al., 2008) no heightened amygdala response was observed. Given that offspring participants displayed impaired activation of the DLPFC in the absence of altered amygdala activity (Manni et al., 2011), abnormal DLPFC activation may reflect a trait marker for MDD and be present prior to the onset of any mood disturbances.

In sum, findings from behavioral and neuroimaging studies suggest that pediatric MDD is associated with a negative interpretation bias when processing facial affect, a deficit in memory for fearful faces, and dysfunction within a specific neural circuit involving the amygdala and prefrontal cortical regions that appears to be engaged by the processing of fearful faces. However, the direction of amygdala activation has varied across studies, meaning with MDD youth the precise role that the amygdala plays in the pathophysiology of MDD remains unclear.

## Face Emotion Processing Abnormalities in Anxious Youth

Anxiety disorders are thought to be among the most prevalent childhood psychiatric disorders, with prevalence rates ranging from 3-24% (Cartwright-Hatton, McNicol, and Doubleday, 2006). Childhood anxiety disorders are chronic, recurrent, and highly impairing, particularly across multiple domains of functioning, including academic performance, social interaction, self-confidence, and the ability to enjoy experiences of everyday life (Bittner et al., 2007; Pine, 1997). Pediatric anxiety disorders are highly comorbid with other psychiatric disorders, including ADHD (0-21%), conduct disorder and oppositional defiant disorder (CD/ODD) (3-13%), and depression (1-20%) (Costello et al., 2004).

### Behavioral Deficits

Evidence for face emotion processing deficits in youth with anxiety disorders is less consistent than for youth with BD, and has primarily focused on social phobia (SP). Social phobia or social anxiety disorder is characterized by discomfort and difficulty in social situations and interpersonal relationships and a fear of being negatively evaluated by others (Clark and Wells, 1995). Like youth with BD, children and adolescents with SP suffer significant emotional distress and impairment in daily functioning, and lack the necessary skills to be socially successful (Beidel, Turner, and Morris, 1999). Youth with SP desire friendships, but are reluctant to engage in social interactions due to fear of embarrassment. Often this leads to isolation and significant emotional distress (Beidel and Turner, 2007). While much of the emotion processing research on both adults and youth with anxiety disorders has involved attentional and appraisal biases (e.g., Asmundson and Stein, 1994; Dalgleish et al., 2003; Hope, Rapee, Heimber, and Dombeck, 1990; In-Albon et al., 2009; Martin et al., 1992; Perez-Edgar et al., 2010; Vasey et al., 2008), less is known regarding the degree to which these biases impact one's ability to perceive explicit real-life social cues such as the facial affect of others. Misclassification of face emotions may contribute to the maintenance of social fear due to high rates of error, long reaction times, a tendency to interpret neutral and positive facial expressions as negative, and little confidence in the accuracy of classification during social exchanges (Melfson and Florin, 2002).

There are mixed findings regarding deficits and negative interpretive biases in facial affect identification among adults with SP. For example, adults with high social anxiety have a heightened tendency to detect negative emotions in facial expressions (Winton, Clark, and Edelman, 1995), and exhibit an attentional bias away from negative facial expressions (Yuen, 1994) compared to adults with low social anxiety; however, these deficits have not been replicated consistently across other samples of socially anxious adults (e.g., Kolassa, Kolassa, Musial, and Miltner, 2007; Kolassa and Miltner, 2006).

There is also limited research on face emotion processing deficits among youth with SP. Simonion and colleagues (2001) compared socially anxious youth (ages 9-15) to healthy controls on their performance on a face emotion recognition task, where subjects were asked to identify one of six emotions (i.e., happiness, sadness, anger, fear, surprise, and disgust) depicted on images from the Pictures of Facial Affect (Ekman and Friesen, 1976). Compared to healthy controls, youth with SP had significantly more errors overall in facial affect recognition, and these deficits were most pronounced for presentations of happiness, sadness, and disgust. These findings support other research indicating that socially anxious youth are less accurate in identifying facial affect (e.g., Jarros et al., 2012) and more likely than controls to misclassify anger as disgust and neutral as sadness (Battaglia et al., 2004). Further, post-hoc analyses indicated that while state anxiety (i.e., anxiety experienced while completing the task) contributed to some of the patients' difficulty in identifying facial emotions, it did not account for enough variance in recognition scores above and beyond whether the child met diagnostic criteria for SP. Therefore, these results suggest that difficulty detecting facial affect may reflect an inherent cognitive deficit among socially anxious youth.

In a recent study, Wong and colleagues (2012) compared facial affect recognition abilities, pre- and post-test anxiety, and social functioning among youth (7-13 years) with (SP), high functioning autism (HFA), or typical development (TD). In particular, they examined the role of emotional intensity in face recognition abilities. Subjects identified facial emotions (i.e., anger, disgust, fear, happy, neutral, or sad) of images selected from the Penn Emotion Recognition set, consisting of three dimensional, high-quality color facial images (Gur et al., 2002). Each emotion (except neutral) was presented with eight different images: four of mild intensity and four of extreme intensity. Recognition accuracy of youth with SP did not significantly differ from either the HFA or TD groups. The lack of difference between the SP and TD groups is contrary to results of previous studies with socially anxious youth (e.g., Battaglia et al., 2004; Simonion et al., 2001) and with a sample comprised of youth with various anxiety disorders (e.g., Easter et al., 2005). Observed differences, however, could be due to variations in methodology across studies (i.e., use of different facial stimuli and variations in length of time the stimulus was presented).

Brunet, Heisz, Mondloch, Shore, and Schmidt (2009) investigated the relationship between temperamental shyness and face scanning behavior in a non-clinical sample of 11-year old children. Social anxiety and shyness are considered to be both empirically and conceptually related and are characterized by the same affective, cognitive, and behavioral deficits in social situations (Schmidt and Buss, 2009). Brunet and colleagues asked subjects to decide whether pairs of faces were the same or different. With the use of an eye tracker, findings indicated that higher rates of shyness were associated with longer dwell time to the eye region and shorter dwell time to the mouth, suggesting that most shy children were not avoiding the eye region. Findings from this study may also indicate hypersensitivity among some shy children to initially use the eyes as a way of detecting social cues and the intentions of others.

Overall, behavioral findings are inconsistent in socially anxious youth: some research indicates that youth with SP exhibit a greater number of facial affect recognition errors than controls, whereas other research shows no differences in face emotion processing ability. Similar to youth with BD, research has demonstrated that youth with SP have a tendency to interpret ambiguous or neutral facial stimuli as negative; however, this finding has not been consistently replicated in the literature.

### Neurocognitive Deficits

The amygdala and VLPFC are regions involved in the perception of threat, where the amygdala facilitates immediate processing of threat and the VLPFC is responsible for later processing associated with emotion regulation (Phillips, Drevets, Rauch, and Lane, 2003). Dysfunction within this neural circuit is implicated in anxiety disorders (Hariri, Mattay, Tessitore, Fera, and Weinberger, 2003). In general, heightened amygdala, insula, and medial PFC activity have been observed during face emotion processing across a range of anxiety disorders (Britton and Rauch, 2009). Limited information is known, however, about the neural substrates of face emotion processing deficits in youth with anxiety disorders and findings are rather inconsistent. Blair and colleagues (2011) examined the degree to which adolescents and adults with SP and healthy comparisons show similar neural deficits in response to facial expressions. Subjects were asked to make gender judgments on faces depicting anger, fear, and neutral expressions.

Results indicated that relative to controls, both patient groups exhibited significantly greater activation of the rostral ACC (when viewing angry faces versus neutral) and increased activation of the amygdala and rostral ACC (when viewing fearful faces versus neutral). Interestingly, there were no differences in activation when viewing angry or fearful faces between the two patient groups. Additionally, severity of SP was associated with increased rostral ACC in adult patients but not adolescent patients compared to healthy controls. These findings suggest that both adults and adolescents with SP share the same neural deficits when processing facial expressions. The fact that neural perturbations (to emotional facial expressions) in adults with SP are also present in adolescents with SP may reflect the presence of persistent abnormalities unique to SP rather than adaptive responses to perturbed development.

Clearly, additional fMRI studies with SP youth are needed to delineate the pathophysiology of face misperception in socially anxious youth.

## Face Emotion Processing Abnormalities in Autistic Youth

Autism spectrum disorders (ASDs) are increasingly prevalent, life-long neurodevelopmental illnesses that include high-functioning autism (HFA), Asperger's Disorder (AD), and pervasive developmental disorder (PDD-NOS). Studies find that 1 in 88 youths will be diagnosed with ASD in the U.S. (ADDM; Autism and Developmental Disabilities Monitoring Network Surveillance Year 2008, Principal Investigators, 2012). ASDs are characterized by significant impairments in communication, repetitive behaviors, and most notably, social interaction (American Psychiatric Association, 2000). Social difficulties include failure to engage in age-appropriate play (Macintosh and Dissanayake, 2006), trouble perceiving nonverbal communication, poor eye contact, deficient affect comprehension and expression, and an inability to understand the emotions of others (Baron-Cohen, Leslie, and Frith, 1985).

Such deficits in social competence are thought to be due to disturbances in cognitive and affective domains of empathy (Baron-Cohen and Wright, 2004), and impairments in visual scan paths of facial stimuli (Klin et al., 2002) and in processing facial affect (Kleinhans et al., 2010).

## Behavioral Deficits

While the ability of both children and adults with ASDs to recognize facial expression has been widely studied, the degree to which individuals with ASDs truly have impaired processing of facial emotions remains unclear. Looking across both adult and pediatric data, when both children and adults with ASDs are given simple orienting tasks (e.g., matching facial expressions, identifying "same or different" expressions) for unambiguous, straightforward facial stimuli with adequate processing time, their performance does not differ from controls (e.g., Gepner et al., 2001; Ozonoff et al., 1990; Piggot et al., 2004). Findings become more mixed when subjects are required to identify the facial expression (e.g., provide a label or match a label to the face), and the age of the subject is important in clarifying trends in the data. Research suggests that before 10 years of age, both low- and high-functioning children with ASDs show greater impairment than controls in overall labeling of basic facial expressions (Lindner and Rosen, 2006; Tantam, Monaghan, Nicholas, and Stirling, 1989). This gap in ability closes, however, by the age of 12 when children with HFA show similar performance in identifying basic facial expressions as TD individuals, and this finding remains rather consistent through adulthood (Capps et al., 1992; Grossman, Klin, Carter, and Volkmar, 2000).

While it would appear that with age individuals with ASDs become more proficient in their ability to identify basic facial emotion, research also suggests that ASD individuals still struggle when facial stimuli are rapidly presented (Critchley et al., 2000) and display more subtle expressions (Humphreys et al., 2007). Indeed, the majority of research investigating emotion recognition in ASDs allows subjects to view the stimuli for as long as necessary prior to making a response and presents exaggerated versions of facial expressions and thus, does not represent the demands of everyday situations in which typically subtle facial expressions must be processed and interpreted, often in a very short time frame.

To address these issues, Rump and colleagues (2009) investigated the ability to recognize facial expressions in young children, adolescents, and adults with ASDs or typical development by controlling for the subtlety of facial expressions and briefly presenting dynamic, gradually shifting facial stimuli. In the first experiment using video clips comparing children with HFA (aged 5-7 years) and controls, the HFA group performed significantly worse on the recognition task across all emotions. Further, TD children were able to correctly classify anger and fear at one full level of subtlety earlier than HFA children, and HFA children typically required the final, easiest level of emotional display (stimuli exhibiting 100% of the emotion) to reliably identify afraid and angry. These results are consistent with other research indicating that, compared to controls, children with HFA are worse at identifying subtle displays of anger, disgust, and surprise (Law-Smith et al., 2010). A second part of this study failed to identify deficits in HFA youth aged 8-17 years. These results indicate that although younger children with HFA (aged 5-7 years) initially struggle with facial recognition (particularly fear and anger), they seem to catch up with their TD counterparts between the ages of 8 and 12 and maintain comparable proficiency through adolescence.

## Eye Tracking Deficits

Researchers have also posited that although individuals with ASDs are able to perform basic emotion recognition tasks, they do so in a more effortful manner that consists of focusing on specific aspects or details of the face rather than capturing and integrating the global meaning of the stimulus (Baron-Cohen, 2003; Frith, 1993; Klin et al., 1999; Tantum et al., 1989). For example, in a pioneer study, Langdell (1978) found that ASD youth performed better than healthy comparisons at recognizing faces of their peers when viewing isolated features of the face, particularly the mouth region. Joseph and Tanaka (2003) found that children with HFA were significantly better at identifying faces from the mouth alone than from the eyes alone, and generally were impaired at judging facial identity from the eyes alone relative to matched comparisons. Overall, there is substantial evidence from behavioral studies suggesting that individuals with ASDs are deficient in face identification abilities and employ abnormal strategies to process faces (e.g., Boucher and Lewis, 1992; Braverman, Fein, Lucci, and Waterhouse, 1989; Davies, Bishop, Manstead, and Tantam, 1994; Hauck, Fein, Maltby, Waterhouse, and Feinstein, 1998; Joseph and Tanaka, 2003; Klin et al., 1999; Ozonoff, Pennington, and Rogers, 1990; Tantam, Monaghan, Nicholson, and Stirling; Wolf et al., 2008). In particular, individuals with ASDs appear to engage in feature-based processing of faces, what has been referred to as poor central coherence (Pellicano, 2010), with a strong focus on the mouth rather than the eyes. Such altered visual exploration of faces may strongly contribute to the significant social difficulties seen in this population.

Eye tracking provides a way for monitoring gaze fixation behaviors while viewing facial stimuli and this method has been used in both adults and youth with ASDs (e.g., Carpenter et al., 2002; Jones et al., 2008; Klin et al., 2002; Pelphrey et al., 2002; Spezio, Adolphs, Hurley, and Piven, 2007; Trepagnier et al., 2002 van der Geest et al. 2002a; van der Geest, et al., 2002b). Results from eye tracking studies have confirmed behavioral findings and have consistently shown that individuals with ASDs fail to process facial stimuli in a holistic fashion and have a tendency to focus on the mouth region rather than the eye region of faces. Further, these findings extend beyond facial identification tasks and also include tasks where individuals with ASDs are processing faces of emotional valence. For example, numerous studies show that HFA individuals look less at the eye region of emotionally expressive faces in comparison to controls (Corden et al., 2008; Pelphrey et al., 2002), and fail to use information from the upper portions of the face effectively during the identification of facial emotion (Baron-Cohen et al., 1997; Gross, 2008; Spezio et al., 2007).

In an eye tracking study where subjects viewed videotapes of complex social situations (displaying socially expressive interactions), Klin and colleagues (2002) measured the percentage of time ASD and TD adolescent males spent viewing the mouth, eyes, body, and objects in the environment. Results demonstrated that relative to TD adolescents, ASD adolescents focused on the eyes two times less and focused on the mouth, body, and objects two times more. Further, greater fixation on objects was correlated with poorer social functioning. Interestingly, however, greater fixation on the mouth was associated with better social functioning and there was no relationship between eye fixation and social skill functioning.

These results could suggest that for youth with ASDs, visually orienting to the eyes does not assist in their efforts to comprehend social situations and therefore, the eye region is not particularly meaningful to them. This is consistent with previous work indicating that youth with ASDs perform better at identifying faces when presented with only mouths than with only eyes (Joseph and Tanaka, 2003). The finding that greater fixation on the mouth was associated with improved social competence may suggest that ASD subjects were focused on speech, an aspect of the visual stimulus that they could comprehend and thus, serve as a channel to better understand social situations. Finally, research indicates that an increased focus on objects suggests a decreased salience of social stimuli (Klin, Schultz, and Cohen, 2000). Therefore, an association between heightened focus on objects and reduced social competence could mean that social stimuli are overall less meaningful or important to ASD youth and therefore, result in a diminished likelihood of understanding the social situation.

## Neurocognitive Deficits

The amygdala has been implicated in the neuropathology of ASDs according to both structural MRI and fMRI studies. Findings from structural MRI are mixed. For example, an enlarged right amygdala at 3-4 years of age is related to poorer clinical outcome among ASD children (Munson et al., 2006), and larger amygdala volumes have been positively correlated to anxiety severity (Juranek et al., 2006) and social impairment (Nacewicz et al., 2006) in ASDs. Interestingly, similar volumetric abnormalities have also been observed in unaffected siblings of children with ASDs (Dalton et al., 2007).

Data from fMRI studies generally show that individuals with ASDs exhibit reduced activation of the amygdala and the OFC, and increased activation and greater reliance on the superior temporal cortex and ACC during the processing of facial emotions compared to controls (Ashwin et al., 2007; Wang et al., 2004). In a study with ASD youth, Corbett et al. (2009) used functional and structural MRI to examine amygdala and fusiform gyrus (FG) activity in a sample of HFA and TD children (aged 8-12 years) while completing a task involving matching facial expressions (i.e., happy, sad, angry, afraid, neutral; "Same feeling?") and facial identity ("Same person?"). Results demonstrated that in comparison to TD youth, children with HFA had reduced amygdala and FG activation while performing the face emotion matching task, even though the HFA group accurately matched the emotions. Instead, HFA youth utilized different brain regions such as superior temporal gyrus to identify facial affect. This is consistent with other work showing that ASD children recruited different neural networks than TD youth during automatic emotion processing even though emotion identification was intact (Wang et al., 2004). Reduced amygdala activation is reflective of previous fMRI research with ASD individuals during the implicit processing of emotions (Critchley et al., 2000), the processing of fearful faces (Ashwin et al., 2007), and making same/different emotion judgments (Baron-Cohen et al., 1999).

Conversely, Corbett et al. (2009) found that TD youth recruited the amygdala during both matching tasks as evidenced by increased bilateral amygdala activation during the emotion matching condition and increased left amygdala activation during the person matching condition. Behaviorally, HFA subjects showed impaired processing on the person matching condition compared to TD subjects. During this condition, HFA subjects trended towards some activation of the right FG and variable activation of the amygdala, although significantly less so than TD subjects.

Interestingly, relative to controls, Dalton et al. (2005) found a significant positive correlation between activation in the amygdala and FG and time spent fixating on the eyes among adolescent males with ASDs while performing both a facial emotion discrimination task (deciding whether a face was emotional or neutral) and a facial recognition task (deciding whether or not the face was familiar). Therefore, reduced eye gaze fixation, which has been extensively reported in the ASD literature (as previously discussed), may account for the hypoactivation of these brain regions often reported in ASD individuals.

Taken together, these results suggest that youth with ASDs recruit other, atypical brain regions when interpreting facial emotions and social information, particularly frontal and parietal regions responsible for intentional attention allocation rather than regions primarily associated with emotion and automatic processing. Compared to TD youth, youth with ASD display a lack of amygdala activation and reduced activation of the FG when matching faces and facial emotion. Although ASD youth can distinguish basic emotions and encode facial stimuli to some degree, they may be unable to allocate appropriate emotional meaning and social salience. This suggests that the amygdala fails to effectively engage in automatic emotional processing and relay socioemotional relevance to other brain regions such as the FG during basic and more complex social situations.

## Direct Comparisons of Face Emotion Processing Abilities Across Diagnoses

It is important to directly compare facial affect recognition abilities across childhood diagnoses in order to truly begin to elucidate the face processing deficits that are specific to different disorders. Surprisingly, however, there is only one study that has examined and compared face emotion processing abilities across multiple diagnoses. Guyer and colleagues (2007) examined face-labeling deficits using the DANVA task (described earlier) in a large sample of BD youth, youth with comorbid ADHD and CD, youth with comorbid MDD and an anxiety disorder, and healthy controls. Bipolar youth displayed significantly more errors when labeling face emotions than both the ADHD/CD and MDD/anxiety patient samples, as well as the controls. Therefore, while other research indicates that youth with anxiety and/or depression may misidentify scared facial expressions (e.g., Easter et al., 2005; Lenti, Giacobbe, and Pegna, 2000; Simonian et al., 2001) and that youth with CD may misidentify angry and sad faces (e.g., Blair, Colledge, Murray, and Mitchell, 2001; Fairchild et al., 2009), in a rare comparison of different patient samples, only BD youth were found to be deficient in face emotion categorization across a range of facial emotional expressions displayed by both children and adults. Additional direct comparisons between different pediatric patient samples are critical to move beyond comparisons of single-sample controls and patients to better elucidate the diagnostic specificity of face emotion processing deficits.

## Treatment of Impaired Face Emotion Processing

Currently, all empirically-supported psychotherapeutic interventions for BD youth are family-based and primarily consist of a group format (Fristad, Gavazzi, and Mackinaw-Koons, 2003; Miklowitz et al., 2004; Pavuluri et al., 2004; Rich and Rosen, 2012). While these interventions result in reduced bipolar symptomatology in youth (i.e., depression and mania), they do not address the debilitating social dysfunction seen in PBD. To date, there are no interventions specifically targeting face emotion processing deficits in PBD. Similarly, there is an absence of research on therapeutic treatment strategies for addressing impaired facial affect recognition in youth with anxiety and depressive disorders.

Most, if not all, of the research concerning the treatment of impaired face emotion processing has derived from the autism literature. As discussed earlier, a large number of studies have demonstrated that children with ASD have impaired processing of emotional facial expressions (Bölte and Poustka, 2006; Golan, Baron-Cohen, Hill, and Golan, 2006), and these deficits are associated with inadequate social functioning in ASD youth (McPartland, Webb, Keehn, and Dawson, 2011). *The Transporters* DVD (Golan et al., 2009) is an empirically-supported treatment for improving facial recognition skills in youth with ASDs. *The Transporters* is an animated series designed to bolster emotion recognition and understanding in autistic youth. The DVD series follows eight characters, depicted as vehicles with real human faces that display a range of basic (i.e., happy, sad, angry, afraid) and complex (i.e., surprised, ashamed, disgusted, joking, jealous, proud, tired, sorry, kind, excited, worried, unfriendly, grumpy) emotions. Treatment occurs through implicit learning of how to identify affect. Golan and colleagues (2009) found that after 4 weeks of watching episodes of *The Transporters* for 20 minutes a day at home with parental supervision, ASD youth improved their emotional vocabulary and emotional recognition compared to ASD controls. Additionally, the intervention group appeared to catch up with their typically developing counterparts on emotion recognition performance.

In a follow-up study (Young and Posselt, 2012), ASD children were randomly assigned to view *The Transporters* DVD or a *Thomas the Tank Engine* DVD, entitled "Thomas Discovers Emotions," that specifically draws attention to emotions or affect. The two DVDs differed in that *The Transporters* places greater emphasis on emotions, its characters depict real human faces on their vehicle bodies, and the backdrop is simple and featureless further influencing the viewer to attend to the characters' faces. *Thomas the Tank Engine*, however, consisted of an exciting and detailed backdrop, encouraging attention to all areas of the screen. Results indicated that compared to ASD children viewing the *Thomas the Tank Engine* DVD, children viewing *The Transporter* DVD showed greater improvement in their ability to identify and label basic and complex facial expressions. Children viewing *Thomas the Tank Engine* did not show any improvement in facial affect recognition. Further, improved social behavior was significantly related to watching *The Transporters*; however, this finding was not unique to *The Transporters* intervention as ASD children viewing *Thomas the Tank Engine* also showed substantial improvement in social functioning.

The Frankfurt Test and Training of Facial Affect Recognition (FEFA) (Bolte et al., 2002) is one of the few empirically-supported treatments for improving face processing skills in ASD individuals. The FEFA is a computerized program that tests and then trains individuals to better identify and understand basic facial emotions. In the FEFA program, faces are displayed on a computer screen, the individual is asked to identify the face emotion, and then feedback informs the individual of the accuracy of his/her response. Importantly, this computer program is therapeutic in that it teaches the individual what specific aspects of the face (i.e., eyes, eyebrows, mouth) signify a specific emotion. Prior research demonstrates that the FEFA reliably measures face emotion recognition deficits in children with autism spectrum disorders (ASD) and attention-deficit hyperactivity disorder (ADHD) (Kuusikko et al., 2009; Sinzig, Morsch, and Lehmkuhl, 2007). In young adults with ASD, when used as an intervention (five weeks, two hours/week), the FEFA program resulted in improved face emotion identification (Bölte et al., 2002; Bölte et al., 2006) and even improved neural functioning in brain regions associated with face emotion processing (i.e., superior parietal lobule and the right medial occipital gyrus) (Bölte et al., 2006). Further research is needed to replicate these findings in ASD youth.

Face emotion processing deficits in youth with ASD have also been addressed as components of larger comprehensive interventions. For example, the group-based Social Competence Intervention (SCI; Stichter et al., 2010) addresses three areas of social cognition that are impaired in ASD youth: emotion recognition, theory of mind (ability to impute the mental states of others; Baron-Cohen et al., 1985), and executive functioning. SCI consists of 20 hours of group therapy conducted twice weekly for 10 weeks and utilizes meta-cognitive strategies, self-monitoring and self-regulation, and exposure and response situations. Although this study did not include a comparison group, the SCI program was effective in increasing social competence in a sample of adolescent males with HFA or AD. In particular, participants displayed improved social abilities, executive functioning, and identification of facial emotions (i.e., varying intensity of happy, sad, angry, fearful).

Given the relationship between face emotion misidentification and social impairments in PBD, a therapy that targets face processing may be an efficacious intervention for improving social functioning in BD youth. In particular, future research should extend previous work with ASD youth and determine if such interventions described above can significantly improve face emotion understanding and identification and enhance social functioning in youth with BD.

## Conclusion

The most consistent behavioral finding involving the processing of face emotion in PBD youth is a tendency to mislabel face emotions and misinterpret neutral face stimuli as more threatening than controls. Further, such labeling deficits have shown to be evident regardless of comorbid diagnoses (e.g., ADHD, CD, MDD, or anxiety) and are also apparent in youth at risk for BD. Given the importance of identifying and processing faces for navigating the social world, these behavioral findings may help explain the social deficits that characterize PBD.

However, the misclassification of facial expressions is not unique to PBD and is found across a number of disorders, including depression, anxiety, and ASDs. For example, face emotion processing deficits in youth with MDD reflect biases in attending to and encoding facial affect (i.e., recall deficits associated with negative expressions such as sad or fearful) rather than a broad dysfunction in identifying facial emotions. Behavioral findings of socially anxious youth are rather inconsistent, where some studies find that socially anxious youth display more facial affect recognition errors than controls, and other studies find no differences in face emotion processing ability. Finally, youth with ASDs are significantly worse at identifying facial expressions, particularly subtle displays and rapid presentations of facial stimuli, compared to controls.

While youth from various diagnostic backgrounds appear to exhibit deficient processing of facial expressions, it is difficult to distinguish specific differences in impaired face emotion processing across these disorders. Although some studies have compared impaired processing between two pediatric patient groups, only one study to date has examined face emotion processing deficits across multiple pediatric diagnostic groups (i.e., PBD, ADHD/CD, anxiety/depressed, and healthy controls). This study found that BD youth had the most errors in labeling facial expressions and were the only subjects in the sample to exhibit this deficit at all. Thus, facial affect processing may be most impaired in youth with BD, but further research with direct comparisons of face emotion processing across clinical groups is needed to support this claim.

To further understand the pathophysiology underlying face emotion processing in PBD, neuroimaging research has identified abnormalities in brain regions thought to play a role in regulating mood and cognition. Recent fMRI studies suggest that impaired face emotion processing in PBD involves perturbed functioning in a distributed fronto-striatal-limbic network, including the prefrontal cortex (PFC), striatum, anterior cingulate cortex (ACC), and amygdala. Of these regions, the nature of deficits is most clear in the amygdala, a critical brain region implicated in the neural network responsible for emotion regulation (Pfeifer, Welge, Strakowski, Adler, and Delbello, 2008). Studies consistently document greater amygdala activation in BD youth relative to controls when processing face emotions. The specific nature of other neural abnormalities in PBD, however, is inconsistent. Studies document both hyper- and hypo-activity of the PFC, striatum, and ACC in response to facial expressions in BD youth. Overall, however, it appears that amygdala activation in response to emotional faces is poorly inhibited by prefrontal regions in PBD.

Compared to youth with BD, results from fMRI studies of youth with ASDs, anxiety, and MDD show similarities and differences in neural deficits while processing face emotions. For example, youth with ASDs have a tendency to exhibit reduced amygdala and OFC activation, and heightened ACC activation compared to controls. Youth with social anxiety display perturbed activation of the ACC compared to controls in response to facial affect, although the direction of activity varies across studies.

Findings from fMRI studies with depressed youth are inconsistent, where some indicate amygdala hyperactivation during processing of emotional faces, whereas others suggest amygdala hypoactivation or no differences in amygdala functioning relative to controls. The most consistent finding in MDD youth is increased amygdala activation in response to fearful faces.

There are numerous explanations for these discrepancies, most notably methodological differences, including the specific types of stimuli used, the cognitive demands placed on subjects, and even the manner in which data is analyzed, such as using a block- versus event-related design. Traditionally, most studies investigating face emotion processing utilized prototypical posed expressions. However, subtle variations in emotion are typically presented in real life situations and people rarely display emotional extremes. More recent investigations of face emotion processing have extended beyond prototypical face expressions and have focused on more detailed explorations of face processing across a range of emotional intensities. In addition, clinical and demographic differences may explain result discrepancies, including gender, age, medication status, comorbid diagnoses, and mood state of participants. Another important factor to consider is ongoing maturation and developmental changes in face emotion processing abilities (Guyer et al., 2008; Herba and Phillips, 2004), and thus, observed differences between varying age groups may be a reflection of development rather deficient functioning.

Although fMRI findings fail to clearly articulate the neural deficits in PBD, they begin to clarify the cognitive and neural mechanisms underlying impaired face emotion processing in youth with BD, and begin to delineate behavioral and neural deficits found in multiple childhood disorders.

Importantly, the brain regions implicated in these studies may help to elucidate not only the pathophysiology of PBD but also start to uncover the nature of disturbed social interactions present in BD youth. Indeed, regions of this fronto-striatal-limbic network are thought to modulate a number of social functions, including the interpretation of social cues and the regulation of emotional and behavioral responses to these cues (Critchley et al., 2000). Therefore, abnormalities in these neural circuits may impair the processing of social information and the regulation of emotional and behavioral reactivity, resulting in poor social functioning that often characterizes PBD.

Evidence from cognitive-based neuroimaging research on PBD should continue to refine the neural substrates of deficient face emotion processing. In particular, longitudinal investigations of BD youth utilizing neuroimaging methods provide a means of evaluating the neurodevelopmental course of illness, identifying changes in neural and cognitive functioning over time, determining the relationship between clinical course and associated cognitive functioning, and further clarifying the continuity between child- and adult-onset BD. In addition, only a few studies have examined disturbed face emotion processing in at-risk individuals and therefore, further work is needed to specify precursors of BD illness and potential markers of risk for the disorder.

Finally, directly examining the behavioral and neural mechanisms underlying PBD and other common childhood psychiatric illnesses will help to differentiate the pathophysiology of these disorders and determine the neural and cognitive correlates unique to each of these illnesses. This will ultimately assist in the refinement of diagnostic tools and aid in identifying targets for pharmacological and psychosocial intervention specific to PBD. While there are currently no empirically-supported treatments for improving impaired face emotion processing in PBD, future research should draw from the ASD treatment literature to develop psychosocial interventions that target face emotion processing deficits in PBD and effectively improve social competency.

## References

Altshuler, L., Bookheimer, S., Proenza, M. A., Townsend, J., Sabb, F., Firestine, A., ... and Cohen, M. S. (2005). Increased amygdala activation during mania: A functional magnetic resonance imaging study. *American Journal of Psychiatry*, *162*, 1211-1213.

Amaral, D., Price, J.L., Pitaken, A., and Carmichael, S. (1992). *The amygdala: Neurobiological aspects of emotion, memory and mental dysfunction.* New York, NY: Wiley-Liss.

American Psychiatric Association. (2000). *Diagnostic and statistical manual of mental disorders* (4th ed., text rev.). Washington, DC: Author.

Angold, A., and Costello, E. J. (1993). Depressive comorbidity in children and adolescents – Empirical, theoretical, and methodological issues. *The American Journal of Psychiatry, 150*, 1779–1791.

Arsenio, W. F., Gold, J., and Adams, E. (2004). Adolescents' emotion expectancies regarding aggressive and nonaggressive events: Connections with behavior problems. *Journal of experimental child psychology*, *89*, 338-355.

Asmundson, G.J.G., and Stein, M.B. (1994). Selective processing of social threat in patients with generalized social phobia: Evaluation using a dot-probe paradigm. *Journal of Anxiety Disorders, 8*, 107-117.

Ashwin, C., Baron-Cohen, S., Wheelwright, S., O'Riordan, M., and Bullmore, E.T. (2007). Differential activation of the amygdala and the 'social brain' during fearful face processing in Asperger Syndrome. *Neuropsychologia 45*, 2–14.

Autism and Developmental Disabilities Monitoring Network Surveillance Year 2008 Principal Investigators. (2012). Prevalence of autism spectrum disorders-Autism and Developmental Disabilities Monitoring Net-work MMWR Surveillance Summary (Vol. 61, pp. 1-19). United States, 2008: Centers for Disease Control and Prevention.

Axelson, D., Birmaher, B., Strober, M., Gill, M. K., Valeri, S., Chiappetta, L., ... and Keller, M. (2006). Phenomenology of children and adolescents with bipolar spectrum disorders. *Archives of General Psychiatry*, *63*, 1139-1148.

Baron-Cohen, S., Leslie, A.M., and Frith, U. (1985). Does the autistic child have a "theory of mind"? *Cognition, 21*, 37-46.

Baron-Cohen, S., and Wright, S. (2004). The empathy quotient: an investigation of adults with Asperger syndrome or high functioning autism, and normal sex differences. *Journal of Autism and Developmental Disabilities, 34*, 163-175.

Battaglia, M., Ogliari, A., Zanoni, A., Villa, F., Citterio, A., Binaghi, F., ... and Maffei, C. (2004). Children's discrimination of expressions of emotions: relationship with indices of social anxiety and shyness. *Journal of the American Academy of Child and Adolescent Psychiatry*, *43*, 358-365.

Beck, A.T., Rush, A.J., Shaw, B.F., Emery, G. (Eds.), 1979. *Cognitive Therapy of Depression*. New York, NY: Guilford.

Beidel, D.C., and Turner, S.M. (2007). *Shy children, phobic adults: the nature and treatment of social anxiety disorder*. Washington, DC: American Psychological Association.

Beidel, D. C., Turner, S. M., and Morris, T. L. (1999). Psychopathology of childhood social phobia. *Journal of the American Academy of Child and Adolescent Psychiatry*, *38*, 643-650.

Birmaher, B., Arbelaez, C., and Brent, D. (2002). Course and outcome of child and adolescent major depressive disorder. *Child and adolescent psychiatric clinics of North America.*

Birmaher, B., Axelson, D., Goldstein, B., Strober, M., Gill, M. K., Hunt, J., ... and Keller, M. (2009). Four-Year Longitudinal Course of Children and Adolescents with Bipolar Spectrum Disorder: The Course and Outcome of Bipolar Youth (COBY) Study. *The American journal of psychiatry*, *166*, 795.

Bittner, A., Egger, H. L., Erkanli, A., Jane Costello, E., Foley, D. L., and Angold, A. (2007). What do childhood anxiety disorders predict?. *Journal of Child Psychology and Psychiatry*, *48*, 1174-1183.

Blader, J.C., and Carlson, G.A. (2007). Increased rates of bipolar disorder diagnoses among U.S. child, adolescent, and adult inpatients, 1996-2004. *Bipolar Disorder: Neurocircuitry and Neurodevelopment, 62*, 107-114.

Blair, R. J. R., Colledge, E., Murray, L., and Mitchell, D. G. V. (2001). A selective impairment in the processing of sad and fearful expressions in children with psychopathic tendencies. *Journal of abnormal child psychology*, *29*, 491-498.

Blair, K.S., Geraci, M., Korelitz, K., Otero, M., Towbin, K.,…Pine, D.S. (2011). The pathology of social phobia is independent of development changes in face processing. *American Journal of Psychiatry, 168*, 1202-1209.

Bölte, S., Feineis-Matthews, S., Leber, S., Dierks, T., Hubl, D., and Poustka, F. (2002). The development and evaluation of a computer-based program to test and to teach the recognition of facial affect. International Journal of Circumpolar Health, *61*, 61-68.

Bölte, S., Hubl, D., Feineis-Matthews, S., Prvulovic, D., Dierks, T., and Poustka, F. (2006). Facial affect recognition training in autism: can we animate the fusiform gyrus? *Behavioral Neuroscience, 120*, 211-216.

Bölte, S., and Poustka, F. (2006). The broader cognitive phenotype of autism in parents: How specific is the tendency for local processing and executive dysfunction?. *Journal of Child Psychology and Psychiatry*, *47*, 639-645.

Boucher, J., and Lewis, V. (1992). Unfamiliar face recognition in relatively able autistic children. *Journal of Child Psychology and Psychiatry, 33*, 843-859.

Bradley, B. P., Mogg, K., and Williams, R. (2005). Implicit and explicit memory for emotion-congruent information in clinical depression and anxiety. *Behaviour Research and Therapy*, *33*, 755-770.

Braverman, M., Fein, D., Lucci, D., and Waterhouse, L. (1989). Affect comprehension in children with pervasive developmental *disorders. Journal of Autism and Developmental Disorders, 19*, 301-16.

Breiter, H. C., Etcoff, N. L., Whalen, P. J., Kennedy, W. A., Rauch, S. L., Buckner, R. L., ... and Rosen, B. R. (1996). Response and habituation of the human amygdala during visual processing of facial expression. *Neuron*, *17*, 875.

Britton, J. C., and Rauch, S. L. (2009). Neuroanatomy and neuroimaging of anxiety disorders. *Oxford handbook of anxiety and related disorders*, 97-110.

Brotman, M., Guyer, A., Lawson, E., Horsey, S., Rich, B., Dickstein, D., ... and Leibenluft, E. (2008a). Facial emotion labeling deficits in children and adolescents at risk for bipolar disorder. *American Journal of Psychiatry*, *165*, 385-389.

Brotman, M.A., Skup, M., Rich, B.A., Blair, K.S., Pine, D.S.,…Leibenluft, E. (2008). Risk for bipolar disorder is associated with face-processing deficits across emotions. *Journal of the American Academy of Child and Adolescent Psychiatry, 47*, 1455-1461.

Capps, L., Yirmiya, N., and Sigman, M. (1992). Understanding of simple and complex emotions in non-retarded children with autism. *Journal of Child Psychology and Psychiatry, 33*, 1169-1182.

Carlson, G.A., Bromet, E.J., Driessens, C., Mojtabai, R., and Schwartz, J.E. (2002). Age at onset, childhood psychopathology, and 2-year outcome in psychotic bipolar disorder. *American Journal of Psychiatry, 159*, 307-309.

Carpenter, M., Pennington, B.F., and Rogers, S.J. (2002). Interrelations among social-cognitive skills in young children with autism. *Journal of Autism and Developmental Disorders, 32*, 91-106.

Case, B.G., Olfson, M., Marcus, S.C., and Siegel, C. (2007). Trends in the inpatient mental health treatment of children and adolescents in U.S. Community hospitals between 1990 and 2000. *Archives of General Psychiatry, 64,* 89-96.

Chen, C. H., Suckling, J., Lennox, B. R., Ooi, C., and Bullmore, E. T. (2011). A quantitative meta-analysis of fMRI studies in bipolar disorder. *Bipolar disorders*, *13*, 1-15.

Chen, C. H., Suckling, J., Ooi, C., Jacob, R., Lupson, V., Bullmore, E. T., and Lennox, B. R. (2010). A longitudinal fMRI study of the manic and euthymic states of bipolar disorder. *Bipolar Disorders*, *12*, 344-347.

Corbett, B. A., Carmean, V., Ravizza, S., Wendelken, C., Henry, M. L., Carter, C., and Rivera, S. M. (2009). A functional and structural study of emotion and face processing in children with autism. *Psychiatry research*, *173*, 196-205.

Corden, B., Chilvers, R., and Skuse, D. (2008). Avoidance of emotionally arousing stimuli predicts social-perceptual impairment in Asperger's syndrome. *Neuropsychologia, 46*, 137-147.

Costello, E. J., Mustillo, S., Erkanli, A., Keeler, G., and Angold, A. (2003). Prevalence and development of psychiatric disorders in childhood and adolescence. *Archives of general psychiatry*, *60*, 837.

Clark, D. M., and Wells, A. (1995). A cognitive model of social phobia. In R.G. Heimberg, M.R. Leibowitz, D.A. Hope, and F.R. Schneier (Eds.). *Social phobia: Diagnosis, assessment, and treatment* (pp. 69-93). New York, NY: Guilford Press.

Critchley, H., Daly, E., Phillips, M., Brammer, M., Bullmore, E., Williams, S., ... and Murphy, D. (2000). Explicit and implicit neural mechanisms for processing of social information from facial expressions: a functional magnetic resonance imaging study. *Human brain mapping*, *9*, 93-105.

Dalgleish, T., Taghavi, R., Neshat-Doost, Moradi, A., Canterbury, R., and Yule, W. (2003). Patterns of processing bias for emotional information across clinical disorders: A comparison of attention, memory, and prospective cognition in children and adolescents with depression, generalized anxiety, and posttraumatic stress disorder. *Journal of Clinical Child and Adolescent Psychology, 32*, 10-21.

Dalton, K.M., Nacewicz, B.M., Alexander, A.L., and Davidson, R.J. (2007). Gaze-fixation, brain activation, and amygdala volume in unaffected siblings of individuals with autism. *Biological Psychiatry, 61*, 512-520.

Dalton, K.M., Nacewicz, B.M., Johnstone, T., Schaefer, H.S., Gernsbacher, M.A.,…Davidson, R.J. (2005). Gaze fixation and the neural circuitry of face processing in autism. *Nature Neuroscience, 8*, 519-526.

Davies, S., Bishop, D., Manstead, A.S.R., and Tantam, D. (1994). Face perception in children with autism and Asperger's syndrome. *Journal of Child Psychology and Psychiatry, 35*, 1033-1057.

Delvecchio, G., Fossati, P., Boyer, P., Brambilla, P., Falkai, P., Gruber, O., ... and Frangou, S. (2012). Common and distinct neural correlates of emotional processing in Bipolar Disorder and Major Depressive Disorder: a voxel-based meta-analysis of functional magnetic resonance imaging studies. *European Neuropsychopharmacology*, *22*, 100-113.

De Sonneville, L. M., Verschoor, C. A., Njiokiktjien, C., Op het Veld, V., Toorenaar, N., and Vranken, M. (2002). Facial identity and facial emotions: Speed, accuracy, and processing strategies in children and adults. *Journal of Clinical and Experimental Neuropsychology, 24*, 200-213.

Dickstein, D. P., Rich, B. A., Roberson-Nay, R., Berghorst, L., Vinton, D., Pine, D. S., and Leibenluft, E. (2007). Neural activation during encoding of emotional faces in pediatric bipolar disorder. *Bipolar disorders*, *9*, 679-692.

Drevets, W. C. (2003). Neuroimaging abnormalities in the amygdala in mood disorders. *Annals of the New York Academy of Sciences*, *985*, 420-444.

Drevets, W.C., Price, J.L., Bardgett, M.E., Reich, T., Todd, R.D., and Raichle, M.E. (2002). Glucose metabolism in the amygdala in depression: Relationship to diagnostic subtype and plasma cortisol levels. *Pharmacological and Biochemical Behavior, 71*, 431-447.

Easter, J., McClure, E. B., Monk, C. S., Dhanani, M., Hodgdon, H., Leibenluft, E., ... and Ernst, M. (2005). Emotion recognition deficits in pediatric anxiety disorders: implications for amygdala research. *Journal of Child and Adolescent Psychopharmacology*, *15*, 563-570.

Egger, H. L., and Angold, A. (2006). Common emotional and behavioral disorders in preschool children: Presentation, nosology, and epidemiology. *Journal of Child Psychology and Psychiatry*, *47*(3-4), 313-337.

Ekman, P., and Friesen, W. (1976). *Pictures of facial affect*. Palo Alto, CA: Consulting Psychologists.

Ekman, P., Sorenson, E. R., and Friesen, W. V. (1969). Pan-cultural elements in facial displays of emotion. *Science*, *164*, 86-88.

Ernst, M., Nelson, E. E., Jazbec, S., McClure, E. B., Monk, C. S., Leibenluft, E., ... and Pine, D. S. (2005). Amygdala and nucleus accumbens in responses to receipt and omission of gains in adults and adolescents. *Neuroimage*, *25*(4), 1279.

Erwin, R. J., Gur, R. C., Gur, R. E., Skolnick, B., Mawhinney-Hee, M., and Smailis, J. (1992). Facial emotion discrimination: I. Task construction and behavioral findings in normal subjects. *Psychiatry Research*, *42*, 231-240.

Fairchild, G., Van Goozen, S. H., Calder, A. J., Stollery, S. J., and Goodyer, I. M. (2009). Deficits in facial expression recognition in male adolescents with early-onset or adolescence-onset conduct disorder. *Journal of Child Psychology and Psychiatry*, *50*(5), 627-636.

Fales, C.L., Barch, D.M., Rundle, M.M., Mintun, M.A., Snyder,…Sheline,Y.I., (2008). Altered emotional interference processing in affective and cognitive-controlled brain circuitry in major depression. *Biological Psychiatry, 63*, 377-384.

Fanselow, M. S., and LeDoux, J. E. (1999). Why we think plasticity underlying Pavlovian fear conditioning occurs in the basolateral amygdala. *Neuron, 23*, 229-232.

Foland-Ross, L. C., Bookheimer, S. Y., Lieberman, M. D., Sugar, C. A., Townsend, J. D., Fischer, J., ... and Altshuler, L. L. (2012). Normal amygdala activation but deficient ventrolateral prefrontal activation in adults with bipolar disorder during euthymia. *Neuroimage, 59*, 738-744.

Fristad, M.A., Gavazzi, S.M., and Mackinaw-Koons, B. (2003). Family psychoeducation: Adjunctive intervention for children with bipolar disorder. *Biological Psychiatry, 53*, 1000-1008.

Garber, J., and Horowitz, J. L. (2002). Depression in children. *Handbook of depression*, 510-540.

Garrett, A.S., Reiss, A.L., Howe, M.E., Kelley, R.G., Singh, M.K.,…Chang, K.D. (2012). Abnormal amygdala and prefrontal cortex activation to facial expressions in pediatric bipolar disorder. *Journal of the American Academy of Child and Adolescent Psychiatry, 51*, 821-831.

Geller, B., Bolhofner, K., Craney, J.L., Williams, M., Delbello, M.P., and Gundersen, K. (2000). Psychosocial functioning in a prepubertal and early adolescent bipolar disorder phenotype. *Journal of the American Academy of Child and Adolescent Psychiatry,* 39, 1543-1548.

Geller, B., Craney, J.L., Bolhofner, K., DelBello, M.P., Williams, M., and Zimerman, B. (2001). One-year recovery and relapse rates of children with a prepubertal and early adolescent bipolar disorder phenotype. *American Journal of Psychiatry, 158*, 303-305.

Geller, B., and Luby, J. (1997). Child and adolescent bipolar disorder: a review of the past 10 years. *Journal of the American Academy of Child and Adolescent Psychiatry, 36*, 1168-1176.

Gepner, B., Deruelle, C., and Grynfeltt, S. (2001). Motion and emotion: A novel approach to the study of face processing by young autistic children. *Journal of Autism and Developmental Disorders, 31*, 37-45.

Golan, O., Baron-Cohen, S., Hill, J. J., and Golan, Y. (2006). The "reading the mind in films" task: Complex emotion recognition in adults with and without autism spectrum conditions. *Society of Neuroscience, 1,* 111-123.

Goldstein, T. R., Miklowitz, D. J., and Mullen, K. (2006). Social skills knowledge and performance among adolescents with bipolar disorder. *Bipolar Disorders, 8*, 350-361.

Gross, T. F. (2008). Recognition of immaturity and emotional expressions in blended faces by children with autism and other developmental disabilities. *Journal of Autism and Developmental Disorders, 38*, 297-311.

Grossman, J. B., Klin, A., Carter, A. S., and Volkmar, F. R. (2000). Verbal bias in recognition of facial emotions in children with Asperger syndrome. *Journal of Child Psychology and Psychiatry, 41*, 369-379.

Gur, R. C., Sara, R., Hagendoorn, M., Marom, O., Hughett, P., Macy, L., ... and Gur, R. E. (2002). A method for obtaining 3-dimensional facial expressions and its standardization for use in neurocognitive studies. *Journal of neuroscience methods, 115*, 137-143.

Guyer, A. E., Lau, J. Y., McClure-Tone, E. B., Parrish, J., Shiffrin, N. D., Reynolds, R. C., ... and Nelson, E. E. (2008). Amygdala and ventrolateral prefrontal cortex function during anticipated peer evaluation in pediatric social anxiety. *Archives of general psychiatry*, *65*(11), 1303.

Guyer, A.E., McClure, E.B., Adler, A.D., Brotman, M.A., Rich, B.A., Kimes, A.S.,…Leibenluft E. (2007). Specificity of facial expression labeling deficits in childhood psychopathology. *Journal of Child Psychology and Psychiatry, 48*, 863-871.

Hariri, A. R., Mattay, V. S., Tessitore, A., Fera, F., and Weinberger, D. R. (2003). Neocortical modulation of the amygdala response to fearful stimuli. *Biological psychiatry*, *53*(6), 494-501.

Hassel, S., Almeida, J. R., Frank, E., Versace, A., Nau, S. A., Klein, C. R., ... and Phillips, M. L. (2009). Prefrontal cortical and striatal activity to happy and fear faces in bipolar disorder is associated with comorbid substance abuse and eating disorder. *Journal of affective disorders*, *118*, 19-27.

Hassel, S., Almeida, J. R., Kerr, N., Nau, S., Ladouceur, C. D., Fissell, K., ... and Phillips, M. L. (2008). Elevated striatal and decreased dorsolateral prefrontal cortical activity in response to emotional stimuli in euthymic bipolar disorder: no associations with psychotropic medication load. *Bipolar disorders*, *10*, 916-927.

Hauck, M., Fein, D., Maltby, N., Waterhouse, L., and Feinstein, C. (1998). Memory for faces in children with autism. *Child Neuropsychology, 4*, 187-198.

Haxby, J.V., Hoffman, E.A., and Gobbini, M.I. (2002). Human neural systems for face recognition and social communication. *Biological Psychiatry, 51*, 59-67.

Herba, C., and Phillips, M. (2004). Annotation: development of facial expression recognition from childhood to adolescence: Behavioural and neurological perspectives. *Journal of Child Psychology and Psychiatry, 45*, 1185-1198.

Hope, D.A., Rapee, R.M., Heimberg, R.G., and Dombeck, M.J. (1990). Representations of the self in social phobia: Vulnerability to social threat. *Cognitive Therapy and Research, 14*, 177-189.

Humphreys, K., Minshew, N., Leonard, G. L., and Behrmann, M. (2007). A fine-grained analysis of facial expression processing in high-functioning adults with autism. *Neuropsychologia, 45*, 685-695.

In-Albon, T., Dubi, K., Rapee, R.M., and Schneider, S. (2009). Forced choice reaction time paradigm in children with separation anxiety disorder, social phobia, and nonanxious controls. *Behaviour Research and Therapy, 47*, 1058-1065.

Jarros, R.B., Salum, G.A., Belem de Silva, C.T., Toazza, R., de Abreu Costa, M.,…Manfro G.G. (2012). Anxiety disorders in adolescence are associated with impaired facial expression recognition to negative valence. *Journal of Psychiatric Research, 46*, 147-151.

Jones, W., Carr, K., and Klin, A. (2008). Absence of preferential looking to the eyes of approaching adults predicts level of social disability in 2-year-old toddlers with autism spectrum disorder. *Archives of General Psychiatry, 65,* 946-954.

Joseph, R.M., and Tanaka, J. (2003). Holistic and part-based face recognition in children with autism. *Journal of Child Psychology and Psychiatry, 44*, 529-542.

Joshi, G., and Wilens, T. (2009). Comorbidity in Pediatric Bipolar Disorder. *Child and Adolescent Psychiatric Clinics of North America, 18,* 291-319.

Juranek, J., Filipek, P.A., Berenji, G.R., Modahl, C., Osann, K., and Spence, M.A. (2006). Association between amygdala volume and anxiety level: magnetic resonance imaging (MRI) study in autistic children. *Journal of Child Neurology 21*, 1051-1058.

Kalmar, J. H., Wang, F., Chepenik, L. G., Womer, F. Y., Jones, M. M., Pittman, B., ... and Blumberg, H. P. (2009). Relation between amygdala structure and function in adolescents with bipolar disorder. *Journal of the American Academy of Child and Adolescent Psychiatry*, *48*, 636-642.

Kanwisher, N., McDermott, J., and Chun, M. M. (1997). The fusiform face area: a module in human extrastriate cortex specialized for face perception. *The Journal of Neuroscience*, *17*, 4302-4311.

Kim, P., Thomas, L.A., Rosen, B.H., Moscicki, A.M., Brotman, M.A.,…Leibenluft, E. (2012). Differing amygdala responses to facial expression in children and adults with bipolar disorder. *American Journal of Psychiatry, 169*, 642-649.

Kleinhans, N.M., Richards, T., Weaver, K., Johnson, L.C., Greenson, J.,…Aylward, E. (2010). Association between amygdala response to emotional faces and social anxiety in autism spectrum disorders. *Neuropsychologia, 48*, 3665-3670.

Klin, A., Jones, W., Schultz, R., Volkmar, F., and Cohen, D. (2002). Visual fixation patterns during viewing of naturalistic social situations as predictors of social competence in individuals with autism. *Arcives of General Psychiatry, 59*, 809-816.

Knapp, M. L., and Hall, J. A. (2009). *Nonverbal communication in human interaction*. Fort Worth, TX: Wadsworth Publishing Company.

Kohler, C. G., Hoffman, L. J., Eastman, L. B., Healey, K., and Moberg, P. J. (2011). Facial emotion perception in depression and bipolar disorder: a quantitative review. *Psychiatry research*, *188*, 303-309.

Kolassa, I. T., Kolassa, S., Musial, F., and Miltner, W. H. (2007). Event-related potentials to schematic faces in social phobia. *Cognition and Emotion*, *21*, 1721-1744.

Kolassa, I. T., and Miltner, W. H. (2006). Psychophysiological correlates of face processing in social phobia. *Brain research*, *1118*, 130-141.

Kuusikko, S., Haapsamo, H., Jansson-Verkasalo, E., Hurtig, T., Mattila, M.L., Ebeling, H.,… Moilanen, I. (2009). Emotion recognition in children and adolescents with autism spectrum disorders. *Journal of Autism and Developmental Disorders, 39*, 938-945.

Langdell, T. (1978). Recognition of faces: An approach to the study of autism. *Journal of Child Psychology and Psychiatry, 19*, 255–268.

Lawrence, N. S., Williams, A. M., Surguladze, S., Giampietro, V., Brammer, M. J., Andrew, C., ... and Phillips, M. L. (2004). Subcortical and ventral prefrontal cortical neural responses to facial expressions distinguish patients with bipolar disorder and major depression. *Biological psychiatry*, *55*, 578-587.

Law-Smith, M.J., Montagne, B., Perrett, D.I., Gill, M., and Gallagher, L. (2010). Detecting subtle facial emotion recognition deficits in high-functioning Autism using dynamic stimuli of varying intensities. *Neuropsychologia, 48*, 2777-2781.

Lenti, C., Giacobbe, A., and Pegna, C. (2000). Recognition of emotional facial expressions in depressed children and adolescents. *Perceptual and Motor Skills*, *91*, 227-236.

Lewinsohn, P. M., Klein, D. N., and Seeley, J. R. (1995). Bipolar disorders in a community sample of older adolescents: prevalence, phenomenology, comorbidity, and course. *Journal of the American Academy of Child and Adolescent Psychiatry*, *34*, 454-463.

Lewinsohn, P.M., Klein, D.N., and Seeley, J.R. (2000). Bipolar disorder during adolescence and young adulthood in a community sample. *Bipolar Disorders, 2*, 281-293.

Lindner, J. L., and Rosén, L. A. (2006). Decoding of emotion through facial expression, prosody and verbal content in children and adolescents with Asperger's syndrome. *Journal of Autism and Developmental Disorders*, *36*, 769-777.

Macintosh, K., and Dissanayake, C. (2006). Social skills and problem behaviours in school aged children with high functioning autism and Asperger's disorder. *Journal of Autism and Developmental Disorder, 36*, 1065-1076.

Malhi, G. S., Lagopoulos, J., Sachdev, P. S., Ivanovski, B., Shnier, R., and Ketter, T. (2007). Is a lack of disgust something to fear? A functional magnetic resonance imaging facial emotion recognition study in euthymic bipolar disorder patients. *Bipolar disorders*, *9*, 345-357.

Martin, M., Williams, R. M., and Clark, D. M. (1992). Does anxiety lead to selective processing of threat-related information? *Behaviour Research and Therapy,29*, 147-160.

McClure, E. B., Treland, J. E., Snow, J., Schmajuk, M., Dickstein, D. P., Towbin, K. E., ... and Leibenluft, E. (2005). Deficits in social cognition and response flexibility in pediatric bipolar disorder. *American Journal of Psychiatry*, *162*, 1644-1651.

McNally, R. J. (1997). Memory and anxiety disorders. *Philosophical Transactions of the Royal Society B: Biological Sciences*, *352*, 1755.

McPartland, J. C., Webb, S. J., Keehn, B., and Dawson, G. (2011). Patterns of visual attention to faces and objects in autism spectrum disorder. *Journal of autism and developmental disorders*, *41*, 148-157.

McWhirter, B.T., and Walters, K.P. (2008). Preventing and treating mood disorders in children and adolescents. In D. Capuzzi, and D. Gross (Eds.), Youth at risk: A prevention resource for counselors, teachers, and parents (pp. 127-153). Alexandria, VA: American Counseling Association.

Melfsen, S., and Florin, I. (2002). Do socially anxious children show deficits in classifying facial expressions of emotions? *Journal of Nonverbal Behavior, 26,* 109-122.

Miklowitz, D.J., George, E.L., Axelson, D.A., Kim, E.Y., Birmaher, B., Schneck, C.,…Brent, D.A. (2004). Family-focused treatment for adolescents with bipolar disorder. *Journal of Affective Disorder, 82S*, S113-S128.

Monk, C., Klein, R., Telzer, E., Schroth, E., Mannuzza, S., Moulton, J., ... and Ernst, M. (2008). Amygdala and nucleus accumbens activation to emotional facial expressions in children and adolescents at risk for major depression. *American Journal of Psychiatry*, *165*, 90-98.

Monk, C. S., McClure, E. B., Nelson, E. E., Zarahn, E., Bilder, R. M., Leibenluft, E., ... and Pine, D. S. (2003). Adolescent immaturity in attention-related brain engagement to emotional facial expressions. *Neuroimage*, *20*, 420-428.

Moreno, C., Laje, G., Blanco, C., Jiang, H., Schmidt, A.B., and Olfson, M. (2007). National trends in the outpatient diagnosis and treatment of bipolar disorder in youth. *Archives of General Psychiatry, 64*, 1032-1039.

Munson, J., Dawson, G., Abbott, R., Faja, S., Webb, S. J., Friedman, S. D., ... and Dager, S. R. (2006). Amygdalar volume and behavioral development in autism. *Archives of general psychiatry*, *63*, 686.

Nacewicz, B. M., Dalton, K. M., Johnstone, T., Long, M. T., McAuliff, E. M., Oakes, T. R., ... and Davidson, R. J. (2006). Amygdala volume and nonverbal social impairment in adolescent and adult males with autism. *Archives of general psychiatry*, *63*, 1417.

Nelson, C.A., Bloom, F.E., Cameron, J.L., Amaral, D., Dahl, R.E., and Pine, D. (2002). An integrative, multidisciplinary approach to the study of brain-behavior relations in the context of typical and atypical development. *Developmental Psychopathology, 14*, 499-520.

Olsavsky, A.K., Brotman, M.A., Rutenberg, J.G., Muhrer, E.J., Deveney, C.M.,…Leibenluft, E. (2012). Amygdala hyperactivation during face emotion processing in unaffected youth at risk for bipolar disorder. *The American Academy of Child and Adolescent Psychiatry, 51*, 294-303.

Ozonoff, S., Pennington, B. F., and Rogers, S. J. (1990). Are there emotion perception deficits in young autistic children? *Journal of Child Psychology and Psychiatry, 31*, 343-361.

Pavuluri, M.N., Graczyk, P.A., Henry, D.B., Carbray, J.A., Heidenreich, J., and Miklowitz, D.J. (2004). Child- and family-focused cognitive-behavioral therapy for pediatric bipolar disorder: Development and preliminary results. *Journal of the American Academy of Child and Adolescent Psychiatry, 43*, 528-537.

Pavuluri, M. N., O'Connor, M. M., Harral, E., and Sweeney, J. A. (2007). Affective neural circuitry during facial emotion processing in pediatric bipolar disorder. *Biological psychiatry*, *62*, 158-167.

Pavuluri, M. N., Passarotti, A. M., Harral, E. M., and Sweeney, J. A. (2009). An fMRI study of the neural correlates of incidental versus directed emotion processing in pediatric bipolar disorder. *Journal of the American Academy of Child and Adolescent Psychiatry*, *48*, 308.

Pellicano, E. (2010). Individual differences in executive function and central coherence predict developmental changes in theory of mind in autism. *Developmental Psychology*, *46*, 530.

Pelphrey, K. A., Sasson, N. J., Reznick, J. S., Paul, G., Goldman, B. D., and Piven, J. (2002). Visual scanning of faces in autism. *Journal of autism and developmental disorders*, *32*, 249-261.

Perez-Edgar, K., Bar-Haim, Y., McDermott, J.M., Gorodetsky, E., Hodgkinson, C.A.,…Fox, N.A. (2010). Variations in the serotonin-transporter gene are association with attention bias patterns to positive and negative emotion faces. *Biological Psychology, 83*, 269-271.

Pfeifer, J. C., Welge, J., Strakowski, S. M., Adler, C., and Delbello, M. P. (2008). Meta-analysis of amygdala volumes in children and adolescents with bipolar disorder. *Journal of the American Academy of Child and Adolescent Psychiatry*, *47*, 1289-1298.

Phillips, M. L., Drevets, W. C., Rauch, S. L., and Lane, R. (2003). Neurobiology of emotion perception I: The neural basis of normal emotion perception. *Biological psychiatry*.

Piggot, J., Kwon, H., Mobbs, D., Blasey, C., Lotspeich, L., Menon, V., ... and Reiss, A. L. (2004). Emotional attribution in high-functioning individuals with autistic spectrum disorder: a functional imaging study. *Journal of the American Academy of Child and Adolescent Psychiatry*, *43*, 473-480.

Pine, D. S. (1997). Childhood anxiety disorders. *Current opinion in pediatrics*, *9*, 329-338.

Pine, D. S., Cohen, P., Gurley, D., Brook, J., and Ma, Y. (1998). The risk for early-adulthood anxiety and depressive disorders in adolescents with anxiety and depressive disorders. *Archives of General Psychiatry*, *55*, 56-64.

Pine, D. S., Lissek, S., Klein, R. G., Mannuzza, S., Moulton, J. L., Guardino, M., and Woldehawariat, G. (2004). Face-memory and emotion: associations with major depression in children and adolescents. *Journal of Child Psychology and Psychiatry*, *45*, 1199-1208.

Roberson-Nay, R., McClure, E. B., Monk, C. S., Nelson, E. E., Guyer, A. E., Fromm, S. J., ... and Pine, D. S. (2006). Increased amygdala activity during successful memory encoding in adolescent major depressive disorder: an fMRI study. *Biological Psychiatry*, *60*, 966-973.

Robinson, J. L., Monkul, E. S., Tordesillas-Gutiérrez, D., Franklin, C., Bearden, C. E., Fox, P. T., and Glahn, D. C. (2008). Fronto-limbic circuitry in euthymic bipolar disorder: evidence for prefrontal hyperactivation. *Psychiatry Research: Neuroimaging*, *164*, 106-113.

Rich, B.A., Grimley, M.E., Schmajuk, M., Blair, K.S., Blair, R.J., and Leibenluft, E. (2008). Face emotion labeling deficits in children with bipolar disorder and severe mood dysregulation. *Developmental Psychopathology, 20,* 529-546.

Rich, B.A., and Rosen, H.R. (2012). Family dysfunction in pediatric bipolar disorder and associated family-based interventions. In E. Trejos-Castillo (Ed.), *Youth: Practices, Perspectives, and Challenges.* New York, NY: NOVA Publishers.

Rich, B.A., Vinton, D., Roberson-Nay, R., Hommer, R., Berghorst, L., McClure, E.,…Leibenluft, E. (2006). Limbic hyperactivation during processing of neutral facial expressions in children with bipolar disorder. *Proceedings of the National Academy of Sciences USA, 103,* 8900-8905.

Rosen, H. R., and Rich, B. A. (2010). Neurocognitive correlates of emotional stimulus processing in pediatric bipolar disorder: a review. *Postgraduate medicine*, *122*, 94-104.

Rump, K.M., Giovannelli, J.L., Minshew, N.J., Strauss, M.S. (2009). The development of emotion recognition in individuals with autism. *Child Development, 80*, 1434-1447.

Schenkel, L. S., Pavuluri, M. N., Herbener, E. S., Harral, E. M., and Sweeney, J. A. (2007). Facial emotion processing in acutely ill and euthymic patients with pediatric bipolar disorder. *Journal of the American Academy of Child and Adolescent Psychiatry*, *46*, 1070-1079.

Schepman, K., Taylor, E., Collishaw, S., and Fombonne, E. (2012). Face emotion processing in depressed children and adolescents with and without comorbid conduct disorder. *Journal of Abnormal Child Psychology, 40*, 583-593.

Schmidt, L. A., and Buss, A. H. (2009). Understanding shyness: Four questions and four decades of research. In K. R. Rubin and R. J. Coplan (Eds.), *The development of shyness and social withdrawal*. New York: Guildford Publications.

Sheline, Y. I., Barch, D. M., Donnelly, J. M., Ollinger, J. M., Snyder, A. Z., and Mintun, M. A. (2001). Increased amygdala response to masked emotional faces in depressed subjects resolves with antidepressant treatment: an fMRI study. *Biological psychiatry*, *50*, 651-658.

Siegle, G. J., Thompson, W., Carter, C. S., Steinhauer, S. R., and Thase, M. E. (2007). Increased amygdala and decreased dorsolateral prefrontal BOLD responses in unipolar depression: related and independent features. *Biological psychiatry*, *61*, 198-209.

Silver, H., Shlomo, N., Turner, T., and Gur, R. C. (2002). Perception of happy and sad facial expressions in chronic schizophrenia: evidence for two evaluative systems. *Schizophrenia research*, *55*, 171-177.

Simonian, S. J., Beidel, D. C., Turner, S. M., Berkes, J. L., and Long, J. H. (2001). Recognition of facial affect by children and adolescents diagnosed with social phobia. *Child Psychiatry and Human Development*, *32*, 137-145.

Sinzig, J., Morsch, D., and Lehmkuhl, G. (2008). Do hyperactivity, impulsivity and inattention have an impact on the ability of facial affect recognition in children with autism and ADHD? *European Child and Adolescent Psychiatry, 17*, 63-72.

Spezio, M. L., Adolphs, R., Hurley, R. S., and Piven, J. (2007). Analysis of face gaze in autism using? Bubbles?. *Neuropsychologia*, *45*, 144-151.

Surguladze, S., Brammer, M. J., Keedwell, P., Giampietro, V., Young, A. W., Travis, M. J., ... and Phillips, M. L. (2005). A differential pattern of neural response toward sad versus happy facial expressions in major depressive disorder. *Biological psychiatry*, *57*,201-209.

Tantam, D., Monaghan, L., Nicholson, II., and Stirling, J. (1989). Autistic children's ability to interpret faces: A research note. *Journal of Child Psychology and Psychiatry and Allied Disciplines, 30*, 623-630.

Thomas, K. M., Drevets, W. C., Dahl, R. E., Ryan, N. D., Birmaher, B., Eccard, C. H., ... and Casey, B. J. (2001). Amygdala response to fearful faces in anxious and depressed children. *Archives of General Psychiatry*, *58*, 1057-1063.

Trepagnier, C., Sebrechts, M. M., and Peterson, R. (2002). Atypical face gaze in autism. *Cyberpsychology and Behavior*, *5*, 213-217.

Usher, J., Leucht, S., Falkai, P., and Scherk, H. (2010). Correlation between amygdala volume and age in bipolar disorder-a systematic review and meta-analysis of structural MRI studies. *Psychiatry research*, *182*, 1-8.

van der Geest, J. N., Kemner, C., Camfferman, G., Verbaten, M. N., and van Engeland, H. (2002a). Eye movements, visual attention, and autism: a saccadic reaction time study using the gap and overlap paradigm. *Biological Psychiatry*, *50*, 614-619.

van der Geest, J. N., Kemner, C., Verbaten, M. N., and van Engeland, H. (2002b). Gaze behavior of children with pervasive developmental disorder toward human faces: A fixation time study. *Journal of Child Psychology and Psychiatry, 43*, 669-678.

Vasey, M. W., El-Hag, N., and Daleiden, E. L. (2008). Anxiety and the Processing of Emotionally Threatening Stimuli: Distinctive Patterns of Selective Attention among High-and Low-Test-Anxious Children. *Child Development*, *67*, 1173-1185.

Wang, A.T., Dapretto, M., Hariri, A.R., Sigman, M., and Bookheimer, S.Y. (2004). Neural correlates of facial affect processing in children and adolescents with autism spectrum disorder. *Journal of the American Academy of Child and Adolescent Psychiatry, 43*, 481–490.

Whalen, P.J., Shin, L.M., Somerville, L.H., McLean, A.A., and Kim, H. (2002). Functional neuroimaging studies of the amygdala in depression. *Seminars in Clinical Psychology, 7,* 234-242.

Wolf, J.M., Tanaka, J.W., Klaiman, C., Cockburn, J., Herlihy, L.,.. Schultz, R.T., (2008). Specific impairment of face-processing abilities in children with autism spectrum disorder using the *Let's Face It!* skills battery. *Autism Research, 1*, 329-340.

Wong, N., Beidel, D.C., Sarver, D.E., and Sims, V. (2012). Facial emotion recognition in children with high functioning autism and children with social phobia. *Child Psychiatry and Human Development, 43*, 775-794.

Winton, E. C., Clark, D. M., and Edelmann, R. J. (1995). Social anxiety, fear of negative evaluation and the detection of negative emotion in others. *Behaviour Research and Therapy*, *33*, 193-196.

Wright, C. I., Fischer, H., Whalen, P. J., McInerney, S. C., Shin, L. M., and Rauch, S. L. (2001). Differential prefrontal cortex and amygdala habituation to repeatedly presented emotional stimuli. *Neuroreport*, *12*, 379-383.

Yaniv, D., Schafe, G. E., LeDoux, J. E., and Richter-Levin, G. A. L. (2000). Perirhinal cortex and thalamic stimulation induces LTP in different areas of the amygdala. *Annals of the New York Academy of Sciences*, *911*, 474-476.

Young, R. L., and Posselt, M. (2012). Using the Transporters DVD as a learning tool for children with autism spectrum disorders (ASD). *Journal of autism and developmental disorders*, *42*(6), 984-991.

Yuen, P. K. (1994). Social anxiety and the allocation of attention: Evaluation using facial stimuli in a dot-probe paradigm. *Unpublished research project, Department of Experimental Psychology, University of Oxford, UK.*

Yurgelun-Todd, D. A., Gruber, S. A., Kanayama, G., Killgore, W. D., Baird, A. A., and Young, A. D. (2002). fMRI during affect discrimination in bipolar affective disorder. *Bipolar Disorders*, *2*, 237-248.

In: Bipolar Disorder
Editor: Nickolas B. Moore

ISBN: 978-1-62618-666-8


*Chapter III*

# Brain-Derived Neurotrophic Factor and Neurocognitive Profiles in the Psychosis Spectrum: Findings in Bipolar Disorder and Schizophrenia

***Anthony O. Ahmed*, Daniel J. Fridberg, Mona Hanna and Peter F. Buckley***

Department of Psychiatry and Health Behavior, Medical College of Georgia, Georgia Regents University, Augusta, GA, US

## Abstract

Background: There has been recent interest in the role of brain-derived neurotrophic factor (BDNF) in the pathophysiology and treatment of bipolar disorder and schizophrenia. BDNF plays a role in neuroplasticity by promoting neuronal growth, survival, differentiation, neurostructure, and neurofunction in several brain areas. Its specific neuroplasticity-related role in affective and non-affective psychoses has shown several commonalities that cast doubts on traditional Kraepelinian distinctions between bipolar disorder and schizophrenia.

Method: We review relevant studies of BDNF gene polymorphisms and expression in people with bipolar disorder and schizophrenia compared to healthy controls that suggest its putative role in etiology, mechanism, and phenotypic expression in both disorders.

Results: Studies suggest that peripheral BDNF is low in people with bipolar disorder and schizophrenia and BDNF concentrations are inversely correlated with symptom

* Correspondence should be addressed to: Anthony O. Ahmed, Ph.D., Department of Psychiatry and Health Behavior, Medical College of Georgia/Georgia Regents University, 997 Saint Sebastian Way, Augusta, GA 30912. Phone: (706)721-7874. Fax: (706)721-1793. E-mail: aahmed@gru.edu; Disclosures: None.

severity. At the DNA level, studies of the Val66Met single nucleotide polymorphisms (SNP) of the BDNF gene suggests that the Met allele is associated with neurocognitive deficits present in both disorders. In contrast, several studies suggest that the Val allele may be associated with symptom severity and the incidence of both bipolar disorder and schizophrenia.

Conclusions: BDNF appears to be a shared biomarker of bipolar disorder and schizophrenia with demonstrable associations with incidence, clinical symptoms, and neurocognitive phenotypes. This state of affairs supports a latent dimension or spectrum model of affective and non-affective psychoses rather than the traditional categorical distinctions. Despite growing evidence of BDNF's role in the psychosis spectrum, questions remain about its reliability and validity as a clinical biomarker and predictor of bipolar disorder and schizophrenia.

# Introduction

There is an ongoing movement to identify reliable biomarkers that would indicate disease risk, presence, and treatment response in psychiatric disorders [1-2]. The search for biomarkers has gained particular momentum in the study of psychotic disorders as interest has shifted towards identifying candidate genes, neuroimages, and the expression of tissue-based proteins [3]. With findings emerging from genetic, neurochemical, and psychopharmacological research, particular interest has been directed towards the role of neurotrophins in the pathophysiology and treatment of affective and non-affective psychotic disorders including bipolar disorder and schizophrenia [4-5]. The neurobiology of bipolar disorder and schizophrenia generally remains unclear. Both disorders have been linked to overlapping vulnerability genes that interact in complex ways with environmental and social learning variables [6]. Although less explored in bipolar disorder relative to schizophrenia, neurodevelopmental models purport that adverse life events in childhood and obstetric complications during gestation contribute to bifurcations in brain development [7-9]. These bifurcations are manifested in both early development and adulthood as ubiquitous neurological aberrations [10-12] that increase responsivity to stressors and increase liability to neuropsychiatric disorders--for example, recently indexed abnormalities in amygdala neurodevelopment in adolescent onset bipolar disorder [13]. There is evidence that suggests that abnormalities in cell migration, synaptic efficiency, neural connectivity, neurotransmitter system, and neural plasticity, present in both bipolar disorder and schizophrenia, may have a neurodevelopmental origin [14-15]. Of particular interest is the role of brain-derived neurotrophic factor (BDNF) and its isoforms on the aforementioned neuronal processes.

In childhood, aberrations in BDNF expression are associated with concomitant aberrations in neurogenesis, maturation, migration, and survival; whereas in late development, reduced BDNF expression is linked to reduced dendritic growth and density, neural outgrowth and connectivity, and synaptic plasticity [16-17]. Several preclinical (animal model) and clinical studies have also emerged that have suggested that abnormalities in BDNF expression in the central nervous system contribute to the signs and symptoms of affective and non-affective psychosis by mediating the maturation and activity of neurotransmitter systems that have been implicated in psychosis [18-20]. This review summarizes the neurochemistry of BDNF and discusses its role in the pathophysiology of both bipolar disorder and schizophrenia. The review will demonstrate that the specific neuroplasticity-related role of BDNF in affective and non-affective psychoses shows several commonalities that cast doubts on traditional Kraepelinian distinctions between bipolar disorder and schizophrenia.

## Basic Neurobiology of BDNF

Neurotrophins are a class of dimeric polypeptides involved in the neuronal growth, survival, differentiation, neurostructure, and neurofunction in several brain areas [21-22]. Several studies have suggested that neurotrophins [along with several other molecules such as the glutamergic, GABAergic, dopaminergic-linked neuregulin, dysbidin, reelin] are involved in neuroplasticity-related functions such as neurogenesis, neuronal migration, positioning, and neurocognitive functions [23-24]. They not only promote growth and differentiation in the nervous system but regulate the resilience of neurons to environmental stressors that contribute to neuropsychiatric illnesses [23,25]. The family of proteins classified as neurotrophins include BDNF, vascular endothelial growth factor (VEGF), nerve growth factor (NGF), neurotrophin-3 (NT-3), neurotrophin-4/5 (NT-4/5), neurotrophin-6 (NT-6), and neurotrophin-7 (NT-7) [26,27]. The most common of these neurotrophic factors is BDNF, which has been now been linked to the neurobiology of both bipolar disorder and schizophrenia [28-29]. Indeed, BDNF activity has been demonstrated in the hippocampus and several other regions of the brain that include the cerebral cortex, striatum, cerebellum, the brain stem, hypothalamus, and the basal ganglia [17].

All neurotrophins are synthesized as pro-isoforms—pro-neurotrophin kDa precursor proteins that are cleaved into mature neurotrophins within the neuron or after the pro-neurotrophin has been transported extracellularly by pro-convertases through dibasic amino acid sites [30]. The secretion process is regulated by neural activity and cellular calcium ion transport [31]. Structurally, the pro-isoform of a neurotrophin has an N-terminal domain that is removed during proteolytic cleavage into the mature isoform. Whereas the neurotrophin precursors bind to $p^{75}$ neurotrophin receptor ($p^{75}$NTR)—a member of the tumor necrosis family (TNF) through the N-terminal domain; the mature, secreted neurotrophins bind to a family of specific protein-kinase neurotrophin receptors—tropomyosine-related kinase (Trk) and lose high affinity for $p^{75}$NTR [31-33]. While different classes of neurotrophins are structurally similar, there are slight structural variations that determine the class of Trk receptors to which neurotrophins bind. BDNF and NT-4 bind to Trk B, NGF to Trk A, whereas NT-3 binds to Trk C [34]. The binding of neurotrophins and pro-neurotrophins to their corresponding receptors activates several receptor-mediated signaling pathways. The binding of mature neurotrophins to their Trk receptors activates mitogen-activated protein kinase (MAPK), phosphatidylinositol 3-kinase (*PI3*-K), and phospholipase C gamma (PLC-γ) signal pathways—all of which are considered survival pathways [26-27, 35-36]. In contrast, pro-neurotrophins, known to have high affinity for $p^{75}$NTR but low affinity for Trk receptors, bind to the earlier and activate apoptotic signal pathways that cause cysteine-aspartic proteases (caspases) and c-Jun N-terminal kinase (JNK) production [37-38]. Caspases are involved in several cellular processes including the regulation of neuronal apoptosis through the cleaving action of effector [executioner] caspases on other proteins in the neuron [39-40]. Caspases have also been linked to survival processes that include differentiation, proliferation, and activation of survivor signals such as the nuclear factor kappa-light-chain-enhancer of activated B cells (NFκB) [41]. The production of JNKs can result in apoptotic and survival processes [e.g., proliferation, differentiation] depending on JNKs activity in activating and inhibiting the action of several other proteins in the neuron including upstream and downstream kinases [42]. The binding of mature neurotrophins to $p^{75}$NTR, to which they have low affinity, also activates survival processes such as NFκB and the Ras homolog gene family, member A [RhoA] signal pathways [4, 32-33, 43]. Both proteins regulate pathways that are involved in the proliferation of neurons and the formation and remodeling of the cytoskeleton.

BDNF is the product of the cleaving action of pro-peptides on the BDNF precursor; a process that could be both intracellular and extracellular [44-46]. This begins when proBDNF is synthesized in the endoplasmic recticulum after which it is cleaved into pro-BDNF. Within the endoplasmic recticulum, pro-BDNF can be cleaved into the mature 14-KDa form (m-BDNF) by the action of furin, an endoprotease [32]. Pro-BDNF may also be transported to the Golgi where it is sorted into secretory vesicles and cleaved into the m-BDNF by proprotein convertases and endoproteases [47]. If it reaches the extracellular milieu, pro-BDNF is cleaved to m-BDNF by plasmin—a tissue plasminogen activator (tPA)-dependent activation—and matrix metalloproteases. Extracellular pro-BDNF can also be endocytosed and cleaved to produce m-BDNF after it binds to $p^{75}$NTR receptors [44-47]. The process of cleaving pro-BDNF to m-BDNF has been linked to late-phase long-term potentiation in the hippocampus and the formation of long-term memory [32, 48]. The use of animal models has been critical in the discovery of the role of BDNF in long-term potentiation—particularly the use of "knock-out" strains. In these studies, a copy of the BDNF gene is "knocked-out" or deleted in healthy rodents such that they become heterozygous for the BDNF gene [49]. The characteristics of knock-out strains are then evaluated in comparison to homozygous strains. Studies have demonstrated that BDNF knock-out mice demonstrate reduced hippocampal volumes and deficits in long-term potentiation when their hippocampal slices are examined and reduced GABAergic and serotonergic neuron-dependent gamma activity in the hippocampus [49-50]. Knock-out mice also demonstrate deficits in cognitive tasks designed to assess their spatial learning and memory functions (e.g., the Morris water maze paradigm) [51]. Similarly, animal studies that have inhibited BDNF activity through the use of function-blocking compounds and antibodies have linked impaired BDNF expression to deficits in maze learning [52-53]. For example, Fiore and colleagues [52] demonstrated that prenatal exposure to methylazoxymethanol acetate during gestation reduced BDNF expression and maze learning deficits in the offspring. Similarly, Angelucci and colleagues [54] demonstrated that chronic administration of D-amphetamine reduces BDNF (and NGF) expression in the occipital cortex and hypothalamus. Castren et al [53] also showed that administration of MK-801, a NMDA receptor antagonist, decreases BDNF expression in the hippocampus and cerebral cortex. Some mice models have focused on inhibiting Trk B receptor functions by creating knock-out strains with altered receptor properties or deleted receptors. In these studies, heterozygous strains have demonstrated inhibited BDNF activity, antidepressant refractory properties to behavioral despair in forced swim, and impaired response to amygdala kindling—a neuroplasticity-based model of complex partial and motor seizures in epilepsy—in which repeated subconvulsive electrical stimulation of the amygdala causes neurons become progressively and permanently excitable [55-56]. The state of neural excitability is mediated by changes in neural transmission and changes in networks that link the amygdala to the hippocampal trisynaptic excitatory circuit, believed to regulate kindling [57].

### Synopsis of the Genetics of BDNF

The complex BDNF gene is located on the short arm of chromosome 11p13 in humans (between base pairs 27,676,439 and 27,743,604) [58]. The gene contains nine 5' exons that include exons I to IXA and one 3' encoding exon, exon IX, for a total of 10 exons. One of the 5' exons binds to the 3' exon after transcription and splicing—therefore there are nine BDNF mRNA forms for translation and expression [59]. The BDNF gene is characterized by several single nucleotide polymorphisms [SNPs] that include the heavily studied rs6265 or Val66Met, and other less researched polymorphisms that include C270T, rs7103411, rs2030324, rs2203877, rs2049045 and rs7124442 [19]. The Val66Met polymorphism is a proregion G196A [guanine-adenine] polymorphism that results in a valine-to-methionine substitution at locus 66. The Val66Met SNP is located in exon VIII [60] and has been linked to inefficient BDNF mRNA transport to dendrites, altered activity-dependent BDNF secretion, and concomitant deficits in synaptic connectivity and neurocognitive functioning [61-63].

## Does the Val66Met Polymorphism Predict the Incidence of Psychotic Disorders?

The BDNF Val66Met polymorphism has been studied with regard to its association with the occurrence of bipolar disorder and schizophrenia. Findings in this area have been mixed especially with regard to bipolar disorder. In two studies, Sklar and colleagues [64] examined the association with bipolar disorder incidence in an initial sample of 136 parent probands and a second sample of 334 parent probands. In both samples, they found that the BDNF polymorphism was significantly associated with bipolar disorder diagnosis in the probands with a greater occurrence of the Val allele in people with bipolar disorder. This was soon replicated in 283 probands diagnosed with bipolar I, II, or schizoaffective disorder, manic type in a study that similarly found an association between the SNP and a bipolar disorder-related diagnosis [65]. Lohoff and colleagues [66] conducted a replication study of the two previous family association studies in 621 people with bipolar disorder and 998 control samples. In their exclusively Caucasian sample, they found a significantly greater occurrence of the Val allele in bipolar patients than the control sample. Green and colleagues [29] conducted another replication study with the largest sample to date of 3062 individuals that included 864 bipolar I patients, 98 bipolar II patients, and 2100 controls. In this sample, there was no association between the Val66Met polymorphism and bipolar disorder status. They did however find an association between the Val allele and bipolar status in individuals with life-time rapid-cycling bipolar disorder relative to controls. In their reanalysis of the Neves-Pereira et al study, Müller et al [67] further confirmed that most of the association found in the earlier study was accounted for by rapid-cycling status. Other small scale studies have also found an association between the Val66Met polymorphism and pediatric-onset bipolar disorder [68-69], but investigations in this area have been inconsistent. Several studies have failed to replicate the association of Val66Met with bipolar disorder [70-75]. Several of these studies were in Asian samples; others were in Scottish and polish samples. It may be that certain biological differences across ethnic groups impact the effect of the Val66Met polymorphism on bipolar incidence.

In schizophrenia, the association with Val66Met has been similarly inconsistent. Neves-Pereira and colleagues [74] examined the association of the Val66Met polymorphism with schizophrenia in 934 probands from Scotland. Of the probands, 321 were diagnosed with schizophrenia or schizoaffective disorder and 263 individuals with bipolar disorder, and 350 healthy controls. They found that there was an association of Val66Met with schizophrenia incidence in their sample with a greater frequency of the Val in people with schizophrenia relative to controls. This relation was absent for their bipolar sample. Rosa and colleagues [76] examined the association of Val66Met with schizophrenia in 94 nuclear families. Their sample confirmed an association between the transmission of the Val allele and the incidence of schizophrenia. Chang et al. [77] examined Val/Met frequencies between 251 people with schizophrenia and 284 healthy controls. Although they obtained no differences across groups in allele frequency distributions, they found that an association between the Val66Met polymorphism and the severity of negative and general psychopathology symptoms measured by the Positive and Negative Syndrome Scale (PANSS). Several studies have however failed to find an association in both Caucasian and Asian samples [78-79]. Nanko et al. [78] examined the association between the Val66Met polymorphism and schizophrenia in a Japanese sample of 178 people with schizophrenia and 332 controls. They found no differences between the groups in their odds of carrying the Val allele. Xu and colleagues [80] similarly found no association in their Han Chinese sample of 275 people with schizophrenia and 297 healthy controls. Meta-analytic reviews of studies that have examined the association of Val66Met with schizophrenia incidence in both Asian and Caucasian samples have concluded that there are no differences in the distributions of the Val allele across schizophrenia and control samples [75, 79-80].

In summary, there is evidence that the Val66Met polymorphism is relevant to the pathophysiology of both bipolar disorder and schizophrenia [66, 81-82] but results have been highly inconsistent with regard to associations with both disorders [75, 79]. Meta-analytic reviews found no association between the Val66Met polymorphism and either bipolar disorder or schizophrenia across aggregated studies, but this may be due to the heterogeneity within both diagnoses with regard to susceptibility loci for illness [83].

## Other Clinical Correlates of the BDNF Val66Met Polymorphism

In clinical and non-clinical samples, the BDNF Val66Met polymorphism has been associated with reduced hippocampal volume, alterations in hippocampal and medial temporal lobe activity, and inefficient memory encoding and processing [84-86]. It has been associated with alterations in amygdala functioning and concomitant deficits in fear conditioning [87]. In a recent meta-analytic review, Molendijk and colleagues [88] demonstrated that although Met allele carriers appeared to demonstrate lower hippocampal volumes than Val/Val homozygotes, there appeared to be a "decline effect" over time, with more recent studies demonstrating smaller effect sizes. A number of studies have linked the Val66Met polymorphism to reductions in white matter structural integrity in non-clinical samples [89].

Some individual studies have suggested that the Met allele may be associated with suicidality in bipolar disorder [90], age of onset in schizophrenia [91], glucose metabolism in both disorders [92], decrease in cerebral gyrification in bipolar disorder [93], brain volume reductions in both bipolar disorder and schizophrenia [94-96] (particularly in the hippocampus [97-98]), and neurocognitive deficits in both disorders [94,99-100].

## Resilience to Stressors and BDNF Expression

Neurodevelopmental models provide an important platform for considering the role of BDNF in the pathophysiology of affective and non-affective psychosis. As prenatal stressors, obstetric complications, and early childhood adverse experiences exert their effect on the developing brain, they contribute to the individual's inherent liability to develop psychiatric illnesses later in life. As espoused by diathesis-stress models, the latent liability is expressed in the presence of environmental stressors [e.g., traumatic experiences, hardship]—a model that works for both bipolar disorder and schizophrenia [101-102]. There is growing evidence from animal and human studies that variations in BDNF expression contribute to the neurobiological substrate of the diatheses of bipolar disorder and schizophrenia [101]. The impact of prenatal stress on BDNF expression has been demonstrated in several studies using rodent models that simulated forms of prenatal stress such as restraint, food deprivation, low temperatures, non-escapable swim, and crowding conditions [103-105]. These studies demonstrate the impact of stressors on both the acute expression of BDNF and its long-term expression [i.e., levels in adulthood]. Acute stress paradigms appear to have an impact on acute BDNF expression; however, the long-lasting effect of prenatal stress is also demonstrated in studies that show differential impact of chronic stressors on BDNF mRNA expression between rats that had experienced prenatal stress and those that had no such prenatal exposure [105]. In one study, rats exposed to prenatal stress demonstrated reduced BDNF expression in their prefrontal cortex and their striatum. In adulthood, they also demonstrated deviant expressions of BDNF relative to "normal" rats during exposure to chronic stress [104]. Similarly, animal models have demonstrated that stressors during the neonatal period induced acutely produce acute decreases in BDNF levels in the hippocampus whereas chronic induction of stressors during this period chronically impact BDNF expression in the frontal areas [106-107]. The impact of stressors on BDNF expression does appear to be moderated by the genetic strain of the animal. For example, Neeley et al [108] demonstrated that three rat strains that differed in their corticosterone (Hypothalamic-Pituitary-Adrenal [HPA axis]) responsivity—Fischer rats (high), Lewis rats (low), and Sprague-Dawley rats (intermediate)—also differed in their level of both pro-BDNF and mature-BDNF following prenatal stress exposure. Prenatal stress had the greatest impact on BDNF expression in Lewis rats, followed by Sprague-Dawley rats. In both rat strains, prenatal stress decreased acute BDNF mRNA expression, concentrations of m-BDNF, and pro-BDNF, and also altered the Trk B receptor and its signal pathway. Prenatal stress had little impact on BDNF signaling in Fischer rats, suggesting that their genetic configuration may confer neuroprotective benefits against prenatal stress. Overall, it appears that stressors during pregnancy and in early development may have acute and long-lasting effects on BDNF expression that may be critical to the neuronal integrity in a way that may heighten the latent psychiatric diathesis. For example, stress may compromise the neuronal architecture of hippocampal structures by decreasing their connectivity, size, and integrity.

Stressors are equally recognized as contributors to the emergence of affective and non-affective psychoses. Several studies provide evidence that stress-response circuits are important in the pathophysiology of schizophrenia and bipolar disorder [109-110]. Studies have shown that people with schizophrenia demonstrate higher baseline cortisol and adrenocorticotrophic hormones relative to controls [111-112]. They also demonstrate increased cortisol response in pharmacological challenge studies; decreased hippocampal sizes and hence poorer hippocampal regulation of HPA axis activity; and abnormalities in glucocorticoid signaling including increased secretion that result in increased dopamine circuits downstream [113, 114-115]. Studies have also demonstrated that people with bipolar disorder demonstrate abnormalities in cortisol response relative to healthy controls—these include cortisol non-suppression in response to dexamethasone and increased response to corticotrophin releasing hormone [114]. There is a clear role for HPA axis responsivity in the relation between stress and BDNF expression. Chronic stressors may increase the expression of glucocorticoids which may attenuate the expression of BDNF mRNA in the hippocampus and other brain structures; thereby interfering with synaptogenesis and neuroplasticity [115]. In addition, Fuchikami and colleagues [103] demonstrated that acute stress may also impact BDNF transcription through glucocorticoid-influenced epigenetic regulation. HPA axis responsivity thus establishes a neurochemical link between the influence of stressors on BDNF expression and their influence on psychiatric symptoms.

Also related to resilience is the degree to which BDNF expression is related to relapse and remission in psychiatric illness. There is evidence that escalating depressive symptoms are associated with decreased serum BDNF levels. It also appears that various antidepressants improved serum BDNF levels along with depressive symptoms in depressed patients [116-118]. As such, it is possible that antidepressants may confer their therapeutic benefits by influencing BDNF activity perhaps by improving neuronal integrity, synaptogenesis at catecholamine receptor sites, and downstream signaling of extracellular signal-regulated kinase (ERK) and cAMP response element-binding protein (CREB) [119]. A number of studies that examined the association between polymorphisms of the BDNF gene and susceptibility to psychiatric illness following life stressors have gone a long way to establish the role of BDNF in resilience. In the first of these studies, Kaufman and colleagues [120] examined the impact of the experience of childhood maltreatment on depressive symptoms in 198 children, 108 of whom had experienced abuse and 87 classified as non-maltreated controls. Kaufman and colleagues also obtained DNA specimens from both groups genotyped for the serotonin transporter gene (5-HTTLPR s/l at locus SLC6A4) and the BDNF gene (Val66Met). The Met variant is usually associated with less BDNF activity than the Val variant of the allele and individuals heterozygous for the allele (i.e., Val/Met individuals) usually demonstrate less efficient BDNF signaling and decreased BDNF expression. Kaufman and colleagues found that there was a three-way interaction between maltreatment status, BDNF, and 5-HTTLPR polymorphisms such that maltreated children who carried the Met allele and two short alleles of 5-HTTLPR (s-carriers) demonstrated higher depression scores than other groups. Wichers and colleagues [121] replicated the Kaufman and colleagues study in a sample of 394 individuals drawn from a female twin study. They obtained findings that generally replicated those of Kaufman and colleagues—a three-way interaction in which Met carriers experienced more depressive symptoms due to childhood, an experience that was even more profound among s-carriers of the 5HTTLPR gene. In a similar study, Kim and colleagues [122] examined the relation between stressful life events, depression, and BDNF and 5-HTTLPR polymorphisms in 732 older adults. After controlling for age, gender, disability, and education, the authors also obtained a significant three-way interaction between stressful life events, BDNF, and 5HTTLPR polymorphisms. Recently, Grabe and colleagues [123] established the role of BDNF in concert with 5HTTLPR in resilience with the largest sample to date (N = 2035). In this study, they also obtained a three-way interaction between childhood abuse, BDNF, and 5HTTLPR polymorphism in the relation with depression. They also found that individuals who experienced abuse, and who were homozygous s/s for 5HTTLPR, only experienced depression when they carried the Val/Val polymorphism and not when they carried the Met allele. Results also revealed that individuals who carried the l allele of 5HTTLPR also experienced depressive symptoms due to abuse when they carried the Met allele. It therefore appears that the BDNF gene polymorphisms are critical to determining the effect of 5HTTLPR polymorphisms on the emergence of depressive symptoms following trauma, such that homozygous s/s status could be either protective or confer risk depending on the BDNF polymorphism.

In summary, there appears to be a relationship between the stress response circuits and BDNF expression in the CNS. HPA axis hypersensitivity to stress and increased secretion of cortisol and glucocorticoids modulate the expression of hippocampal BDNF mRNA and neuroplasticity. Second, the BDNF gene in the form of the Val66Met SNP and its expression appears to contribute to the biological substrate of the diathesis of psychotic disorders. BDNF regulates the impact of childhood abuse, life stressors, and other adverse environmental experiences on clinical symptoms and neuroplasticity.

## BDNF as a Biomarker in the Psychosis Spectrum: Findings in Schizophrenia and Bipolar Disorder

Several studies have examined the degree of BDNF expression in people with schizophrenia and bipolar disorder relative to healthy controls. These studies include those that examined post-morten brain tissue and others that obtained serum, plasma, or cerebrospinal fluid concentrations of BDNF in live individuals with the assumption that concentrations in these media reflect their frank expressions in the CNS. Studies of live individuals can further be classified into those that examined people with chronic schizophrenia and individuals experiencing their first episode (medication-naïve samples).

### Postmortem Studies in Schizophrenia and Bipolar Disorder

The published post-mortem studies in patients with schizophrenia and bipolar disorder have largely focused their investigations on the prefrontal cortex, and to a lesser extent, the hippocampus; although one study did examine the cerebellum. Four post-mortem studies have examined BDNF mRNA expression levels in the prefrontal cortex. Weickert and colleagues [124] examined post-mortem brain samples of 23 individuals with schizophrenia compared with a control sample of 26 individuals matched by age, race, tissue pH, postmortem interval, and brain size. They found that individuals with schizophrenia demonstrated reduced BDNF mRNA and protein in their dorsolateral prefrontal cortex (DLPFC) relative to the control group. They also found that BDNF expression was especially low in layers II, V, and VI of the DLPFC of people with schizophrenia. Similarly, Hashimoto and colleagues [125] examined postmortem brain samples of 15 individuals with schizophrenia and compared their prefrontal cortex concentrations of BDNF and TrkB mRNA to a matched control sample. They found that people with schizophrenia had lower concentrations of BDNF and TrkB mRNA in their prefrontal cortex relative to the control sample. Pillai [126] compared the BDNF and Sprouty2 post-mortem DLPFC concentrations of 35 people with schizophrenia, 31 with bipolar disorder, and 34 control samples. Sprouty2 is believed to regulate the signaling of growth factors in the CNS. Pillai found that people with schizophrenia and bipolar disorder demonstrated reduced concentrations of both BDNF and Sprouty2 in their DLPFC compared to the control group but there were no significant differences between the diagnostic groups. Issa and colleagues [127] measured cortisol and BDNF levels in the prefrontal cortex of 15 people with schizophrenia compared with 15 matched controls. They found that whereas PFC cortisol concentrations were higher in patients with schizophrenia, their BDNF concentrations were lower relative to the control group. They also found modest inverse correlations between cortisol and BDNF concentrations.

A few studies have also examined BDNF concentrations in the hippocampus using post-mortem samples. Unlike studies that focused on the PFC, there has been less consistency in findings obtained from this area. Comparing schizophrenia patients to controls, Takahashi and colleagues [128] found that BDNF levels were elevated in the hippocampus of people with schizophrenia but their TrkB receptors were reduced in the same brain region. Dunham and colleagues [129] compared 15 people with schizophrenia, 15 with bipolar disorder, and 15 with major depressive disorder to a control sample of 15 individuals in their levels of ProBDNF expression in the hippocampus. Although they found no change in the schizophrenia group, both mood disorder groups demonstrated reductions in their right hippocampus. People with schizophrenia also demonstrated reductions in their $p^{75}$ receptors in both their right and left hippocampus. Ray and colleagues [130] similarly compared the three diagnostic subgroups and a control group on the levels of BDNF mRNA, TrkB expression in hippocampus. They found that whereas people with bipolar disorder demonstrated reductions in BDNF mRNA expression in the cornu ammonis 4 (CA4) region of the hippocampus and reduced expression of the TrkB receptor in the entorhinal cortex, people with schizophrenia demonstrated reductions in both the protein and in the receptor in the CA4 region.

## Serum and Plasma Studies in First-Episode Psychosis Patients

There have been a number of studies that examined the serum or plasma concentrations of BDNF in first-episode, drug-naive schizophrenia patients. Buckley and colleagues [131] obtained plasma BDNF samples from 14 drug naïve, first episode patients, and 15 control subjects that were matched for age and gender. They compared the plasma concentrations of both groups and found that first episode patients demonstrated substantially lower BDNF expressions with concentrations that were about 5 standard deviation (SD) units lower. There has been only one other study of first-episode patients that also obtained plasma concentrations. Pillai and colleagues [132] also compared 34 first-episode schizophrenia patients to 36 age-matched controls on their plasma and cerebrospinal fluid (CSF) BDNF concentrations. They found that BDNF concentrations were lower for first-episode patients in both media; however, they obtained effect size differences that were substantially lower than that obtained by Buckley and colleagues. In schizophrenia patients, plasma BDNF concentrations were .53 SD units lower and CSF BDNF concentrations were .74 SD units lower. They also found that plasma BDNF concentrations were correlated with CSF concentrations. In both studies, plasma BDNF concentrations were correlated with the severity of psychotic symptoms.

Many more studies of first-episode patients have focused on serum BDNF concentrations. Rizos and colleagues [133] compared serum BDNF levels of 32 medication-naïve schizophrenia patients with 15 control subjects matched for age, marital status, education, gender, and employment status. The patient group demonstrated reduced concentrations of serum BDNF with concentrations that were 1.32 SD units lower than control group concentrations. Jindal et al. [134] compared the serum BDNF concentrations of 24 medication-naïve schizophrenia patients to 41 control subjects matched by age and gender. In this study, first-episode schizophrenia patients demonstrated BDNF concentrations that were about .55 SD units lower than control subjects. In contrast, there were no statistically significant differences between patients with non-schizophrenia psychosis (i.e., Major Depressive Disorder and Psychotic Disorder NOS) and control subjects in their degree of BDNF expression. Further, they found no correlation between BDNF levels and ratings on the positive and Negative Syndrome Scale (PANSS). There was however evidence from the study that BDNF expression may be distributed in a dimensional way across diagnostic subgrouping with people with schizophrenia-related psychosis expressing the lowest amount of BDNF and people with non-schizophrenia psychosis falling in between schizophrenia groups and healthy controls. Chen and colleagues [135] compared BDNF levels from 88 drug-naïve first-episode patients with those from 90 control subjects matched by age and gender. In their sample, the schizophrenia group demonstrated BDNF levels that were lower by .92 SD units. They also obtained a positive correlation between BDNF concentrations and positive symptoms of schizophrenia. They found that people with the paranoid schizophrenia subtype demonstrated significantly higher levels of BDNF than people classified in the undifferentiated and "combined" subtypes, indicating that BDNF concentrations may differ according to diagnostic subtype of the illness.

## Serum and Plasma Studies in Chronic Schizophrenia Patients

Several studies have examined BDNF serum expression in chronic patients with schizophrenia undergoing antipsychotic treatment with very little examination of plasma concentrations. In one of the only plasma studies in chronic schizophrenia patients to date, Yoshimura and colleagues [136] compared plasma BDNF concentrations of 89 patients, all of whom were switched to risperidone for at least a week before plasma draws. Their plasma

BDNF levels, which were compared to those of a healthy control sample of 103 individuals matched by age and gender, were about .45 SD units lower than those of the control sample.

Tan and colleagues [137] measured and compared serum BDNF levels in 81 people with schizophrenia with a control sample of 45 individuals matched by age and sex. There was a .63 SD separation between the patient group and the control group with the patient group demonstrating reduced BDNF concentrations. Grillo and colleagues [138] obtained BDNF samples from 44 patients with schizophrenia, 20 of whom had been on clozapine for an average of 13.4 years and 24 who had been receiving first generation antipsychotics for 13.5 years. Compared to a control sample of 25 people, the patient sample demonstrated decreases in serum BDNF levels (lower by 1.36 SD units). They also found that patients on clozapine had marginally higher BDNF levels than those on first generation antipsychotics but the difference did not achieve statistical significance. They also found a strong positive correlation between clozapine dosage and serum BDNF levels. Ikeda and colleagues compared serum samples they obtained from 74 patients with schizophrenia taking several antipsychotics and 87 healthy controls matched by age, gender, BMI, and smoking status. Schizophrenia patients demonstrated reduced BDNF levels relative to controls with group separations of .65 SD units. Piridar and colleagues [139] examined the BDNF levels of 22 schizophrenia patients at baseline and following six weeks of antipsychotic treatment relative to an equaled-sized control group matched by age and sex. Most of the patients (n = 17) had been taking risperidone, whereas the minority had been taking olanzapine and clozapine. At baseline, schizophrenia patients demonstrated lower serum BDNF levels than the control group (lower by 1.78 SD units); they however found no correlation between serum BDNF concentrations and the severity of psychotic symptoms. In addition, they also found that despite improvements in psychiatric symptoms following medication treatment, there was no change in serum BDNF concentration. Toyooka and colleagues [140] examined two samples of 34 patients with schizophrenia, the majority of who were receiving haloperidol and levomepromazine treatment, and analyzed their whole blood and serum concentrations of BDNF. They compared the serum BDNF levels of patients to that of the corresponding control sample (n=35) and determined that patients had decreased BDNF levels that were .85 SD units less than controls. In the largest sample used to date, Xiu and colleagues [141] compared the serum BDNF levels of 364 people with schizophrenia to an age and gender-matched control group of 323 individuals. Most patients with schizophrenia were on clozapine and risperidone, although others were on perphenazine, haloperidol, and chlorpromazine. In all, the patient group demonstrated decreased serum BDNF levels that were .93 SD units lower than those of the control group. Vinogradov and colleagues [142] demonstrated that 56 patients with schizophrenia had lower serum concentrations of BDNF relative to 16 age, gender, and education-matched controls (lower by .60 SD units]. They also showed that cognitive remediation intervention geared toward alleviating neurocognitive deficits normalized serum BDNF expression after 50 hours (10 weeks) of cognitive training.

Findings in this literature have not been all unanimous. Reis and colleagues [143] compared the serum BDNF levels of 40 patients who had been ill for an average of about 32.4 years to a control sample of 20 individuals matched by age and gender. Most of the patients had been receiving haloperidol, whereas others were receiving chlorpromazine, levomepromazine, and trifluorperazine. Surprisingly, the patient group demonstrated increased serum BDNF levels that were 1.78 SD units greater than those of the control group. In Macklin et al's [144] study, there were no differences between 20 schizophrenia patients,

20 bipolar patients, and an age and gender matched control group of 14 individuals in their serum BDNF concentrations.

## Serum and Plasma Studies in Bipolar Disorder

There have been several studies of serum BDNF in bipolar patients. Many of these studies examine BDNF levels in patients who were receiving medications. Medicated samples may introduce noise to determining the degree of BDNF expression in clinical samples; given that medications such as mood stabilizers and antidepressants may improve BDNF expression [145-146]. As such, some studies have also examined BDNF expression in non-medicated patients with bipolar disorder. Machado-Vieira and colleagues [147] examined the plasma BDNF concentrations of 30 medication-naïve individuals who met criteria for DSM-IV manic episode and compared their plasma concentrations to those of an equal-sized control group matched by age and gender. They found that the mean plasma BDNF concentration of the patient group was .964 SD units lower than that of the control group. They also found that there was an inverse correlation between plasma BDNF concentrations and the severity of mania symptoms. Tramontina and colleagues [148] examined and compared serum BDNF concentration of 10 individuals with acute mania with those of an age and gender-matched control group. Nine of the patients were treated with Lithium and one of them received electroconvulsive therapy. The authors found that patients with bipolar disorder demonstrated decreased BDNF during acute mania relative to controls. Following treatment, patients experienced a significant increase in their BDNF levels and there were no statistically significant differences between patients and controls in their BDNF concentrations. Cunha and colleagues [149] compared the serum BDNF levels of 85 currently medicated bipolar disorder patients classified by current symptom phases—of whom 21 were depressed, 32 manic, and 32 euthymic] to a healthy control sample of 32 people matched by age, gender, and education. They found that serum BDNF levels were lowest for patients in the manic and depressive phases than patients in the euthymic phase and healthy controls. Moreover, the severity of mania and depression was negatively correlated with serum BDNF levels. Monteleone and colleagues [150] obtained serum BDNF levels of 24 patients with unipolar depression, 17 patients with bipolar I disorder, 11 patients with bipolar II disorder, and 11 unipolar disorder patients and those of a control group of 22 people. Fifteen of the patients were medication-free whereas others had been off medications for at least a month. The authors found that all of their patient groups demonstrated equivalent serum BDNF concentrations. The patient group demonstrated reduced BDNF concentrations relative to the control group that was about .48 SD units lower. Further, there were no significant differences between medication-free patients and patients receiving medications on the serum BDNF concentrations. De Oliviera and colleagues [151] also compared medicated and medication-free bipolar patients to determine if there were any differences in their serum BDNF levels. In their study, they obtained BDNF concentrations of 22 medicated bipolar patients, 22 medication-free patients, and a control group of 22 individuals. They found that the patient groups, regardless of their medication status demonstrated lower serum BDNF levels than the control group. Further, there were no differences in BDNF concentrations between medicated and medication-free patients although medication-free patients demonstrated slightly lower BDNF concentrations. The entire patient group demonstrated reduced BDNF concentrations relative to controls with depressed patients demonstrating slightly lower BDNF concentrations than manic patients. Gama and colleagues [152] compared the serum BDNF levels of 30 euthymic bipolar patients most of whom were taking lithium and/or valproate with 26 healthy controls. Much like the Cunha and colleagues' study, Gama and colleagues found no significant differences between patients with euthymic bipolar disorder and healthy controls on their BDNF levels.

Overall, these studies demonstrate that first-episode psychosis and chronic schizophrenia are associated with reduced expression of serum and plasma concentrations of BDNF. Similarly, people with bipolar disorder demonstrate reduced BDNF levels regardless of their medication status (medication-free versus medicated) and episode phase (depressive versus manic episodes). Concentrations appear to be lower in medicated-free patients compared to medicated patients, although most studies did not find significant differences. Manic and depressive phases of illness appear to be associated with decreased BDNF expression; however euthymic illness phases did not appear to be associated with BDNF expression. It may be that BDNF is a putative episode marker in bipolar illness, such that its expressions are normalized in euthymia, whereas its concentrations are negatively correlated with the symptom severity in depressive and manic phases.

## BDNF and Neurocognition in Schizophrenia and Bipolar Disorder

Next we consider more closely the role of BDNF in neurocognition in bipolar disorder and schizophrenia. Both disorders are characterized by well-documented deficits in several neurocognitive domains such as attention, working memory, processing speed, planning, problem-solving, and other executive functions [153-154]. The phenomenology of neurocognitive deficits has been long characterized in schizophrenia—they are present in the prodromal phase, during the first psychotic episode, and are present among unaffected family members. There has been relatively less attention paid to investigating or characterizing neurocognitive deficits in people with bipolar disorder and there have been fewer articles in the literature dealing with deficits in these diagnostic group compared to literature on neurocognitive deficits in people with schizophrenia [153]. There is evidence that people with bipolar disorder experience similar neurocognitive deficits as people with schizophrenia, although it also appears that deficits are less severe in bipolar disorder [155-157]. It has been argued that neurocognitive profiles across schizophrenia and mood spectrum disorders may be best conceptualized as a dimensional phenotype ranging in severity within and across both diagnostic spectra [158]. Considering a set of evidence—that diagnosis does not fully account for variances in neurocognitive performance; that neurocognitive deficits are present in family members of both diagnosis; and that severity differences are minimal in people with schizophrenia and bipolar disorder with a history of psychosis, Simonsen and colleagues [158] suggested that a history of psychosis rather than clinical diagnosis may better explain differences in neurocognitive impairments in patient samples.

Given BDNF's role in neurogenesis, neuroplasticity, and other survival-related functions, it is important to consider the impact of the BDNF gene and its expression in the CNS on concomitant neurocognition in people with bipolar disorder and schizophrenia. A number of studies have examined the association between the BDNF gene Val66Met polymorphism on neurocognitive functioning in schizophrenia and bipolar disorder. Egan and colleagues [62] examined the association between allelic variations and neurocognitive functioning in 641 people that included 133 healthy controls, 203 people with schizophrenia, and 305 unaffected siblings of people with schizophrenia. The authors found that across groups, Met allele carriers tended to perform worse on a measure of episodic memory and immediate recall (Wechsler Memory Scale) relative to Val/Val homozygotes. The performance of heterozygote Val/Met individuals tended to fall between those of Val/Val and Met/Met individuals, with Val/Val individuals performing the best. In a replication in a Chinese sample, Tan and colleagues [159] compared 108 individuals with chronic schizophrenia to 145 controls on their performance on the WMS Logical Memory subscale. The patient and control samples were also genotyped to identify the relative BDNF Val/Met allele frequencies, which were not significantly different across the groups. As in the Egan and colleagues' study, they found an association between the Val66Met polymorphism and memory performance with the allelic variation accounting for 5.5% of the variance in memory performance. People who carried the Met allele (both homozygous and heterozygous) performed worse than Val/Val homozygous individuals on the Logical Memory test. Ho and colleagues [160] compared the neurocognitive performance of 294 patients with schizophrenia spectrum disorders and 144 healthy controls across several domains including verbal memory, processing speed/attention, problem solving, language, and visuospatial abilities. They found a significant association between the Val66Met polymorphism and verbal memory and visuospatial abilities but not other cognitive domains. In both patients and healthy controls, Met carriers demonstrated lower scores on tasks of verbal memory and visuospatial reasoning. In the same study, the authors demonstrated that patients and healthy controls carrying the Met allele also demonstrated reduced gray matter volumes in their temporal and occipital lobes relative to Val/Val homozygous individuals. Within the patient group, carriers of the Met allele demonstrated reduced volumes in their left parahippocampal gyrus and left supramarginal gyrus, areas known to play roles in verbal memory and visual control respectively. Other studies have examined the association of serum BDNF and neurocognition. Carlino and colleagues [161] examined the association between serum BDNF levels and neurocognitive performance in attention, memory, processing speed, and perceptual-motor skills. Their study focused on three isoforms of the BDNF protein in 40 patients with schizophrenia and 40 healthy controls including pro-BDNF, m-BDNF, and the 28 kDa form, truncated-BDNF. They found that the ratio of serum truncated-BDNF to the total BDNF concentration was inversely proportional to neurocognitive performance such that low truncated-BDNF levels contributed to poorer neurocognitive performance. In their study of the benefits of cognitive remediation for people with schizophrenia, Vinogradov and colleagues [142] obtained baseline serum BDNF and neurocognitive test performance of 56 people with schizophrenia and 16 healthy controls. Although there were no associations between serum BDNF and neurocognition at baseline within or between groups; following cognitive training, improvements in neurocognitive performance was associated with an increase in serum BDNF concentrations. The association of the BDNF Val66Met polymorphism and BDNF expression with neurocognition has been similarly demonstrated in bipolar disorder. Rybakowski and colleagues [162] examined the prefrontal neurocognitive functioning of 111 patients with bipolar disorder, 129 patients with schizophrenia, and 160 health controls and its association with the Val66Met polymorphism. Neurocognitive functioning was assessed with the Wisconsin Card Sort Test (WCST) and the N-back test. They found that neurocognitive performance was impaired in the patient groups relative to controls with schizophrenia patients performing worse than bipolar patients. In people with schizophrenia, there were only significant differences between Met and non-Met carriers in the N-back percentage correct index with Met carriers performing worse than Val/Val homozygote individuals. People with bipolar disorder who carried the Met allele performed worse on three WCST indices—perseveration errors, percentage of conceptual level responses, and number of correctly completed categories. Rybakowski and colleagues suggested that given that the N-Back test relies on basic visuomotor coordination and the WCST relies primarily on planning and mental flexibility, it may be that BDNF is implicated in the early phases of information processing in schizophrenia and in the later phases in bipolar disorder. Dias and colleagues [163] obtained serum BDNF levels and neurocognitive performance scores of 65 patients with Bipolar I disorder and 50 healthy controls. Although they found no differences in serum BDNF between patients and controls, they found a correlation between BDNF levels and performance in verbal fluency in both bipolar patients and healthy controls. Not all studies have confirmed a relationship between BDNF and neurocognition in bipolar disorder. Tramontina et al [164] examined the association of the Val66Met polymorphism with executive function as measured by the WCST in 64 patients with bipolar disorder. The authors found no differences between the Met allele carriers and individuals who were Val/Val homozygotes on most indices of executive functioning. The Val/Val group produced more non-perseveration errors than Met carriers. Chou et al. [165] examined BDNF concentrations and administered measures of attention, memory, and executive functions in 23 patients in euthymic bipolar I disorder and 33 healthy controls. While the authors obtained differences on some indicators of facial memory and executive function, there were no robust differences between groups across neuroconitive measures. There were also no differences in BDNF concentrations between the patient and the control sample. As such, there was no correlation found between BDNF concentrations and neurocognitive scores. It may be that the relation between BDNF and neurocognition in bipolar disorder is nonexistent for the euthymic type, given that BDNF levels in this group of patients remains fairly comparable to those of healthy controls across several studies. It is also likely that any possible deficits in facial memory and executive function indicators in euthymic bipolar disorder are better explained by other factors. In summary, the Val66Met polymorphism and its expression levels in the serum appear to be associated with neurocognitive functioning in schizophrenia and bipolar disorder. While studies in people with schizophrenia have produced consistent evidence of an association, findings in bipolar disorder are slightly less robust. There have also been relatively fewer studies of the BDNF association with neurocognition in samples of people with bipolar disorder than schizophrenia.

## Prospects and Problems of BDNF as a Putative Biomarker

The research literature on the role of BDNF in bipolar disorder and schizophrenia is growing quickly. As the literature currently stands, there are a number of conclusions that can be drawn about the role of BDNF in these disorders.

1) Symptoms and Course: Several studies suggest that BDNF plays a role in the pathophysiology of bipolar disorder and schizophrenia. However, the association between the Val66Met polymorphism and either disorder was poorly replicated across studies. In contrast, studies of BDNF expression levels suggest that there is an association with ratings of symptoms in schizophrenia. Similarly, some studies have found correlations between BDNF levels and severity of depressive and manic symptoms in people with bipolar disorder. BDNF levels appear reduced in bipolar patients during manic and depressive episodes but not during euthymic episodes. There is also evidence from studies that the Val66Met polymorphism is associated with the clinical profile of schizophrenia and bipolar patients including suicidality, glucose metabolism, and neurocognitive deficits. Overall, the results across studies appear more robust for schizophrenia than bipolar disorders, but there are relatively fewer studies of BDNF in bipolar disorder than in schizophrenia. BDNF research remains in relative infancy as much work needs to be done to establish its viability as a biomarker of affective and non-affective psychosis. To establish the construct validity of BDNF as a biomarker for psychosis, the process of extracting and measuring peripheral BDNF must be standardized and its reliability ascertained so that variability in assays across studies could be eliminated as a confound contributing to inconsistent findings. The process of establishing the nomological network of this putative biomarker for bipolar disorder would require clearer demonstration of its covariation with bipolar illness phases by examining fluctuations in serum or plasma BDNF concentrations longitudinally through symptom phases. Existing studies to date have only compared bipolar patients in different phases with control samples. While such studies are informative, they say little about whether peripheral BDNF is a harbinger of illness phase (and hence a possible predictor) or an episode footprint.
2) Diagnosis: The question of whether BDNF assays can be incorporated into the standard clinical assessment of bipolar disorder and schizophrenia and used as an indicator for rendering diagnostic decisions is one that remains of interest. We remain cautiously skeptical about such an endeavor given that the biomarker status of BDNF in bipolar disorder and schizophrenia has yet to be resolved. Much like other biomarkers, the diagnostic efficiency of BDNF as an indicator of mood episodes, psychosis status, and treatment effects remains an open question. In one study, Fernandes and colleagues (168) evaluated the utility of serum BDNF as a potential indicator of clinical diagnosis in a sample that comprised 40 patients with bipolar disorder, 10 with major depressive disorder, and 30 health controls. Using receiver operating characteristics (ROC) analysis, they obtained high diagnostic accuracy of .94 for classifying individuals into respective groups using serum BDNF, which was lowest in bipolar patients, as a marker. They were also able to identify a cutoff that had strong sensitivity and specificity for the bipolar group. The result of their study is promising for considering the adjunctive benefit of BDNF in psychiatric diagnosis. The study sample size was small, however, and the study would clearly benefit from replication. Moreover, as with all biomarker candidates, the practicality of their use in clinical settings is limited by the absence of expertise in the interpretation of such data in real-world clinical settings.

3) Treatment Response: In addition, much needs to be learned about the impact of the BDNF gene and its expression on treatment response in bipolar disorder and schizophrenia. Given the association of the Met allele with variables such as neurocognitive deficits, suicidality, brain volume reductions, and glucose metabolism, its impact on the efficacy of psychopharmacological and psychosocial interventions is of interest. It may be that people carrying the Met allele may be less responsive to treatments due to neurocognitive deficits, or may be more prone to relapse and rehospitalization due to their higher levels of suicidality relative to non-carriers of the allele. Similarly, the association of the Met allele with disturbed glucose metabolism may render Met allele carriers poor candidates for medications with high proclivity to induce metabolic dysfunction. With regard to neurocognition, it may be of interest to determine if the Val66Met polymorphism predicts responsiveness to treatments geared towards remediating cognitive deficits in bipolar disorder and schizophrenia. Addressing these empirical questions may serve to tailor particular treatments to individuals for whom they would be most likely efficacious.
4) Neurocognition: Val66Met appears to be an important biomarker of neurocognition in bipolar disorder and schizophrenia. The association of Val66Met with neurocognitive performance scores is consistent with views about the contribution of BDNF to neuronal processes that are linked to neurocognition. For example, the impact of the Val66Met polymorphism can be seen in the activity of BDNF in the hippocampus and parahippocampus where activity dependent secretion and trafficking of BDNF contributes to synaptogenesis during long-term potentiation. People who carry the Met allele demonstrate reduced activity-dependent secretions during the encoding of memory information, which likely contributes to memory impairments [62, 85]. The results of association analyses were not consistent across studies with some studies finding no association between the Val66Met polymorphism and neurocognitive performance. It is noteworthy that a recent meta-analysis that aggregated the results of several studies of the BDNF Val66Met and neurocognition association in clinical and non-clinical samples concluded that there was no consistent association [166]. Of course there are several factors that could contribute to inconsistent findings besides the absence of an actual relationship. Neurocognitive test performance is still relatively far down along the causal chain linking genetic causes to the observable phenotype (neurocognition). In contrast, neuroimaging data and other intermediate phenotypes are closer to the genetic causes. As such it may be that several intermediate phenotypes interact along the causal chain to impact neurocognitive performance and by extension, its genetic penetrance [167].
5) The Psychosis Spectrum: The association of the BDNF gene and its peripheral expression with phenotypes of bipolar disorder and schizophrenia share commonalities that in our view support a dimensional model of the psychosis phenotype. Bipolar disorder and schizophrenia are similarly predicted by the Val66Met polymorphism (although findings are not greatly consistent) and the peripheral expressions of BDNF are correlated with ratings of psychopathology. Neurocognitive dysfunction appears to be predicted by BDNF Val66Met in both disorders. Moreover, several studies that examined BDNF expression levels in both disorders relative to controls appear to support no more than severity differences

between people with bipolar disorder and schizophrenia. Our view of a dimension that includes bipolar disorder and schizophrenia is also supported by findings in neuroimaging research that suggests that people with bipolar disorder and people with schizophrenia are often qualitatively similar regard to neurostructural and neurofunctional abnormalities [169]. The similarities in their patterns of neurocognitive deficits found in both disorders [153-154] and their overlapping genetic origins further supports a dimensional view of these traditionally distinguished disorders.

## Conclusion

The BDNF gene and its peripheral expression appear to play a role in the pathophysiology of bipolar disorder and schizophrenia. Studies examining the association of BDNF with several aspects of the phenomenology of bipolar disorder and schizophrenia have been generally mixed. However, some studies have linked BDNF to psychopathology in bipolar disorder and schizophrenia. The widely studied Val66Met polymorphism of the BDNF gene has been linked to the incidence of illness, neurocognitive functioning, and aspects of treatment response in both disorders. The shared associations of bipolar disorder and schizophrenia with BDNF cast some doubt about the traditional Kraepelinian distinction of both disorders, instead lending credence to an affective–non-affective psychosis spectrum. Although BDNF appears to be a promising biomarker of bipolar disorder and schizophrenia, the preponderance of mixed findings and several remaining questions temper enthusiasm about its use for clinical practice.

## References


[1] Singh I, Rose N. Biomarkers in psychiatry. *Nature*. 2009 Jul 8;460(7252):202–7.

[2] Lakhan SE, Vieira K, Hamlat E. Biomarkers in psychiatry: drawbacks and potential for misuse. *International Archives of Medicine*. 2010 Jan 12;3(1):1.

[3] Lakhan SE, Kramer A. Schizophrenia genomics and proteomics: are we any closer to biomarker discovery? *Behavioral and Brain Functions*. 2009 Jan 7;5(1):2.

[4] Buckley PF, Mahadik S, Pillai A, Terry A Jr. Neurotrophins and schizophrenia. *Schizophr. Res*. 2007 Aug;94(1-3):1–11.

[5] Post RM. Role of BDNF in bipolar and unipolar disorder: clinical and theoretical implications. *J Psychiatr Res*. 2007 Dec;41(12):979–90.

[6] Walss-Bass C, Escamilla MA, Raventos H, Montero AP, Armas R, Dassori A, et al. Evidence of genetic overlap of schizophrenia and bipolar disorder: linkage disequilibrium analysis of chromosome 18 in the Costa Rican population. *Am. J. Med. Genet. B Neuropsychiatr. Genet*. 2005 Nov 5;139B(1):54–60.

[7] Akabaliev V, Sivkov S, Mantarkov M, Ahmed-Popova F. Minor physical anomalies in patients with bipolar I disorder and normal controls. *Journal of Affective Disorders*. 2011 Dec;135(1–3):193–200.

[8] Fatemi SH, Folsom TD. The Neurodevelopmental Hypothesis of Schizophrenia, Revisited. *Schizophr. Bull.* 2009 May 3;35(3):528-548.

[9] Murray RM, Sham P, Van Os J, Zanelli J, Cannon M, McDonald C. A developmental model for similarities and dissimilarities between schizophrenia and bipolar disorder. *Schizophr. Res*. 2004 Dec 1;71(2-3):405–16.

[10] Cannon TD, Van Erp TGM, Bearden CE, Loewy R, Thompson P, Toga AW, et al. Early and late neurodevelopmental influences in the prodrome to schizophrenia: contributions of genes, environment, and their interactions. *Schizophr Bull.* 2003;29(4):653–69.

[11] Cannon M, Murray RM. Neonatal origins of schizophrenia. *Arch. Dis. Child.* 1998 Jan;78(1):1–3.

[12] Meehl PE. Schizotaxia revisited. *Arch. Gen. Psychiatry.* 1989 Oct;46(10):935–44.

[13] Bitter SM, Mills NP, Adler CM, Strakowski SM, DelBello MP. Progression of amygdala volumetric abnormalities in adolescents after their first manic episode. *J Am Acad Child Adolesc Psychiatry.* 2011 Oct;50(10):1017–26.

[14] Kapczinski F, Frey BN, Kauer-Sant'Anna M, Grassi-Oliveira R. Brain-derived neurotrophic factor and neuroplasticity in bipolar disorder. *Expert Rev Neurother*. 2008 Jul;8(7):1101–13.

[15] Krebs MO, Guillin O, Bourdell MC, Schwartz JC, Olie JP, Poirier MF, et al. Brain derived neurotrophic factor (BDNF) gene variants association with age at onset and therapeutic response in schizophrenia. *Mol. Psychiatry*. 2000 Sep;5(5):558–62.

[16] Jones KR, Fariñas I, Backus C, Reichardt LF. Targeted disruption of the BDNF gene perturbs brain and sensory neuron development but not motor neuron development. *Cell*. 1994 Mar 25;76(6):989–99.

[17] Mayeur S, Silhol M, Moitrot E, Barbaux S, Breton C, Gabory A, et al. Placental BDNF/TrkB Signaling System is Modulated by Fetal Growth Disturbances in Rat and Human. *Placenta*. 2010 Sep;31(9):785–91.

[18] De Sousa RT, Van de Bilt MT, Diniz BS, Ladeira RB, Portela LV, Souza DO, et al. Lithium increases plasma brain-derived neurotrophic factor in acute bipolar mania: a preliminary 4-week study. *Neurosci. Lett*. 2011 Apr 20;494(1):54–6.

[19] Pillai A, Buckley PF. Reliable biomarkers and predictors of schizophrenia and its treatment. *Psychiatr. Clin. North Am*. 2012 Sep;35(3):645–59.

[20] Grande I, Kapczinski F, Stertz L, Colpo GD, Kunz M, Cereser KM, et al. Peripheral brain-derived neurotrophic factor changes along treatment with extended release quetiapine during acute mood episodes: an open-label trial in drug-free patients with bipolar disorder. *J Psychiatr Res.* 2012 Nov;46(11):1511–4.

[21] Huang EJ, Reichardt LF. NEUROTROPHINS: Roles in Neuronal Development and Function. *Annual Review of Neuroscience*. 2001;24(1):677–736.

[22] Sofroniew MV, Howe CL, Mobley WC. Nerve growth factor signaling, neuroprotection, and neural repair. *Annu. Rev. Neurosci.* 2001;24:1217–81.

[23] Dodd S, Maes M, Anderson G, Dean OM, Moylan S, Berk M. Putative neuroprotective agents in neuropsychiatric disorders. Prog. Neuropsychopharmacol. *Biol. Psychiatry.* 2013 Apr 5;42:135–45.

[24] Arévalo JC, Wu SH. Neurotrophin signaling: many exciting surprises! *Cell. Mol. Life Sci*. 2006 Jul;63(13):1523–37.

[25] Karatsoreos IN, McEwen BS. Psychobiological allostasis: resistance, resilience and vulnerability. *Trends Cogn. Sci.* (Regul. Ed.). 2011 Dec;15(12):576–84.

[26] Skaper SD. The neurotrophin family of neurotrophic factors: an overview. *Methods Mol. Biol.* 2012;846:1–12.

[27] Skaper SD. The biology of neurotrophins, signalling pathways, and functional peptide mimetics of neurotrophins and their receptors. *CNS Neurol Disord Drug Targets*. 2008 Feb;7(1):46–62.

[28] Green MJ, Matheson SL, Shepherd A, Weickert CS, Carr VJ. Brain-derived neurotrophic factor levels in schizophrenia: a systematic review with meta-analysis. *Mol. Psychiatry*. 2011 Sep;16(9):960–72.

[29] Green EK, Raybould R, Macgregor S, Hyde S, Young AH, O'Donovan MC, et al. Genetic variation of brain-derived neurotrophic factor (BDNF) in bipolar disorder: case-control study of over 3000 individuals from the UK. *Br J Psychiatry*. 2006 Jan;188:21–5.

[30] Teng KK, Felice S, Kim T, Hempstead BL. Understanding Proneurotrophin Actions: Recent Advances and Challenges. *Dev Neurobiol*. 2010 Apr;70(5):350–9.

[31] Huang EJ, Reichardt LF. Trk receptors: roles in neuronal signal transduction. Annu. Rev. Biochem. 2003;72:609–42.

[32] Lu B, Pang PT, Woo NH. The yin and yang of neurotrophin action. *Nat. Rev. Neurosci.* 2005 Aug;6(8):603–14.

[33] Nykjaer A, Lee R, Teng KK, Jansen P, Madsen P, Nielsen MS, et al. Sortilin is essential for proNGF-induced neuronal cell death. *Nature*. 2004 Feb 26;427(6977):843–8.

[34] Segal RA. Selectivity in neurotrophin signaling: theme and variations. *Annu. Rev. Neurosci.* 2003;26:299–330.

[35] Jeanneteau F, Deinhardt K, Miyoshi G, Bennett AM, Chao MV. The MAP kinase phosphatase MKP-1 regulates BDNF-induced axon branching. *Nat. Neurosci.* 2010 Nov;13(11):1373–9.

[36] Mullen LM, Pak KK, Chavez E, Kondo K, Brand Y, Ryan AF. Ras/p38 and PI3K/Akt but not Mek/Erk signaling mediate BDNF-induced neurite formation on neonatal cochlear spiral ganglion explants. *Brain Res*. 2012 Jan 9;1430:25–34.

[37] Mast TG, Fadool DA. Mature and precursor brain-derived neurotrophic factor have individual roles in the mouse olfactory bulb. *PLoS ONE*. 2012;7(2):e31978.

[38] Ichim G, Tauszig-Delamasure S, Mehlen P. Neurotrophins and cell death. Experimental *Cell Research*. 2012 Jul 1;318(11):1221–8.

[39] Chowdhury I, Tharakan B, Bhat GK. Caspases - an update. Comp. Biochem. Physiol. B, *Biochem. Mol. Biol.* 2008 Sep;151(1):10–27.

[40] Coleman M. Molecular signaling how do axons die? *Adv. Genet.* 2011;73:185–217.

[41] Lamkanfi M, Festjens N, Declercq W, Vanden Berghe T, Vandenabeele P. Caspases in cell survival, proliferation and differentiation. *Cell Death Differ*. 2007 Jan;14(1):44–55.

[42] Bode AM, Dong Z. The functional contrariety of JNK. M*ol. Carcinog.* 2007 Aug;46(8):591–8.

[43] Sun Y, Lim Y, Li F, Liu S, Lu J-J, Haberberger R, et al. ProBDNF Collapses Neurite Outgrowth of Primary Neurons by Activating RhoA. *PLoS ONE*. 2012 Apr 27;7(4):e35883.

[44] Matsumoto T, Rauskolb S, Polack M, Klose J, Kolbeck R, Korte M, et al. Biosynthesis and processing of endogenous BDNF: CNS neurons store and secrete BDNF, not pro-BDNF. *Nat. Neurosci.* 2008 Feb;11(2):131–3.

[45] Greenberg ME, Xu B, Lu B, Hempstead BL. New Insights in the Biology of BDNF Synthesis and Release: Implications in CNS Function. *J. Neurosci.* 2009 Oct 14;29(41):12764–7.

[46] Yang J, Siao C-J, Nagappan G, Marinic T, Jing D, McGrath K, et al. Neuronal release of proBDNF. *Nat. Neurosci.* 2009 Feb;12(2):113–5.

[47] Barker PA. Whither proBDNF? *Nature Neuroscience*. 2009;12(2):105–6.

[48] Lu Y, Christian K, Lu B. BDNF: a key regulator for protein synthesis-dependent LTP and long-term memory? *Neurobiol Learn Mem.* 2008 Mar;89(3):312–23.

[49] Huang Y, Morozov A. Hippocampal Deletion of BDNF Gene Attenuates Gamma Oscillations in Area CA1 by Up-Regulating 5-HT3 Receptor. *PLoS ONE*. 2011 Jan 26;6(1):e16480.

[50] Korte M, Carroll P, Wolf E, Brem G, Thoenen H, Bonhoeffer T. Hippocampal long-term potentiation is impaired in mice lacking brain-derived neurotrophic factor. *Proc. Natl. Acad. Sci. U.S.A.* 1995 Sep 12;92(19):8856–60.

[51] Heldt SA, Stanek L, Chhatwal JP, Ressler KJ. Hippocampus-specific deletion of BDNF in adult mice impairs spatial memory and extinction of aversive memories. *Mol. Psychiatry*. 2007 Jul;12(7):656–70.

[52] Fiore M, Korf J, Antonelli A, Talamini L, Aloe L. Long-lasting effects of prenatal MAM treatment on water maze performance in rats: associations with altered brain development and neurotrophin levels. *Neurotoxicol Teratol*. 2002 Apr;24(2):179–91.

[53] Castrén E, Da Penha Berzaghi M, Lindholm D, Thoenen H. Differential effects of MK-801 on brain-derived neurotrophic factor mRNA levels in different regions of the rat brain. *Exp. Neurol.* 1993 Aug;122(2):244–52

[54] Angelucci F, Mathé AA, Aloe L. Brain-derived neurotrophic factor and tyrosine kinase receptor TrkB in rat brain are significantly altered after haloperidol and risperidone administration. *J. Neurosci. Res*. 2000 Jun 15;60(6):783–94.

[55] Jones NC, Lee HE, Yang M, Rees SM, Morris MJ, O'Brien TJ, et al. Repeatedly stressed rats have enhanced vulnerability to amygdala kindling epileptogenesis. *Psychoneuroendocrinology*. 2013 Feb;38(2):263–70.

[56] Friedman WJ. Proneurotrophins, Seizures, and Neuronal Apoptosis. Neuroscientist. 2010 Jun 1;16(3):244–52.

[57] Matveeva EA, Vanaman TC, Whiteheart SW, Slevin JT. Asymmetric Accumulation of Hippocampal 7S SNARE Complexes Occurs Regardless of Kindling Paradigm. *Epilepsy Res*. 2007 Mar;73(3):266–74.

[58] Houlihan LM, Harris SE, Luciano M, Gow AJ, Starr JM, Visscher PM, et al. Replication study of candidate genes for cognitive abilities: the Lothian Birth Cohort 1936. *Genes Brain Behav*. 2009 Mar;8(2):238–47.

[59] Zheng F, Zhou X, Luo Y, Xiao H, Wayman G, Wang H. Regulation of Brain-Derived Neurotrophic Factor Exon IV Transcription through Calcium Responsive Elements in Cortical Neurons. *PLoS ONE*. 2011 Dec 9;6(12):e28441.

[60] Liu Q-R, Walther D, Drgon T, Polesskaya O, Lesnick TG, Strain KJ, et al. Human brain derived neurotrophic factor (BDNF) genes, splicing patterns, and assessments of

associations with substance abuse and Parkinson's Disease. *Am. J. Med. Genet. B Neuropsychiatr. Genet.* 2005 Apr 5;134B(1):93–103.

[61] Chen Z-Y, Patel PD, Sant G, Meng C-X, Teng KK, Hempstead BL, et al. Variant brain-derived neurotrophic factor (BDNF) (Met66) alters the intracellular trafficking and activity-dependent secretion of wild-type BDNF in neurosecretory cells and cortical neurons. *J. Neurosci.* 2004 May 5;24(18):4401–11.

[62] Egan MF, Kojima M, Callicott JH, Goldberg TE, Kolachana BS, Bertolino A, et al. The BDNF val66met polymorphism affects activity-dependent secretion of BDNF and human memory and hippocampal function. *Cell.* 2003 Jan 24;112(2):257–69.

[63] Hashimoto R, Moriguchi Y, Yamashita F, Mori T, Nemoto K, Okada T, et al. Dose-dependent effect of the Val66Met polymorphism of the brain-derived neurotrophic factor gene on memory-related hippocampal activity. *Neurosci. Res.* 2008 Aug;61(4):360–7.

[64] Sklar P, Gabriel SB, McInnis MG, Bennett P, Lim Y-M, Tsan G, et al. Family-based association study of 76 candidate genes in bipolar disorder: BDNF is a potential risk locus. Brain-derived neutrophic factor. *Mol. Psychiatry.* 2002;7(6):579–93.

[65] Neves-Pereira M, Mundo E, Muglia P, King N, Macciardi F, Kennedy JL. The Brain-Derived Neurotrophic Factor Gene Confers Susceptibility to Bipolar Disorder: Evidence from a Family-Based Association Study. *Am J Hum Genet. 2002 Sep;71(3):651–5.*

[66] Lohoff FW, Sander T, Ferraro TN, Dahl JP, Gallinat J, Berrettini WH. Confirmation of association between the Val66Met polymorphism in the brain-derived neurotrophic factor (BDNF) gene and bipolar I disorder. *Am. J. Med. Genet. B Neuropsychiatr. Genet.* 2005 Nov 5;139B(1):51–3.

[67] Müller DJ, Luca VD, Sicard T, King N, Strauss J, Kennedy JL. Brain-derived neurotrophic factor (BDNF) gene and rapid-cycling bipolar disorder Family-based association study. *BJP.* 2006 Oct 1;189(4):317–23.

[68] Strauss J, Barr CL, George CJ, Devlin B, Vetró A, Kiss E, et al. Brain-derived neurotrophic factor variants are associated with childhood-onset mood disorder: confirmation in a Hungarian sample. *Mol. Psychiatry.* 2005 Sep;10(9):861–7.

[69] Geller B, Badner JA, Tillman R, Christian SL, Bolhofner K, Cook EH Jr. Linkage disequilibrium of the brain-derived neurotrophic factor Val66Met polymorphism in children with a prepubertal and early adolescent bipolar disorder phenotype. *Am J Psychiatry.* 2004 Sep;161(9):1698–700.

[70] Hong C-J, Huo S-J, Yen F-C, Tung C-L, Pan G-M, Tsai S-J. Association study of a brain-derived neurotrophic-factor genetic polymorphism and mood disorders, age of onset and suicidal behavior. *Neuropsychobiology.* 2003;48(4):186–9.

[71] Nakata K, Ujike H, Sakai A, Uchida N, Nomura A, Imamura T, et al. Association study of the brain-derived neurotrophic factor (BDNF) gene with bipolar disorder. *Neurosci. Lett.* 2003 Jan 30;337(1):17–20.

[72] Kunugi H, Iijima Y, Tatsumi M, Yoshida M, Hashimoto R, Kato T, et al. No association between the Val66Met polymorphism of the brain-derived neurotrophic factor gene and bipolar disorder in a Japanese population: a multicenter study. *Biol. Psychiatry.* 2004 Sep 1;56(5):376–8.

[73] Skibinska M, Hauser J, Czerski PM, Leszczynska-Rodziewicz A, Kosmowska M, Kapelski P, et al. Association analysis of brain-derived neurotrophic factor (BDNF)

gene Val66Met polymorphism in schizophrenia and bipolar affective disorder. *World J. Biol. Psychiatry*. 2004 Oct;5(4):215–20.

[74] Neves-Pereira M, Cheung JK, Pasdar A, Zhang F, Breen G, Yates P, et al. BDNF gene is a risk factor for schizophrenia in a Scottish population. *Mol. Psychiatry*. 2005 Feb;10(2):208–12.

[75] Kanazawa T, Glatt SJ, Kia-Keating B, Yoneda H, Tsuang MT. Meta-analysis reveals no association of the Val66Met polymorphism of brain-derived neurotrophic factor with either schizophrenia or bipolar disorder. *Psychiatr. Genet.* 2007 Jun;17(3):165–70.

[76] Rosa A, Cuesta MJ, Fatjó-Vilas M, Peralta V, Zarzuela A, Fañanás L. The Val66Met polymorphism of the brain-derived neurotrophic factor gene is associated with risk for psychosis: evidence from a family-based association study. *Am. J. Med. Genet. B Neuropsychiatr. Genet.* 2006 Mar 5;141B(2):135–8.

[77] Chang H-A, Lu R-B, Shy M-J, Chang C-C, Lee M-S, Huang S-Y. Brain-derived neurotrophic factor Val66Met polymorphism: association with psychopathological symptoms of schizophrenia? *J Neuropsychiatry Clin Neurosci*. 2009;21(1):30–7.

[78] Nanko S, Kunugi H, Hirasawa H, Kato N, Nabika T, Kobayashi S. Brain-derived neurotrophic factor gene and schizophrenia: polymorphism screening and association analysis. *Schizophr. Res.* 2003 Aug 1;62(3):281–3.

[79] Naoe Y, Shinkai T, Hori H, Fukunaka Y, Utsunomiya K, Sakata S, et al. No association between the brain-derived neurotrophic factor (BDNF) Val66Met polymorphism and schizophrenia in Asian populations: Evidence from a case-control study and meta-analysis. *Neurosci. Lett.* 2007 Mar 26;415(2):108–12.

[80] Xu M-Q, St Clair D, Ott J, Feng G-Y, He L. Brain-derived neurotrophic factor gene C-270T and Val66Met functional polymorphisms and risk of schizophrenia: A moderate-scale population-based study and meta-analysis. *Schizophrenia Research*. 2007 Mar;91(1–3):6–13.

[81] Rybakowski JK. BDNF gene: functional Val66Met polymorphism in mood disorders and schizophrenia. *Pharmacogenomics*. 2008 Nov;9(11):1589–93.

[82] Wang Z, Li Z, Chen J, Huang J, Yuan C, Hong W, et al. Association of BDNF gene polymorphism with bipolar disorders in Han Chinese population. *Genes Brain Behav*. 2012 Jul;11(5):524–8.

[83] De Luca V, Strauss J, Semeralul M, Huang S, Li PP, Warsh JJ, et al. Analysis of BDNF Val66Met allele-specific mRNA levels in bipolar disorder. *Neurosci. Lett.* 2008 Aug 22;441(2):229–32.

[84] Hajek T, Kopecek M, Höschl C. Reduced hippocampal volumes in healthy carriers of brain-derived neurotrophic factor Val66Met polymorphism: meta-analysis. *World J. Biol. Psychiatry*. 2012 Mar;13(3):178–87.

[85] Kauppi K, Nilsson L-G, Adolfsson R, Lundquist A, Eriksson E, Nyberg L. Decreased medial temporal lobe activation in BDNF (66)Met allele carriers during memory encoding. *Neuropsychologia*. 2012 Dec 2;

[86] Molendijk ML, Bus BAA, Spinhoven P, Kaimatzoglou A, Oude Voshaar RC, Penninx BWJH, et al. A systematic review and meta-analysis on the association between BDNF val(66)met and hippocampal volume--a genuine effect or a winners curse? *Am. J. Med. Genet. B Neuropsychiatr. Genet.* 2012 Sep;159B(6):731–40.

[87] Carballedo A, Morris D, Zill P, Fahey C, Reinhold E, Meisenzahl E, et al. Brain-derived neurotrophic factor Val66Met polymorphism and early life adversity affect hippocampal volume. *Am. J. Med. Genet. B Neuropsychiatr. Genet.* 2013 Jan 22;

[88] Molendijk ML, Van Tol M-J, Penninx BWJH, Van der Wee NJA, Aleman A, Veltman DJ, et al. BDNF val66met affects hippocampal volume and emotion-related hippocampal memory activity. *Transl Psychiatry*. 2012;2:e74.

[89] Tost H, Alam T, Geramita M, Rebsch C, Kolachana B, Dickinson D, et al. Effects of the BDNF val(66)met polymorphism on white matter microstructure in healthy adults. *Neuropsychopharmacology*. 2013 Feb;38(3):525–32.

[90] Kim B, Kim CY, Hong JP, Kim SY, Lee C, Joo YH. Brain-derived neurotrophic factor Val/Met polymorphism and bipolar disorder. Association of the Met allele with suicidal behavior of bipolar patients. *Neuropsychobiology*. 2008;58(2):97–103.

[91] Numata S, Ueno S-I, Iga J-I, Yamauchi K, Hongwei S, Ohta K, et al. Brain-derived neurotrophic factor (BDNF) Val66Met polymorphism in schizophrenia is associated with age at onset and symptoms. *Neurosci. Lett.* 2006 Jun 19;401(1-2):1–5.

[92] Burghardt K j., Pop-Busui R, Bly M j., Grove T b., Taylor S f., Ellingrod V l. The Influence of the Brain-Derived Neurotropic Factor Val66Met -Genotype and HMG-CoA Reductase Inhibitors on Insulin Resistance in the Schizophrenia and Bipolar Populations. *Clinical and Translational Science.* 2012;5(6):486–90.

[93] Mirakhur A, Moorhead TWJ, Stanfield AC, McKirdy J, Sussmann JED, Hall J, et al. Changes in gyrification over 4 years in bipolar disorder and their association with the brain-derived neurotrophic factor valine(66) methionine variant. *Biol. Psychiatry.* 2009 Aug 1;66(3):293–7.

[94] Matsuo K, Walss-Bass C, Nery FG, Nicoletti MA, Hatch JP, Frey BN, et al. Neuronal correlates of brain-derived neurotrophic factor Val66Met polymorphism and morphometric abnormalities in bipolar disorder. *Neuropsychopharmacology*. 2009 Jul;34(8):1904–13.

[95] Chepenik LG, Fredericks C, Papademetris X, Spencer L, Lacadie C, Wang F, et al. Effects of the brain-derived neurotrophic growth factor val66met variation on hippocampus morphology in bipolar disorder. *Neuropsychopharmacology*. 2009 Mar;34(4):944–51.

[96] Takahashi T, Suzuki M, Tsunoda M, Kawamura Y, Takahashi N, Tsuneki H, et al. Association between the brain-derived neurotrophic factor Val66Met polymorphism and brain morphology in a Japanese sample of schizophrenia and healthy comparisons. *Neurosci. Lett.* 2008 Apr 11;435(1):34–9.

[97] Koolschijn PCMP, Van Haren NEM, Bakker SC, Hoogendoorn MLC, Hulshoff Pol HE, Kahn RS. Effects of brain-derived neurotrophic factor Val66Met polymorphism on hippocampal volume change in schizophrenia. *Hippocampus.* 2010 Sep;20(9):1010–7.

[98] Smith GN, Thornton AE, Lang DJ, Macewan GW, Ehmann TS, Kopala LC, et al. Hippocampal volume and the brain-derived neurotrophic factor Val66Met polymorphism in first episode psychosis. *Schizophr. Res*. 2012 Feb;134(2-3):253–9.

[99] Carlino D, Leone E, Di Cola F, Baj G, Marin R, Dinelli G, et al. Low serum truncated-BDNF isoform correlates with higher cognitive impairment in schizophrenia. *J Psychiatr Res*. 2011 Feb;45(2):273–9.

[100] Dias VV, Brissos S, Frey BN, Andreazza AC, Cardoso C, Kapczinski F. Cognitive function and serum levels of brain-derived neurotrophic factor in patients with bipolar disorder. *Bipolar Disord.* 2009 Sep;11(6):663–71.

[101] Brietzke E, Mansur RB, Soczynska J, Powell AM, McIntyre RS. A theoretical framework informing research about the role of stress in the pathophysiology of bipolar disorder. *Prog. Neuropsychopharmacol. Biol. Psychiatry.* 2012 Oct 1;39(1):1–8.

[102] Jones SR, Fernyhough C. A new look at the neural diathesis--stress model of schizophrenia: the primacy of social-evaluative and uncontrollable situations. *Schizophr Bull. 2007* Sep;33(5):1171–7.

[103] Fuchikami M, Morinobu S, Kurata A, Yamamoto S, Yamawaki S. Single immobilization stress differentially alters the expression profile of transcripts of the brain-derived neurotrophic factor (BDNF) gene and histone acetylation at its promoters in the rat hippocampus. *Int. J. Neuropsychopharmacol.* 2009 Feb;12(1):73–82.

[104] Fumagalli F, Bedogni F, Perez J, Racagni G, Riva MA. Corticostriatal brain-derived neurotrophic factor dysregulation in adult rats following prenatal stress. *Eur. J. Neurosci.* 2004 Sep;20(5):1348–54.

[105] Yuluğ B, Ozan E, Gönül AS, Kilic E. Brain-derived neurotrophic factor, stress and depression: a minireview. *Brain Res. Bull.* 2009 Mar 30;78(6):267–9.

[106] Tsankova NM, Berton O, Renthal W, Kumar A, Neve RL, Nestler EJ. Sustained hippocampal chromatin regulation in a mouse model of depression and antidepressant action. *Nat. Neurosci.* 2006 Apr;9(4):519–25.

[107] Sierksma ASR, Vanmierlo T, De Vry J, Raijmakers MEA, Steinbusch HWM, Van den Hove DLA, et al. Effects of prenatal stress exposure on soluble Aβ and brain-derived neurotrophic factor signaling in male and female APPswe/PS1dE9 mice. *Neurochem. Int.* 2012 Oct;61(5):697–701.

[108] Neeley EW, Berger R, Koenig JI, Leonard S. Prenatal stress differentially alters brain-derived neurotrophic factor expression and signaling across rat strains. *Neuroscience.* 2011 Jul 28;187:24–35.

[109] Belvederi Murri M, Pariante CM, Dazzan P, Hepgul N, Papadopoulos AS, Zunszain P, et al. Hypothalamic-pituitary-adrenal axis and clinical symptoms in first-episode psychosis. *Psychoneuroendocrinology.* 2012 May;37(5):629–44.

[110] Van der Werf-Eldering MJ, Riemersma-van der Lek RF, Burger H, Holthausen EAE, Aleman A, Nolen WA. Can variation in hypothalamic-pituitary-adrenal (HPA)-axis activity explain the relationship between depression and cognition in bipolar patients? *PLoS ONE.* 2012;7(5):e37119.

[111] Mondelli V, Dazzan P, Hepgul N, Di Forti M, Aas M, D'Albenzio A, et al. Abnormal cortisol levels during the day and cortisol awakening response in first-episode psychosis: the role of stress and of antipsychotic treatment. *Schizophr. Res.* 2010 Feb;116(2-3):234–42.

[112] Valiengo LL, Soeiro-de-Souza MG, Marques AH, Moreno DH, Juruena MF, Andreazza AC, et al. Plasma cortisol in first episode drug-naïve mania: differential levels in euphoric versus irritable mood. *J Affect Disord.* 2012 Apr;138(1-2):149–52.

[113] Winkel R van, Stefanis NC, Myin-Germeys I. Psychosocial Stress and Psychosis. A Review of the Neurobiological Mechanisms and the Evidence for Gene-Stress Interaction. *Schizophr Bull.* 2008 Nov 1;34(6):1095–105.

[114] Daban C, Vieta E, Mackin P, Young AH. Hypothalamic-pituitary-adrenal axis and bipolar disorder. *Psychiatr. Clin. North Am.* 2005 Jun;28(2):469–80.

[115] Kumamaru E, Numakawa T, Adachi N, Yagasaki Y, Izumi A, Niyaz M, et al. Glucocorticoid prevents brain-derived neurotrophic factor-mediated maturation of synaptic function in developing hippocampal neurons through reduction in the activity of mitogen-activated protein kinase. *Mol. Endocrinol.* 2008 Mar;22(3):546–58.

[116] Aydemir O, Deveci A, Taneli F. The effect of chronic antidepressant treatment on serum brain-derived neurotrophic factor levels in depressed patients: a preliminary study. *Prog. Neuropsychopharmacol. Biol. Psychiatry.* 2005 Feb;29(2):261–5.

[117] Matrisciano F, Bonaccorso S, Ricciardi A, Scaccianoce S, Panaccione I, Wang L, et al. Changes in BDNF serum levels in patients with major depression disorder (MDD) after 6 months treatment with sertraline, escitalopram, or venlafaxine. *J Psychiatr Res.* 2009 Jan;43(3):247–54.

[118] Lee H-Y, Kim Y-K. Plasma brain-derived neurotrophic factor as a peripheral marker for the action mechanism of antidepressants. *Neuropsychobiology.* 2008;57(4):194–9.

[119] Schmidt HD, Duman RS. Peripheral BDNF produces antidepressant-like effects in cellular and behavioral models. *Neuropsychopharmacology.* 2010 Nov;35(12):2378–91.

[120] Kaufman J, Yang B-Z, Douglas-Palumberi H, Grasso D, Lipschitz D, Houshyar S, et al. Brain-derived neurotrophic factor-5-HTTLPR gene interactions and environmental modifiers of depression in children. *Biol. Psychiatry.* 2006 Apr 15;59(8):673–80.

[121] Wichers M, Kenis G, Jacobs N, Mengelers R, Derom C, Vlietinck R, et al. The BDNF Val(66)Met x 5-HTTLPR x child adversity interaction and depressive symptoms: An attempt at replication. *Am. J. Med. Genet. B Neuropsychiatr. Genet.* 2008 Jan 5;147B(1):120–3.

[122] Kim J-M, Stewart R, Kim S-W, Yang S-J, Shin I-S, Kim Y-H, et al. Interactions between life stressors and susceptibility genes (5-HTTLPR and BDNF) on depression in Korean elders. *Biol. Psychiatry.* 2007 Sep 1;62(5):423–8.

[123] Grabe HJ, Schwahn C, Mahler J, Appel K, Schulz A, Spitzer C, et al. Genetic epistasis between the brain-derived neurotrophic factor Val66Met polymorphism and the 5-HTT promoter polymorphism moderates the susceptibility to depressive disorders after childhood abuse. Prog. Neuropsychopharmacol. *Biol. Psychiatry.* 2012 Mar 30;36(2):264–70.

[124] Weickert CS, Hyde TM, Lipska BK, Herman MM, Weinberger DR, Kleinman JE. Reduced brain-derived neurotrophic factor in prefrontal cortex of patients with schizophrenia. *Molecular Psychiatry.* 2003;8(6):592–610.

[125] Hashimoto T, Bergen SE, Nguyen QL, Xu B, Monteggia LM, Pierri JN, et al. Relationship of Brain-Derived Neurotrophic Factor and Its Receptor TrkB to Altered Inhibitory Prefrontal Circuitry in Schizophrenia. *J. Neurosci.* 2005 Jan 12;25(2):372–83.

[126] Pillai A. Decreased expression of Sprouty2 in the dorsolateral prefrontal cortex in schizophrenia and bipolar disorder: a correlation with BDNF expression. *PLoS ONE.* 2008;3(3):e1784.

[127] Issa G, Wilson C, Terry Jr. AV, Pillai A. An inverse relationship between cortisol and BDNF levels in schizophrenia: Data from human postmortem and animal studies. *Neurobiology of Disease.* 2010 Sep;39(3):327–33.

[128] Takahashi M, Shirakawa O, Toyooka K, Kitamura N, Hashimoto T, Maeda K, et al. Abnormal expression of brain-derived neurotrophic factor and its receptor in the corticolimbic system of schizophrenic patients. *Mol. Psychiatry*. 2000 May;5(3):293–300.

[129] Dunham JS, Deakin JFW, Miyajima F, Payton A, Toro CT. Expression of hippocampal brain-derived neurotrophic factor and its receptors in Stanley consortium brains. *Journal of Psychiatric Research*. 2009 Sep;43(14):1175–84.

[130] Thompson Ray M, Weickert CS, Wyatt E, Webster MJ. Decreased BDNF, trkB-TK+ and GAD67 mRNA expression in the hippocampus of individuals with schizophrenia and mood disorders. *J Psychiatry Neurosci.* 2011 May;36(3):195–203.

[131] Buckley PF, Pillai A, Evans D, Stirewalt E, Mahadik S. Brain derived neurotropic factor in first-episode psychosis. *Schizophr. Res*. 2007 Mar;91(1-3):1–5.

[132] Pillai A, Kale A, Joshi S, Naphade N, Raju MSVK, Nasrallah H, et al. Decreased BDNF levels in CSF of drug-naive first-episode psychotic subjects: correlation with plasma BDNF and psychopathology. *Int. J. Neuropsychopharmacol.* 2010 May;13(4):535–9.

[133] Rizos EN, Rontos I, Laskos E, Arsenis G, Michalopoulou PG, Vasilopoulos D, et al. Investigation of serum BDNF levels in drug-naive patients with schizophrenia. *Progress in Neuro-Psychopharmacology and Biological Psychiatry.* 2008 Jul 1;32(5):1308–11.

[134] Jindal RD, Pillai AK, Mahadik SP, Eklund K, Montrose DM, Keshavan MS. Decreased BDNF in patients with antipsychotic naïve first episode schizophrenia. *Schizophr. Res*. 2010 Jun;119(1-3):47–51.

[135] Chen DC, Wang J, Wang B, Yang SC, Zhang CX, Zheng YL, et al. Decreased levels of serum brain-derived neurotrophic factor in drug-naïve first-episode schizophrenia: relationship to clinical phenotypes. *Psychopharmacology* (Berl.). 2009 Dec;207(3):375–80.

[136] Yoshimura R, Hori H, Sugita A, Ueda N, Kakihara S, Umene W, et al. Treatment with risperidone for 4 weeks increased plasma 3-methoxy-4-hydroxypnenylglycol (MHPG) levels, but did not alter plasma brain-derived neurotrophic factor (BDNF) levels in schizophrenic patients. Prog. Neuropsychopharmacol. *Biol. Psychiatry*. 2007 Jun 30;31(5):1072–7.

[137] Tan YL, Zhou DF, Cao LY, Zou YZ, Zhang XY. Decreased BDNF in serum of patients with chronic schizophrenia on long-term treatment with antipsychotics. *Neurosci. Lett.* 2005 Jul 1;382(1-2):27–32.

[138] Grillo RW, Ottoni GL, Leke R, Souza DO, Portela LV, Lara DR. Reduced serum BDNF levels in schizophrenic patients on clozapine or typical antipsychotics. *J Psychiatr Res*. 2007 Feb;41(1-2):31–5.

[139] Pirildar S, Gönül AS, Taneli F, Akdeniz F. Low serum levels of brain-derived neurotrophic factor in patients with schizophrenia do not elevate after antipsychotic treatment. Prog. Neuropsychopharmacol. *Biol. Psychiatry*. 2004 Jul;28(4):709–13.

[140] Toyooka K, Asama K, Watanabe Y, Muratake T, Takahashi M, Someya T, et al. Decreased levels of brain-derived neurotrophic factor in serum of chronic schizophrenic patients. *Psychiatry Res*. 2002 Jul 31;110(3):249–57.

[141] Xiu MH, Hui L, Dang YF, Hou TD, Zhang CX, Zheng YL, et al. Decreased serum BDNF levels in chronic institutionalized schizophrenia on long-term treatment with

typical and atypical antipsychotics. *Prog. Neuropsychopharmacol. Biol. Psychiatry*. 2009 Nov 13;33(8):1508–12.

[142] Vinogradov S, Fisher M, Holland C, Shelly W, Wolkowitz O, Mellon SH. Is serum brain-derived neurotrophic factor a biomarker for cognitive enhancement in schizophrenia? *Biol. Psychiatry*. 2009 Sep 15;66(6):549–53.

[143] Reis HJ, Nicolato R, Barbosa IG, Prado PHT do, Romano-Silva MA, Teixeira AL. Increased serum levels of brain-derived neurotrophic factor in chronic institutionalized patients with schizophrenia. *Neuroscience Letters*. 2008 Jul 11;439(2):157–9.

[144] Mackin P, Gallagher P, Watson S, Young AH, Ferrier IN. Changes in brain-derived neurotrophic factor following treatment with mifepristone in bipolar disorder and schizophrenia. *Aust N Z J Psychiatry*. 2007 Apr;41(4):321–6.

[145] Sen S, Duman R, Sanacora G. Serum brain-derived neurotrophic factor, depression, and antidepressant medications: meta-analyses and implications. *Biol. Psychiatry*. 2008 Sep 15;64(6):527–32.

[146] Malhi GS, Tanious M, Das P, Coulston CM, Berk M. Potential Mechanisms of Action of Lithium in Bipolar Disorder : Current Understanding. *CNS Drugs*. 2013 Feb 1;

[147] Machado-Vieira R, Dietrich MO, Leke R, Cereser VH, Zanatto V, Kapczinski F, et al. Decreased plasma brain derived neurotrophic factor levels in unmedicated bipolar patients during manic episode. *Biol. Psychiatry*. 2007 Jan 15;61(2):142–4.

[148] Tramontina JF, Andreazza AC, Kauer-Sant'anna M, Stertz L, Goi J, Chiarani F, et al. Brain-derived neurotrophic factor serum levels before and after treatment for acute mania. *Neurosci. Lett.* 2009 Mar 13;452(2):111–3.

[149] Cunha ABM, Frey BN, Andreazza AC, Goi JD, Rosa AR, Gonçalves CA, et al. Serum brain-derived neurotrophic factor is decreased in bipolar disorder during depressive and manic episodes. *Neurosci. Lett.* 2006 May 8;398(3):215–9.

[150] Monteleone P, Serritella C, Martiadis V, Maj M. Decreased levels of serum brain-derived neurotrophic factor in both depressed and euthymic patients with unipolar depression and in euthymic patients with bipolar I and II disorders. *Bipolar Disord*. 2008 Feb;10(1):95–100.

[151] De Oliveira GS, Cereser KM, Fernandes BS, Kauer-Sant'Anna M, Fries GR, Stertz L, et al. Decreased brain-derived neurotrophic factor in medicated and drug-free bipolar patients. *J Psychiatr Res*. 2009 Sep;43(14):1171–4.

[152] Gama CS, Andreazza AC, Kunz M, Berk M, Belmonte-de-Abreu PS, Kapczinski F. Serum levels of brain-derived neurotrophic factor in patients with schizophrenia and bipolar disorder. *Neurosci. Lett.* 2007 Jun 8;420(1):45–8.

[153] Green MF. Cognitive impairment and functional outcome in schizophrenia and bipolar disorder. *J Clin Psychiatry*. 2006;67 Suppl 9:3–8; discussion 36–42.

[154] Goldberg JF, Chengappa KNR. Identifying and treating cognitive impairment in bipolar disorder. *Bipolar Disord*. 2009 Jun;11 Suppl 2:123–37.

[155] Hill SK, Reilly JL, Harris MSH, Rosen C, Marvin RW, Deleon O, et al. A comparison of neuropsychological dysfunction in first-episode psychosis patients with unipolar depression, bipolar disorder, and schizophrenia. *Schizophr. Res*. 2009 Sep;113(2-3):167–75.

[156] Jabben N, Arts B, Van Os J, Krabbendam L. Neurocognitive functioning as intermediary phenotype and predictor of psychosocial functioning across the psychosis

continuum: studies in schizophrenia and bipolar disorder. *J Clin Psychiatry.* 2010 Jun;71(6):764–74.

[157] Krabbendam L, Arts B, Van Os J, Aleman A. Cognitive functioning in patients with schizophrenia and bipolar disorder: a quantitative review. *Schizophr. Res.* 2005 Dec 15;80(2-3):137–49.

[158] Simonsen C, Sundet K, Vaskinn A, Birkenaes AB, Engh JA, Faerden A, et al. Neurocognitive dysfunction in bipolar and schizophrenia spectrum disorders depends on history of psychosis rather than diagnostic group. *Schizophr Bull.* 2011 Jan;37(1):73–83.

[159] Tan YL, Zhou DF, Cao LY, Zou YZ, Wu GY, Zhang XY. Effect of the BDNF Val66Met genotype on episodic memory in schizophrenia. *Schizophrenia Research.* 2005 Sep 15;77(2–3):355–6.

[160] Ho B-C, Milev P, O'Leary DS, Librant A, Andreasen NC, Wassink TH. Cognitive and magnetic resonance imaging brain morphometric correlates of brain-derived neurotrophic factor Val66Met gene polymorphism in patients with schizophrcnia and healthy volunteers. *Arch. Gen. Psychiatry.* 2006 Jul;63(7):731–40.

[161] Carlino D, Leone E, Di Cola F, Baj G, Marin R, Dinelli G, et al. Low serum truncated-BDNF isoform correlates with higher cognitive impairment in schizophrenia. *J Psychiatr Res.* 2011 Feb;45(2):273–9.

[162] Rybakowski JK, Borkowska A, Skibinska M, Szczepankiewicz A, Kapelski P, Leszczynska-Rodziewicz A, et al. Prefrontal cognition in schizophrenia and bipolar illness in relation to Val66Met polymorphism of the brain-derived neurotrophic factor gene. *Psychiatry Clin. Neurosci.* 2006 Feb;60(1):70–6.

[163] Dias VV, Brissos S, Frey BN, Andreazza AC, Cardoso C, Kapczinski F. Cognitive function and serum levels of brain-derived neurotrophic factor in patients with bipolar disorder. *Bipolar Disord.* 2009 Sep;11(6):663–71.

[164] Tramontina JF, Yates D, Magalhães PV da S, Trentini C, Sant'anna MK, Fries GR, et al. Brain-derived neurotrophic factor gene val66met polymorphism and executive functioning in patients with bipolar disorder. *Rev Bras Psiquiatr.* 2009 Jun;31(2):136–40.

[165] Chou Y-H, Wang S-J, Lirng J-F, Lin C-L, Yang K-C, Chen C-K, et al. Impaired cognition in bipolar I disorder: the roles of the serotonin transporter and brain-derived neurotrophic factor. *J Affect Disord.* 2012 Dec 20;143(1-3):131–7.

[166] Mandelman SD, Grigorenko EL. BDNF Val66Met and cognition: all, none, or some? A meta-analysis of the genetic association. *Genes Brain Behav.* 2012 Mar;11(2):127–36.

[167] Rose EJ, Donohoe G. Brain vs Behavior: An Effect Size Comparison of Neuroimaging and Cognitive Studies of Genetic Risk for Schizophrenia. *Schizophr Bull.* 2012 Apr 12;

[168] Fernandes BS, Gama CS, Kauer-Sant'Anna M, Lobato MI, Belmonte-de-Abreu P, Kapczinski F. Serum brain-derived neurotrophic factor in bipolar and unipolar depression: a potential adjunctive tool for differential diagnosis. *J Psychiatr Res.* 2009 Oct;43(15):1200–4.

[169] Costafreda SG, Fu CHY, Picchioni M, Toulopoulou T, McDonald C, Kravariti E, et al. Pattern of neural responses to verbal fluency shows diagnostic specificity for schizophrenia and bipolar disorder. *BMC Psychiatry.* 2011;11:18.

In: Bipolar Disorder
Editor: Nickolas B. Moore

ISBN: 978-1-62618-666-8


*Chapter IV*

# Understanding Lived Experience and Personal Recovery in People with Bipolar Disorder: A Qualitative Literature Review

***Sara E. Lapsley[1], Vytas Velyvis[2], Anna Ivanova[3], Rachelle Hole[4] and Erin E. Michalak*[5]***

[1]Department of Education, Counselling Psychology, University of British Columbia, Vancouver, BC, Canada
[2]York University, Adler International Learning, Toronto, ON, Canada
[3]Centre for Addiction and Mental Health, Toronto, ON, Canada
[4]School of Social Work, University of British Columbia, Vancouver, BC, Canada
[5]Department of Psychiatry, University of British Columbia, Vancouver, BC, Canada

## Abstract

Objective: The concept of personal recovery (PR) as defined by those who live with mental illness has gained significant momentum and has been adopted as a key principle in mental health services internationally (Slade, 2009b). The philosophy of PR views living with mental illness as a dynamic journey with an emphasis on hope, self-determination, and quality of life despite the presence of symptoms (Anthony, 2000; Deegan, 1996). This differs from the clinical definition of recovery (CR), which focuses on improvements in functional outcomes and may view mental illness as chronic and refractory (Slade, 2009b). Research on PR has largely focused on people living with

* Correspondence and requests for reprints should be addressed to: Erin E. Michalak, Department of Psychiatry, University of British Columbia, 2255 Wesbrook Mall, Vancouver, BC, Canada V6T 2A1, Tel: +1-604-827 3393. Fax: +1-604-822-7792. E-mail: erin.michalak@ubc.ca.

schizophrenia or mixed diagnostic samples. Over the past decade, however, there has been increasing interest in understanding PR in those who live with bipolar disorder (BD). A review of qualitative literature that captures the lived experience of those with BD and their views on PR will consolidate the knowledge to date in order to inform clinical practice, the direction of future research, and the self-management strategies of those affected by BD.

Methods: A systematic review of qualitative studies focusing on the topic of PR in people with BD was conducted. Data compilation consisted of two parallel searches of identified databases by two independent researchers. Approximately 1000 original studies were identified, of which 24 met the following inclusion criteria for review: peer reviewed qualitative studies involving samples of people living with BD (mixed diagnosis samples were not eligible for inclusion), studies employing a psychosocial perspective, and studies published in English. A thematic analysis of the studies under review was completed, resulting in a descriptive narrative which identifies and interprets the main concepts and conclusions in the qualitative findings.

Results: Four overarching themes were identified: the negative impact of BD; ambivalence in relation to living with BD, personal transformation as a result of lived experience, and wellness strategies that highlighted behaviours or practices that contribute to recovery in BD. Our literature review found that the lived experience of BD encompasses both positive and negative aspects. Coping and symptom management may present challenges, there may be ambivalence about the diagnosis of BD and its treatment, and self-esteem may be impaired. However, purpose, hope, and wellness seemed more achievable when the traditional definition of CR was broadened to include a PR perspective, which allowed people to transcend the otherwise seemingly contradictory experiences associated with BD.

**Keywords:** Bipolar disorder, psychosocial recovery, qualitative, review

# Introduction

Bipolar disorder (BD) is a complex mental health condition characterized by pronounced mood shifts, ranging from periods of clinical depression through to extreme elation, grandiosity or irritability (Goodwin and Jamison, 1990). The severity of symptoms, course of the illness, and functional outcomes are variable across individuals (Michalak, Hole, Holmes, Velyvis, Austin, Pesut, and Hou, 2012). The condition is relatively common and has a lifetime prevalence of approximately 3.9% in the general population (Kessler et al., 2005). Less conservative estimates have suggested that up to 8% of the population may experience some milder forms of BD or sub-syndromal manic symptoms (Judd et al., 2003). Up to a half-million Canadians live with BD (Schaffer, Cairney, Cheung, Veldhuizen, and Levitt, 2006). The literature on outcomes in people with BD often paints a bleak picture, indicating that the condition can be associated with significant mortality and co-morbidity (Ösby, Brandt, Correia, Ekbom, and Sparen, 2001). BD is also frequently cited as being the sixth leading cause of disability in the world in the 18-44 year age range (Murray and Lopez, 1997). Poor treatment adherence and high rates of relapse are commonly cited, with an estimated 40% of people relapsing within 1 year, 60% over 2 years, and there is a 73% risk of relapse after 5 years (Tohen et al., 2000; Gitlin, Swendsen, Heller, and Hammen, 1995). Impairment in psychosocial functioning and quality of life (QoL) between mood episodes are described as typical, with marked functional deficits (such as problems returning to the workforce) often endured after recovery from acute mood episodes (Chengappa et al., 2005; Ozer, Ulusahin, Batur, Kabakci, and Saka, 2002; Robb, Cooke, Devins, Young, and Joffe, 1997).

Qualitative research suggests that people with BD often live with subjective distress and face considerable challenges related to symptom management, loss of jobs and relationships, stigma, acceptance of their diagnosis, repeated hospitalizations, and feelings of hopelessness (Lim, Nathan, O'Brien-Malone, and Williams, 2004). Accordingly, 6-10% are at high risk for suicide (Nordentoft, Mortensen, and Pedersen, 2011). Although BD is predominantly viewed as a chronic mental illness from which there is little hope of recovery (Harding, Zubin, and Strauss, 1987), more recent literature is beginning to acknowledge the potentially positive attributes associated with BD. These include increased spirituality, creativity, empathy and resilience (Galvez, Thommi, and Ghaemi, 2011), as well as the attainment of ambitious goals (Johnson, 2005). As BD can be described as both painful and life-enhancing, there may be confusion among affected individuals, their supporters, and clinicians about how to cope with the wide range of experiences related to BD.

The literature in the area of BD and schizophrenia is largely comprised of quantitative studies that focus on the biological causes of the conditions and biomedical approaches to treatment. The biomedical approach defines recovery from mental illness as an invariant and linear progression, measured by concrete variables such as number of hospitalizations, reduction of symptoms, and global functioning (Slade, 2009b). This outcome-oriented definition of clinical recovery (CR) from mental illness is at odds with recovery as defined by the people who make use of mental health services. Over the last two decades there has been a shift in the mental health field from a focus on pathology, chronicity, and decline, towards a dynamic and holistic understanding of recovery coined by (Slade, 2009a) as Personal Recovery (PR), though this philosophy is often referred to simply as "Recovery". The most current working definition describes PR as, "a process of change through which individuals improve their life and wellness, live a self-directed life, and strive to reach their full potential" (SAMHSA, 2011, "SAMHSA News Release," para 2). In contrast to CR, PR suggests that a good quality of life can be achieved despite the presence of symptoms (Anthony, 2000; Deegan, 1996), and may involve developing a sense of identity, hope, social support, empowerment and meaning in life (Andresen, Caputi, and Oades, 2006). PR is considered to be a dynamic process, rather than an end in itself. The journey of recovery is unique to each individual in both its progress over time and the ways in which it is pursued (Pitt, Killbride, Nothard, Welford, and Morrison, 2007). The PR approach suggests that there is capacity for significantly restored functioning, though curing the illness is not the ultimate goal (G. Deegan, 2003; P. Deegan, 1988, 1996).

The PR model has gained significant momentum and is being refined and adopted as best practice internationally in the treatment of mental illness (Slade, 2009b). Previously in populations with mental illness, the absence of negative events such as hospitalizations or exacerbation of symptoms were considered the exemplar of good outcome. With a broadened understanding that includes PR, these hallmarks of stability are not necessarily sufficient to capture the possibilities for an improved QoL. It has been noted that many people with schizophrenia can recover substantially, or even fully, over time (Forchuk, Jewell, Tweedell, and Steinnagel, 2003; Harding, Zubin, and Strauss, 1992), leading to the suggestion that the primary goal of treatment should be based on the fundamentals of PR (Davidson, 2003).

While considerable research has explored the concept of PR in samples of people living with schizophrenia - or in mixed samples of people with various mental health conditions (e.g. Davidson and Strauss, 1992; Young, Green, and Estroff, 2008) - research into resiliency, hope, self-management, wellness, QoL, and recovery in BD has been sparse. There may be several reasons for why the research literature relating to PR has tended to shy away from referring to specific diagnoses. The most obvious rationale may be that an emphasis on psychiatric labels may be perceived by service users as reflecting a paternalistic and biologically deterministic outlook that undermines hope, self-efficacy and empowerment - the key ingredients of the recovery framework (Chadwick, 1997; Frese, Stanley, Kress, and Vogel-Scibilia, 2001; Glover, 2005; Slade, 2009b). That being said, over the past decade there has been increasing attention to PR in the BD literature. Studies using quantitative and qualitative methods, as well as subjective accounts by those who live with BD, have captured rich and varied perspectives. The philosophy of PR continues to gain momentum among those with BD, their supporters, health care practitioners, researchers, and policy makers.

This review aims to consolidate the findings on participants' subjective experiences of BD and how they perceive and engage in their own PR. Ideally the themes that emerge from the studies under review will be helpful in understanding the issues that are important to those with BD, and identify factors that contribute to a successful journey of recovery.

# Methods

A narrative review of qualitative studies focusing on the topic of PR in BD was conducted. A systematic literature search commenced in October 2010 and was completed in December, 2012. A comprehensive list of published research was compiled in order to provide a summary and descriptive interpretation of the findings in qualitative literature that has explored PR in participants who live with BD. Narrative approaches are a flexible way to assess qualitative literature (Mays, Pope, and Popay, 2005, "Narrative Approaches," para 2). As a result, they are able to accommodate studies that may employ different methodological or theoretical approaches, or different research questions (Mays, et al., 2005, Narrative Synthesis," para 4). Although there is no standardized way to perform this method, a logical process is often evident, and generalizability may be established if the studies demonstrate a "proximal similarity" (Mays et al., 2005, "Narrative Reviews," para 5). Thematic analysis is often used in narrative reviews to organize and identify the most important themes, and may involve counting or ranking themes using content analysis techniques (Mays et al., 2005, "Thematic Analysis," para 1). The goal of such a review is to identify, consolidate, and interpret the main concepts and conclusions across studies (Mays et al., 2005, "Narrative Approaches," para 1).

## Compilation of Studies

Parallel database searches were conducted independently (Fink, 2005) by two of the co-authors (SL, AI). Databases searched included: Medline, PsycINFO, CINAHL, EMBASE, AgeLine, Cochrane Database of Systematic Reviews, Database of Abstract Reviews of Effects; Web of Science, CHANGELINE and DARE. The search terms used were: "bipolar disorder", "manic depression", "hypomania", and "mania" in combination with one or more of the following: "recovery", "collaborative recovery model", "mental health recovery", "recovery oriented services" or "social functional recovery".

### Search Outcome

The initial search produced a preliminary list of publications (~1000) that was then explored for eligibility. The inclusion criteria were peer-reviewed qualitative studies of adults diagnosed with BD (mixed diagnostic samples were not eligible for inclusion), that employed a psychosocial perspective, and were published in English. No date range limitations were applied to the search. The final list included 24 studies with publication dates ranging from 1995 to 2012.

### Data Abstraction

The first stage of analysis involved an eligibility assessment of the articles and the identification of relevant key concepts pertaining to PR in BD. The reviewing authors (SL and AI) independently read the complete list of selected articles and summarized the key information. These findings were then merged by SL in consultation with the remaining co-authors. A summary of the extracted information pertaining to methods (i.e., research question, sample, and analytic approach) and key research findings is presented in Table 1. Reference sections of the extracted articles were reviewed and additional relevant studies were added. Although the studies varied somewhat in their focus and analytical approach, overall they demonstrated a proximal similarity (Mays et al., 2005) in that they used a qualitative method that explored the experience of living with BD and individuals' personal perceptions of PR.

The second stage of analysis involved identifying and classifying descriptive codes for the findings of each qualitative study. In consultation with the co-authors, SL developed a coding key of the findings across all compiled studies. When these descriptive codes were clustered, four themes were identified. Sub-codes from the fourth theme were organized according frequency (see Table 2).

Finally, the third stage of analysis involved developing a descriptive summary of the literature reviewed, in order to capture a rich description of the content, context, and prominent themes (Mays et al., 2005) in the collective subjective experience of the participants' experience of BD and PR.

## Results

Four overarching themes were identified across the studies under review. Three of these were related to the participants' experiences of living with BD and their understandings of recovery while the fourth focused on the strategies that participants used to stay well with BD. Theme one focused on the *negative impact* of BD, as subjects spoke of significant distress related to active symptoms and the experience of stigma.

**Table 1.**

| Research Question | Sample | Analytic Approach | Themes Identified | Strategies |
|---|---|---|---|---|
| Open-ended questions were asked about the participants' everyday life context as it related to informational search and need, and their self-management informational needs and activities. (Pollack, 1995) | BD (type not indicated) ($N = 33$) | Conceptual coding; Constant comparative method | Striving for Stability occurs in four phases: i) realization of a need ii) information seeking iii) critical juncture in treatment iv) self-management techniques; multitude of barriers both internal and external. Greatest barrier was the denial of illness and need for treatment. | Informing themselves about the disorder; social support, motivation to get well, self-management through information, motivation, and the ability to apply the knowledge required. |
| Interviews focused on six core areas related to self-management of BD: understanding BD, managing daily life; living in society; relating to others; relating to self; self-management. (Pollack, 1996a) | BD (type not indicated) ($N = 33$) | Grounded theory | Barriers to successful self-management included internal factors (e.g. self-esteem, binging behaviour) and external factors (e.g. social problems, medications); components of successful self-management were identified. | Maintaining relationships; living in society; medication; education; therapy; stress management; relationship with self and others; adhering to a plan that includes medication, education, therapy, and methods for dealing with stress. |
| Interviews focused on six core areas related to self-management of BD: understanding BD, managing daily life; living in society; relating to others; relating to self; self-management. (Pollack, 1996b) | BD (type not indicated) ($N$=33) | Grounded theory | Information-Seeking Motivations: self-management; understanding BD; managing daily life; living in society; relating to self and others. | Willingness to learn from others; perceived benefits of groups; understanding personal responsibility; reading, talking with professionals, attending groups, having hope, desire to live, increased knowledge, and sense of self-satisfaction. |
| Participants were asked questions about identity, cause, time-line, consequences and control/cure of BD. (Pollack and Aponte, 2001) | BD (type not indicated) ($N = 15$) | Content analysis | Coming to terms with diagnosis (experienced as a series of phases likened to Elizabeth Kubler-Ross); importance of personal metaphors; ambivalence about the medical model; denial of diagnosis led to non-adherence and relapse. | Incorporation of creative, strengths-based, and faith-based practices into treatment; medication, actions to improve sense of control improve quality of life; following a treatment plan. |

| Research Question | Sample | Analytic Approach | Themes Identified | Strategies |
| --- | --- | --- | --- | --- |
| Asked about course of BD and impact it had on employment opportunities, factors situations or events that had impact in getting and securing employment. (Tse and Yeats, 2002) | BD (type not indicated) ($N = 67$) | Grounded theory framework | Individual factors; work ethic; professional and community supports; social upbringing and attitudes; available support; systemic factors (e.g. societal attitudes and government policies); stage of recovery; importance of goodness-of-fit to work setting. | People coped with working through: self-determination; having a professional qualification; faith in God; self-management; social support; supportive boss and colleagues; accommodations; right timing in returning to work. |
| What is it like for you to have BD? What sorts of problems/issues do you face in your daily lives? How do you respond to these problems/issues? (Lim et al. 2004) | BD type I ($N = 18$) | Phenomenological approach | Instability; upheaval; disruptions; loss and deficit; view of future as uncertain and hopeless; permanent changes; isolation and rejection. | Striving for stability in life. |
| What does staying well mean to you? (Russell and Browne, 2005) | BD (type not indicated) ($N = 100$) | Thematic analysis | Staying well meant: more control and choices regarding illness, rejecting label of BD, not seeing illness as a character flaw or weakness, living free of symptoms, behaving normally. | Acceptance of diagnosis; mindfulness, identifying triggers and recognizing warning signs, managing sleep and stress, engaging in treatment; educating self and others through books, seminars and internet sources; Stay Well plans and advance directives; learning from personal experience; time with loved ones; accessing support; healthy lifestyle choices (e.g. diet, limiting caffeine and alcohol). |
| What do you need to have good quality of life? Has BD impacted on these areas? Asked to rank order three areas that they thought were most important in determining their QoL. (Michalak, et al., 2006) | BD type I, II, or BD spectrum ($N = 35$); caregivers ($N = 5$); healthcare professionals ($N = 13$) | Qualitative analysis | Social support; physical and mental health; financial health and independence; basic needs and vocation; stigma and disclosure; identity; spirituality (esp. distinguishing healthy religiosity from mania). | Importance of establishing a routine; building self-esteem; coping with stigma; treatment tailored to individual needs. |

**Table 1. (Continued)**

| Research Question | Sample | Analytic Approach | Themes Identified | Strategies |
|---|---|---|---|---|
| Questions were based on the Perceptions-Practicalities Framework. General questions were followed by prompts based on the theory. Participants were also asked about illness and treatment perceptions, and non-adherence to medication. (Clatworthy et al., 2007) | BD (type not indicated) ($N = 16$) | Themes were coded according to Self-regulation model and Necessity Concerns framework | Positive and negative consequences of disorder; denial of diagnosis; perceived need for medication; patients beliefs about BD affected treatment adherence; side-effects and toxicity contributed to non-adherence; difficulty accepting the long-term need for medication; confidence in efficacy of medication. | Adherence linked to acceptance and sense of control over illness. |
| Narratives were generated by participants about how they managed their BD without the use of psychotropic medications. (Mehl-Madrona, 2007) | BD (type not indicated) ($N = 24$) | Dimensional Analysis; Modified Grounded Theory | Some participants managed successfully without the use of medications. Belief that a cure is possible; belief in themselves; questioning of medical model while simultaneously recognizing the need for help; flexible; willing to make lifestyle changes. | Alliances with health care providers; willing to seek help and examine their lives; self-reliance coupled with collaboration with health care providers; meditative and reflective practices (e.g. yoga, prayer, meditation); involvement with others; personal transformation; active efforts to strengthen the belief that a cure is possible. |
| What do you need to have good quality of life? Participants were then asked to describe in more detail whether and how their BD had impacted upon each of these areas. (Michalak et al., 2007) | BD type I, II, or BD spectrum ($N = 35$); caregivers ($N = 5$); healthcare professionals ($N = 13$) | Qualitative analysis | Independence; routine, stigma and disclosure; identity, social support and spirituality. | Maintaining a structured routine, regular sleep, diet, and exercise; autonomy; self-sufficiency, esp. financial; acceptance, faith and spirituality. |
| Participants were asked to describe how they constructed and experienced BD and how BD impacted development of sense of self. (Inder et al., 2008) | BD type I, II, or NOS ($N = 15$) | Thematic analysis | BD negatively impacted relationships and was perceived as disruptive to everyday life; felt BD affected others perceptions of them; development of self was negatively impacted resulting in confusion, contradiction and self-doubt. | Self-acceptance; integrating experience and sense of self. |

| Research Question | Sample | Analytic Approach | Themes Identified | Strategies |
|---|---|---|---|---|
| What is your view of your illness? What is your view of the future? (Jönsson et al., 2008) | BD type I or II ($N$ = 18) | Content analysis | Accepting the illness; striving for understanding; insights into one's ability to feel well; managing the illness; taking responsibility; reintegrating into society; personal growth and perspectives; hopeful vs. uncertain future; meaning in existence; insecure in oneself and one's abilities; difficulties day-to-day due to symptoms. | Planning and life-style changes to reduce stress; taking medications; social support; positive thinking; helping others with BD; filling a role in society; taking responsibility; strategies to manage insecurities in everyday life; healthy routines. |
| What has been the impact of BD on your life? What is your experience of working with others with BD and your experience of group psychotherapy? (O'Connor et al., 2008) | BD (type not indicated) ($N = 11$) | Interpretative phenomenological analysis | Treatment of BD (users had both good and bad experiences); comparison with and perception of others; learning from the group; universality and socialization, not alone, others have similar experiences; negative experience with police and hospitals. | Medications; collaborative and trusting relationships with health care providers; group therapy provided self-esteem, learning; coping strategies, normalizing experience; camaraderie, increased sense of control, and acceptance of diagnosis; CBT; education about BD. |
| Participants were asked to discuss their subjective experiences, difficulties or issues of concern about BD in written form. (Proudfoot et al., 2009) | BD (type not indicated) all diagnosed within the last year ($N$ = 26) | Phenomenological and lived experience framework. | Ambivalence about: medication, mania, diagnosis; challenges were in identifying prodromes, self-doubt and identity, stigma; uncertainty about future; coming to terms with diagnosis. | Daily mood charting; recognizing warning signs and triggers; interactions with Peer Support Workers normalized experience and facilitated coping. |
| Would you like to tell me about your experiences of living with BD? Participants were then further prompted to say more about what those experiences meant to them. (Rusner et al., 2009) | BD (type not indicated) ($N = 10$) | Whole-parts-whole-structure | Intensity and complexity of living with BD, both good and bad aspects of life are experience more fully; challenge to understand disorder and how it is entwined with one's being; creativity; spirituality; self-contempt and negative affect; to fight against the illness is to fight against the self. | Self-reflection, healthy personal relationships, healthy relationship with self. |

**Table 1. (Continued)**

| Research Question | Sample | Analytic Approach | Themes Identified | Strategies |
|---|---|---|---|---|
| Could you describe what's going on in your life when you're feeling well? How do friends, family and co-workers affect your ability to stay well? How do you know it is the right time to start using self-management strategies? (Wang et al., 2009) | BD type I or II ($N = 9$) | Inductive approach | Viewing the condition through a more positive framework (hope, inner peace); importance of taking medication; maintaining harmony; selective disclosure. | Emotional coping strategies to maintain harmony with self and others; spiritual beliefs; collaborative relationships with health-care professionals. |
| Questions were asked about participants' experiences of BD and their understanding of what it meant to them to have BD. (Inder et al., 2010) | BD type I, II or NOS ($N = 15$) | Thematic analysis | Experiencing a variety of unpleasant symptoms (e.g. low or elevated mood; psychosis); making sense of the symptoms; receiving diagnosis; questioning diagnosis; experience of treatment as both good and bad; ambivalent acceptance; lack of trust in health care practitioners; difficulty accepting medication. | Seeking help; educating themselves about BD; diagnosis was experienced as helpful by some. |
| Participants were asked about the approaches they used to remain well, and about their view of life before and after diagnosis, as well as any positive aspects of having experienced BD. (Mansell et al., 2010) | BD type I ($N = 13$) two years free of hospitalization and relapse | Interpretive phenomenological analysis | Ambivalent about monitoring against mania (excitement vs. stability); medication; distinction of prior illness vs. current wellness; sense of identity following diagnosis; helpful approaches: understanding; acceptance of diagnosis; insight coming from lived experience; life-style; social support, social change. | Avoiding activities that led to states of elevation; not defining themselves by the illness; acceptance of BD; striving for stability; routine; sleep; diet; engaging in relationships with others; improvement in social skills; gathering information about BD. |
| What strategies have you found most helpful in managing BD? How do friends, family and co-workers affect your ability to stay well? (Suto et al., 2010) | BD type I or II ($N = 32$) | Thematic analysis | Six themes captured various wellness strategies. | Sleep, diet, exercise, self-monitoring, early intervention plan, reflective and meditative practices, self-responsibility; positive relationships with health-care practitioners and personal relationships; understanding BD; connecting with and educating others. |

| Research Question | Sample | Analytic Approach | Themes Identified | Strategies |
|---|---|---|---|---|
| Participants were asked about their experience of mental health symptoms and how they coped, how they would describe recovery, what they and their supporters did to promote recovery, what hindered their recovery, and what they saw as having contributed to positive changes in their lives. (Veseth et al., 2012) | BD I and II (*N*=13) | Hermeneutical-phenomenological | Ambivalence about the experience of mania; finding balance amidst mood symptoms; paying attention to signals from the self and others; the importance of self-care. | Meaningful activities (e.g. gardening, pursuing spirituality, cooking); being aware of triggers and warning signs; setting limits with self (e.g. reducing activities). |
| Participants were asked about the impact of BD on their lives; work, school, relationships; sense of self and direction in life. (Crowe et al., 2012) | BD I and II; (*N*=21) | Thematic analysis | Difficulty in managing symptoms; experience of other people's responses and social stigma; feeling a loss of personal autonomy; out of control, overwhelmed and flawed. | None |
| As part of a larger discussion on a web-based intervention program, participants were asked about their experiences of personal recovery and their self-management strategies. (Todd et al., 2012) | BD I and II; (*N*=12) | Thematic analysis | Recovery is about personal fulfillment rather than absence of symptoms; Importance of taking personal responsibility for wellness; development of self-management strategies; overcoming barriers such as stigma and negativity. | Increasing activity when depressed; decreasing activity when manic; exercise; relaxing and unwinding; seeking support of family and friends. |
| What strategies have helped your recovery? What strategies have hindered your recovery? How have you experienced recovery? (Michalak et al., 2012) | BD I and II; family members of those living with BD (*N*=19) | Thematic analysis | The importance of using recovery language that is reflective of complex experience; shifting from a perspective that focusses on illness to one that emphasizes wellness and quality of life; managing BD using a range of complex skills and taking responsibility for empowering the self; accepting losses; dealing with external and internal stigma; personal transformation, growth, and rebuilding one's life. | Exercise; taking medication; seeking support from family and friends; educating self and others about the disorder; learning about themselves as a person. |

**Table 2.**

| Found Theme | Frequency Count |
|---|---|
| *Negative Aspects of BD* | 43 |
| *Ambivalence* | 9 |
| *Personal Transformation:* | |
| Meaning and Insight | 15 |
| Self and Identity | 26 |
| Shifting the Frame | 8 |
| *Wellness Strategies:* | |
| Help-seeking and Engaging in Treatment | 23 |
| Self-management and Sense of Control | 19 |
| Healthy Relationships and Social Support | 15 |
| Vocation: Role in Society | 13 |
| Educating Self and Others | 11 |
| Physical Care | 11 |
| Stability and Routine | 10 |
| Spiritual and Creative Practice | 9 |
| Diagnosis and Acceptance | 9 |
| Medications | 6 |

Theme two identified the *ambivalence* that participants felt in relation to living with BD, which manifested as experiencing aspects of the illness as both good and bad. Theme three identified the elements of *personal transformation* that evolved as a result of living with BD. Theme four, *wellness strategies*, highlighted behaviours or practices that contributed to PR in people with BD. Some studies aimed to identify specific wellness strategies with their interview questions, (e.g. Mansell, Powell, Pedley, Thomas, and Jones, 2010; Michalak, Yatham, Kolesar, and Lam, 2006; Michalak, Yatham, Maxwell, Hale, and Lam, 2007; Russell and Browne, 2005) while in others, the wellness strategies emerged spontaneously from open-ended questions (e.g. Pollack and Aponte, 2001; Rusner, Carlsson, Brunt, and Nyström, 2009). The wellness strategies and the frequency with which they were mentioned are presented in Table 2.

## The Negative Impact of BD

One of the major over-arching themes found was regarding the potential *negative impact* of BD. Symptoms of BD such as depression and mania were described as distressing and challenging to cope with by some participants (Inder et al., 2010; Jönsson, Wijk, Skärsäter, and Danielson, 2008). For some, living with these symptoms resulted in disruption, loss, and instability (Lim, et al.,2004; Crowe et al., 2012). Some participants described how BD symptoms affected their relationship with themselves resulting in self-doubt (Inder et al., 2008; Proudfoot et al., 2009; Crowe et al., 2012), insecurity (Jönsson et al., 2008) and self-contempt (Rusner et al., 2009). A number of participants spoke of the negative impact that BD had on their relationships with others, resulting in a sense of isolation and rejection (Lim et al., 2004). Some felt that others perceived them differently after they disclosed their diagnosis of BD (Inder et al., 2008; Michalak et al., 2007), and discussed the noticeable impact of stigma in their day-to-day life (Michalak et al., 2006; Michalak, et al., 2007; Proudfoot et al., 2009; Todd, Jones, and Lobban, 2012). Others described poor experiences within the medical system and a consequent lack of trust in health care practitioners (Inder et al., 2010; O'Connor, Gordon, Graham, Kelly, O'Grady-Walshe, 2008; Todd et al., 2012). A number of participants found it difficult to accept their diagnosis of BD and the need for long-term treatment with medication. Lack of acceptance was associated with medication non-adherence and relapse (Clatworthy, Bowskill, Rank, Parham, and Horne, 2007; Pollack and Aponte 2001). Faced with these internal and external barriers (Pollack, 1996a; Pollack, 1996b), it is not surprising that some participants expressed that they felt uncertain and hopeless about their future (Jönsson et al., 2008; Lim et al., 2004; Proudfoot et al., 2009).

### The Ambivalence of Living with BD

The second theme that emerged was the presence of feelings of ambivalence towards various aspects of living with BD. Some participants perceived the intensity of life with BD as both a gift and a challenge (Rusner et al., 2009). There were instances of ambivalence towards receiving the diagnosis of BD and some participants expressed frustration at being misdiagnosed in the past. To them, receiving the correct diagnosis was a relief, providing a helpful framework through which to view their previous behaviours and challenges (Inder et al., 2010; Proudfoot et al., 2009). Others described reacting to their diagnosis with feelings of shock or anger (Inder et al., 2010; Pollack and Aponte, 2001), corresponding to the phases of grief conceptualized by Kubler-Ross (Pollack and Aponte, 2001). Some participants who had initially accepted their diagnosis went on to subsequently question it and experienced doubt as their symptoms abated (Inder et al., 2010). While many participants acknowledged that medication helped maintain their mental health, the side effects and negative beliefs about being medicated also contributed to feelings of ambivalence (Mansell et al., 2010; Proudfoot et al., 2009). In some cases, ambivalence about diagnosis and the need for medication was also found to fluctuate in rhythm with the person's mood state (Clatworthy et al., 2007; Inder et al., 2010).

There was particular ambivalence about the experience of mania, and this was identified as a considerable challenge (Todd et al., 2012). Mania was experienced as extremely pleasurable and productive in the early stages by some (Inder et al., 2010; Mansell et al., 2010; Proudfoot et al., 2009; Veseth, Binder, Borg, and Davidson, 2012). Some participants felt angry when others tried to intervene in their manic mood state, and had difficulty making changes that might prevent further elevation (Todd et al., 2012). Others described terror at the thought that a manic episode might be imminent (Proudfoot et al., 2009), and were aware of the downsides that come with a manic state (Todd et al., 2012).

Ambivalence was also evident in the conflicting feelings and thoughts about receiving treatment. Some participants expressed feeling disrespected by their health care providers, and consequently found it difficult to establish trust (Inder et al., 2010). A number of participants felt the traditional biomedical model practiced by psychiatrists and doctors was alienating and not helpful in their process of recovery (Clatworthy et al., 2007; Mehl-Madrona, 2007; Pollack and Aponte, 2001). At the same time, participants across most studies identified positive relationships with health care providers as crucial to their ongoing wellness (O'Connor et al., 2008; Suto, Murray, Hale, Amari, and Michalak, 2010). Both negative and positive relationships with treatment providers were apparent in the narratives of the participants, indicating that even individual experiences within the medical system were not uniform.

## Personal Transformation and BD

Personal transformation was an overarching theme that refers to the positive impact that BD may have on subjective perceptions of the self and perception of one's place in the world. Three sub-themes were nested within this category: Meaning and insight, self and identity, and new perspectives.

Meaning and insight: For some participants, personal transformation was enhanced by finding meaning in their suffering and developing insight into their own experiences with BD. Participants spoke of an expanded world-view (Jönsson et al., 2008) and some grew to appreciate the intensity of BD as rich lived experience (Rusner et al., 2009). In Mehl-Madrona's study (2007), participants engaged in the construction of personal narratives and metaphors (also Pollack and Aponte, 2001) that brought about healing and a sense of transformation. The integration of lived experience of BD (Inder et al., 2008) resulted in participants having meaningful insights into their own life history (Mansell et al., 2010).

Delf and identity: The transformative aspects of BD seemed to be underpinned by a healthy relationship to the self. Elements of a strong sense of self included self-acceptance (Inder et al., 2008) and self-esteem (Michalak et al., 2006; Todd et al., 2012). Managing insecurities and focusing on the positive contributed to a strong sense of self in some cases (Jönsson et al., 2008), as did an emphasis on self-determination and personal responsibility (Suto et al., 2010; Tse and Yeats, 2002; Michalak et al., 2012; Todd et al., 2012). Some participants stated that they did not define themselves by their BD (Mansell et al., 2010), and refused to see it as a character flaw or moral weakness (Russell and Browne, 2005).

New perspectives: For some, the process of personal transformation involved changing how life with BD was perceived. Participants spoke of placing a greater emphasis on pursuing wellness and quality of life rather than focusing on the pathology of BD (Michalak et al., 2012) and on seeing the positive aspects of life with BD (Todd et al., 2012). Some participants identified that the current PR parlance was not accurate or helpful to them as they felt it conveyed the expectations of a CR approach. They felt that language which reflects the idiosyncratic and complex lived experience of BD should be adopted (Michalak et al., 2012). Embracing new perspectives also involved rejecting external and internal stigma (Michalak et al., 2012), and other negative messages related to BD (Todd et al., 2012). Perhaps most importantly, participants spoke of believing in their ongoing ability to recover (Todd et al., 2012).

## Wellness Strategies

Several of the studies focused on populations who were successfully living well with BD (Mansell et al., 2010; Michalak 2006, 2007; Russell and Browne, 2005). These participants described numerous *wellness strategies* they used to cope with the challenges of BD. The frequency of each type of found strategy is presented below (see Table 2 for frequency information). The importance of self-care was emphasized by participants (Michalak et al., 2012; Veseth et al., 2012) and self-management was conceptualized as an “art” that involved employing complex skills and varied strategies unique to the individual (Michalak et al., 2012).

Help seeking and engaging in treatment: The most frequently reported strategy was help seeking and engaging in treatment. This involved building collaborative relationships with health care providers (Wang, Tse, Michalak, and Depp, 2009), and modalities such as group therapy or cognitive behavior therapy (O’Connor et al., 2008; Pollack, 1996b). In Michalak et al. (2006), participants spoke about the importance of receiving treatment that was tailored to their individual needs. Health care practitioners who used strengths-based, creative, and spiritual approaches were appealing to some (Pollack and Aponte, 2001). Peer support was also identified by some as helpful and facilitated coping with BD symptoms (Proudfoot et al., 2009). A positive and trusting relationship with the health care provider was also very important to people who lived with BD (Mehl-Madrona, 2007; O’Connor et al., 2008; Suto et al., 2010; Wang et al., 2009).

Self-management and sense of control: The second most frequently mentioned wellness strategy was related to self-monitoring the course of BD (Pollack and Aponte, 2001; Russell and Browne, 2005; Veseth et al., 2012; Todd et al., 2012). Techniques adopted by participants included daily mood charting and developing the ability to recognize early warning signs and triggers (Proudfoot et al., 2009; Russell and Browne, 2005; Suto et al., 2010). Early intervention plans and advance directives, which lay out a procedure to be followed should a person become ill, were important to participants who lived well with BD (Russell and Browne, 2005; Suto et al., 2010).

Healthy relationships and social support: Thirdly, participants identified healthy relationships and social support as important to their PR (Jönsson et al., 2008; Mansell, et al., 2010; Michalak et al., 2006; Michalak et al., 2007; Pollack, 1996a; Rusner et al., 2009; Russell and Browne, 2005; Suto et al., 2010; Tse and Yeats, 2002; Wang et al., 2009; Michalak et al., 2012; Todd et al., 2012). Engaging with others and working on developing social skills were specifically mentioned as ways to actively facilitate supportive relationships (Mansell et al., 2010). In Wang et al.’s study (2009) of members of the New Zealand Chinese community living with BD, participants described the importance of compromise in order to maintain harmony with their families, who were their main support system.

Vocation and role in society: The need for a vocation and a role in society emerged as key to the recovery process. Financial stability and the ability to live independently was important to many participants (Michalak et al., 2006; Michalak et al., 2007). Others described the act of taking responsibility for their lives and reintegrating into society as a wellness strategy (Jönsson et al., 2008). Looking specifically at work and vocation issues, Tse and Yeats (2002) found that goodness-of-fit to work setting, supportive colleagues, and a well-timed return to work were all deemed by participants as important to successfully embracing a satisfying vocation..

Educating the self and others: Participants described the importance of informing themselves and others about BD (e.g. Inder et al., 2010; Mansell et al., 2010; Russell and Browne, 2005; Suto et al., 2010; Michalak et al., 2012). Pollack’s (1996b) study specifically looked at how people with BD sought information. The participants described their motivation for educating themselves as stemming from a need to manage their condition, fit into society, and build healthy relationships. People informed themselves via books, internet sites, chat rooms, and psychoeducational groups (Pollack, 1996b).

stability and routine: The need for a sense of stability was another wellness theme in several of the studies (Lim et al., 2004; Mansell et al., 2010; Pollack, 1995). The importance of a structured daily routine was mentioned as being key to developing stability (Michalak et al., 2006; Michalak et al., 2007; Pollack, 1996a). Reducing stress contributed to stability (Jönsson et al., 2008), as did deliberate avoidance of activities that might lead to mood elevation (Mansell et al., 2010; Proudfoot et al., 2009; Veseth et al., 2012; Todd et al., 2012;).

physical care: Several studies mentioned wellness strategies related to physical self-care such as a healthy diet, exercise, and managing sleep and stress (Michalak et al., 2006; Michalak et al., 2007; Pollack, 1996a; Russell and Browne, 2005; Suto et al., 2010).

spiritual and creative practice: Participants spoke about the role of healthy spirituality in staying well (Michalak et al., 2006; Michalak et al., 2007; Rusner et al., 2009). Specifically, faith in God was important to some participants (Tse and Yeats, 2002; Wang et al., 2009). Reflective and meditative practices such as tai-chi, yoga, gardening and journaling were also identified as helpful (Mehl-Madrona, 2007; Suto et al., 2010; Veseth et al., 2012). Surprisingly, despite a demonstrated link between creativity and BD disorder (Murray and Johnson, 2010), just one study specifically mentioned creativity as important to maintaining wellness (Rusner et al., 2009).

diagnosis and acceptance: Some participants struggled with ambivalence around their diagnosis. However, coming to terms with their diagnosis of BD was an important aspect of achieving and maintaining wellness for many (Clatworthy et al., 2007; Mansell et al., 2010; Michalak et al., 2007; Pollack and Aponte, 2001; Proudfoot et al., 2009; Russell and Browne, 2005).

medication: Similarly, though some participants described ambivalence at the thought of needing to take medication, participants in a number of studies identified medication as a key component of keeping their BD under control (Clatworthy et al., 2007; Jönsson et al., 2008; O'Connor et al., 2008, Pollack, 1996a; Pollack and Aponte, 2001; Wang et al., 2009; Michalak et al., 2012).

In sum, participants across studies described diversity in their experiences with BD. Some talked about the negative impact that BD had on their lives, and areas where they had mixed or conflicting feelings. However, others expressed that their rich lived experience of BD resulted in personal transformation and a healthy relationship with the self. Across the studies, numerous strategies were identified that people with BD used to achieve and maintain wellness.

# Discussion

Although our search focused on the topic of personal recovery in those with BD, the four found themes mapped on to the categories of clinical recovery (CR) and personal recovery (PR), coined by Slade (2009a). This is not surprising as there is a symbiotic relationship between issues of CR and PR, in that changes in clinical outcomes affect PR and vice versa.

## Themes Related to and Affecting Clinical Recovery in BD

The factors related to CR in BD are evident in the negative impact and unpredictability of both manic and depressive relapse, the severe impact on social and role functioning, the effects of social and internalized stigma, and the resulting ambivalence with respect to accuracy of diagnosis, severity, and treatment adherence. This review highlighted the extent to which ambivalence permeates interpretations of clinical experience, the choices of coping responses and treatment decisions, and even impacts the self-concept and social relationships in people with BD.

A number of studies reviewed underscored that the experience of mood symptoms related to both depression and mania are distressing, and are often perceived as a major cause of significant life problems including social and role disruption or loss, and consequent social isolation (e.g., Inder et al., 2008; Lim et al., 2004; Proudfoot et al., 2009; Crowe et al., 2012) in work and personal relationships. These experiences can have insidious negative effects on how those living with BD come to view themselves and their future. In addition to the negative effects of symptoms, much of what was described in this review actually pertains to the result of societal and self-stigma. Self-rejection, self-doubt, and insecurity about the self (e.g., "who am I?") created major internal obstacles (e.g., Inder et al., 2008; Jönsson et al., 2008; Proudfoot et al., 2009; Rusner et al., 2009; Crowe et al., 2012). Not infrequently, negative self-concepts in relation to BD seemed to be perceived as reflected in the attitudes and assumptions of others, which, in turn, provided rational justification to maintain social distance from significant others, work, and even health care professionals (e.g., Inder et al., 2008, Inder et al., 2010; Lim et al., 2004; O'Connor et al., 2008; Proudfoot et al., 2009).

Corrigan (2007) explains the process by which societal stigma can accompany the experience of being given a diagnosis. Independent of the presence or absence of BD symptoms, even being diagnosed with a serious mental illness can set in motion a number of potentially problematic and self-sustaining difficulties which include: self-stigma, not accepting treatment because of the fear of being labelled a "mental patient" (i.e., label avoidance), and blocked life goals due to actual discrimination itself (Corrigan, 2007). There is some evidence that health professionals' attitudes can also be stigmatizing and pessimistic, in turn potentially having a negative effect on expectations of hope for recovery for service users, and setting the stage for learned-helplessness, self-defeating behaviours and self-stigmatizing beliefs (Hugo, 2001; Jorm, Koreten, Jacomb, Christensen, and Hendersen, 1999). Indeed, themes identified in our review of qualitative BD recovery literature seem to fit these same problems noted by Corrigan (2007), Hugo (2001) and others in the mental health stigma literature.

The theme of ambivalence was related to the perceived unreliability and "stages of acceptance" of the diagnosis for some, while conversely for others, BD diagnosis meant relief, associated with finding the "correct" medical condition that could explain their circumstances and thus increase their hope for clinical improvement. Ambivalence around diagnosis was also matched by ambivalence regarding accepting and participating in medical treatment, as well as assessing the negative impact of the condition itself. For example, some felt that their hypomanic experiences were positive and productive, while others were terrified of the onset of even mild symptoms, for fear of impending full blown episodes. Consequently, they responded with hyper-vigilance and social withdrawal as necessary coping mechanisms. If pleasure seeking is seen as normative and a positive way of experiencing life by most people in society, then choosing to categorize all pleasurable experiences as potentially indicative of an oncoming manic episode creates a dilemma for those with BD which explains part of the ambivalence identified in this review. Choosing the appropriate coping response can result in either averting disaster and further social and functional upheaval, or it can artificially maintain an anhedonic and depressed existence which is typical of those diagnosed with BD (Judd et al., 2002). The complex array of mechanisms underlying ambivalence may be a unique phenomenological experience to the BD population compared to others who live with serious mental illness.

A CR approach suggests that the relative presence or absence of clinical symptomatology is inextricably linked to functional recovery outcomes. Thus, according to this clinical model of recovery, one cannot be truly "recovered" if one is still experiencing-or can expect to experience-recurrences in symptoms of illness (Davidson, Tondora, Lawless, O'Connell, and Rowe, 2009). The participants seemed to be faced with the dubious choice of either accepting a life of chronic emotional, psychological, and social instability despite best clinical treatment, or, to reject the diagnosis and treatment altogether while trying to manage by themselves, often unsatisfactorily. With few exceptions, these dichotomous choices (i.e., to accept the diagnosis/treatment or completely reject it) are founded in conceptual traps based in black and white thinking, which necessarily result in unsatisfactory outcomes that further feed ambivalence (e.g., Lim et al., 2004; Jönsson et al., 2008; Proudfoot et al., 2009). While definitely a legitimate focus of attention for both clinicians and service-users, an unfortunate by-product of exclusive focus on clinical outcomes is that it promotes persistent unrealistic expectations and consequent pessimistic prognoses (Davidson et al., 2009; Hugo, 2001; Jorm et al.,, 1999; Slade, 2009b). Instead, it may be more helpful to transcend such a polarization by adopting the principles that resonate with a PR approach.

## Themes Related to and Affecting Personal Recovery in BD

In contrast to the traditional, outcome-oriented definition of CR is the person-centred approach to recovery (PR) coined by Slade (2009a). Andresen, Oades, and Caputi (2003) described four domains that were important to mental health service users in their journey of PR. These included hope, meaning in life (i.e., personal goals and purpose in life), taking personal responsibility for one's own life, and reconnecting with or redefining one's identity or selfhood. Similarly, Slade (2009b) described the PR framework as reflected by four tasks including: developing a positive identity, developing a personally satisfying meaning of experiences, taking personal responsibility through self-management and addressing well-being, and acquiring valued social roles. Davidson et al. (2009) would also add the important but related components of overcoming stigma, and becoming an empowered citizen and role model. These personal recovery approaches show considerable overlap, and yet all differ from CR in that personal PR is not related to a clinical or functional outcome per se, but instead a *process* without an endpoint. It also presumes that individuals are autonomous agents capable of *choosing* treatment approaches to help them cope and *live with* their mental health condition within a model of collaborative decision-making (Davidson et al., 2009). It is through this new lens of PR that we interpret the following two themes found in our literature review of PR in BD: positive self-transformation, and the development of wellness strategies.

Based on our review, an important component of PR for many with BD was learning how to accept, and even appreciate the benefits of the rich emotional experiences associated with the condition. More importantly, some of these emotional experiences were accepted as an integral part of their developing self-concept and even a valued part of their lives for some (e.g., Inder et al., 2008; Mansell et al., 2010; Rusner et al., 2009; Russell and Browne, 2005). For others, actively affirming their own personal strengths and developing their identity and self-esteem was an important ingredient in their PR journey (e.g., Inder et al., 2008; Jönsson et al.,2008; Michalak et al., 2006; Michalak et al., 2012; Todd et al., 2012). Consistent with several models of recovery (e.g., Oades, et al., 2005), our review also underscored that the development of a new and healthy relationship to the self seems to be symbiotically reinforced by the pursuit and attainment of personally relevant and meaningful goals. Integrating lived experience of BD with newly embraced roles and abilities is one means of transcending dichotomous thinking about clinical recovery.

A range of wellness strategies emerged that were integral to the participants self-care and PR (Michalak et al., 2012; Veseth et al., 2012). Those described included both clinical strategies such as mood symptom monitoring, preparation of personalized relapse prevention strategies, stimulation reduction, psychoeducation, CBT, and group therapy (Clatworthy et al., 2007; Mansell et al., 2010; Pollack and Aponte, 2001; Proudfoot et al., 2009; Russell and Browne, 2005), as well as strategies aligned with a psychosocial and PR approach. Our review suggests that CR strategies are not incompatible with PR. It is important to note that the most frequently endorsed wellness strategies are reflective of an engagement with current evidence-based treatment. However, consistent with the PR model, less traditional wellness strategies were also important. Many of these emanate from the individuals themselves, and are not necessarily delivered through the health care system. Strategies such as practicing spirituality is one example of a highly personal wellness goal (e.g., Mehl-Madrona, 2007; Michalak et al., 2006; Michalak et al., 2007; Rusner et al., 2009; Suto et al., 2010; Tse and Yeats, 2002; Wang et al., 2009). Engaging in a healthy lifestyle also involves choices unique to the individual, and was endorsed as important to PR in BD (e.g., Michalak et al., 2006; Michalak et al., 2007; Pollack, 1996a; Russell and Browne, 2005; Suto et al., 2010). For others, however, PR meant abandoning medication and reliance upon clinical services altogether (Mehl-Madrona, 2007). Healthy social relationships, the pursuit of a meaningful vocation and participation in social roles that facilitated community engagement were identified as an integral part of wellness (e.g., Jönsson et al., 2008; Mansell, et al., 2010; Michalak et al., 2006; Michalak et al., 2007; Pollack, 1996a; Rusner et al., 2009; Russell and Browne, 2005; Suto et al., 2010; Tse and Yeats, 2002; Wang et al., 2009). All of the strategies, whether they fell within or outside of the spectrum of traditional health care practice, reflected the participants' own choices and decisions about what worked best for them in achieving and maintaining their personal wellness.

## Limitations

This review has several limitations that may constrain interpretation of the results. First, this is a review of studies which used multiple sample sizes, a range of qualitative approaches, and different interview questions, some which focused less directly on the topic of PR. Although there is considerable consistency in the findings, the results cannot be generalized and can only point to further research and possible new approaches to clinical care and self-management strategies. Secondly, the nature of qualitative data involves rich narratives and overlapping themes that may not be easily quantified or fully captured in a review such as this. The frequency of the wellness strategies are only a guideline and the ranking presented here may privilege one over the other in an arbitrary way. Certainly they may not reflect the particular needs of any one individual. Thirdly, one-person narratives describing lived experience of BD were deliberately excluded in favour of peer-reviewed studies with larger sample sizes. Individual narratives are in keeping with a philosophy of PR, and it may be that more themes and wellness strategies would have emerged had these been included. It is suggested that future reviews of PR in BD specifically target these published one-person narratives to further expand and clarify some of the found themes.

## Clinical Implications

This review may assist health care practitioners in gaining a deeper understanding of the tremendous negative impact of BD, in terms of distressing symptoms as well as the stigma-both external and internal-that those who live with BD face. Similarly, it may be helpful for clinicians to be aware of the extent to which those with BD struggle with ambivalence, especially in regards to the experience of mania. Clinicians may find it useful to explore the issue of ambivalence if they identify it in their client, in order to promote balance in mood states as an ideal. The possible benefits of BD, as reflected by the voices of the participants in the reviewed studies, may be of interest to clinicians and service users. Health care practitioners can assist the journey of recovery by assisting clients in seeing the positive aspects of life with BD and to promote new perspectives that might contribute to personal transformation and enhanced integration of difficult life experiences. Finally, the emphasis on self-care (Michalak et al., 2012; Veseth et al., 2012) and the wealth of self-management strategies shared by participants can form the basis of a treatment plan that may contribute to increased quality of life for those who are affected by BD.

## Conclusion

The integration of traditional clinical approaches with a breadth of non-clinical wellness strategies (e.g. spirituality, creativity), and the importance of establishing meaningful relationships and social roles are all consistent with the general PR literature (Davidson et al., 2009; Slade, 2009b). As such, extant PR models seem quite capable of accommodating those with lived experience of BD. However, the theme of ambivalence, particularly in regards to manic mood states, was more pronounced in BD PR literature. The theme of ambivalence is an intriguing area of future research, as participants identified the “seduction of mania” (Torrey and Knable, 2002) as irresistible at times, despite unwanted consequences. Few other serious mental health conditions elicit such strong positive reactions in addition to the suffering caused by symptoms. Sometimes this resulted in additional confusion and ambivalence, while other participants embraced these as positive and valid personal experiences that contributed to a rich and meaningful life experience. The theme of personal transformation may be applicable to recovery in numerous populations, and it is well articulated in the literature reviewed here. The possibility of creating meaning from suffering and developing a healthy relationship to the Self provides a beacon of hope amidst the chaos of BD symptoms that diminish QoL. As both research and practice move forward, it may be beneficial to continue to look at BD specifically, in order to further ascertain the unique challenges and strengths experienced by those with BD as they engage in a dynamic and self-determined journey of PR.

*In memory of Dan Blaugrund.

# References

*References marked with an asterisk indicate studies included in the narrative review.*

Andresen, R., Oades, L., and Caputi, P. (2003). The experience of recovery from schizophrenia: Towards an empirically validated stage model. *Australian and New Zealand Journal of Psychiatry, 37*, 586-594.

Andresen, R., Caputi, P., and Oades, L. (2006). Stages of recovery instrument: Development of a measure of recovery from serious mental illness. *The Australian and New Zealand Journal of Psychiatry, 40*, 972-980.

Anthony, W. (2000). A recovery-oriented service system: Setting some system level standards. *Psychiatric Rehabilitation Journal, 24*, 159-168.

Chadwick, P. K. (1997). *Schizophrenia: The positive perspective*. London: Routledge.

Chengappa, K., Hennen, J., Baldessarini, R., Kupfer, D., Yatham, L., Gershon, S., … Tohen, M. (2005). Recovery and functional outcomes following olanzapine treatment for bipolar I mania. *Bipolar Disorders, 7*, 68-76. doi:10.1111/j.1399-5618.2004.00171.x.

*Clatworthy, J., Bowskill, R., Rank, T., Parham, R., and Horne, R. (2007). Adherence to medication in bipolar disorder: A qualitative study exploring the role of patients' beliefs about the condition and its treatment. *Bipolar Disorders, 9*, 656–664. doi:10.1111/j.1399-5618.2007.00434.x

Corrigan, P. (2007). How clinical diagnosis might exacerbate the stigma of mental illness. *Social Work, 52*, 31-39.

* Crowe, M., Inder, M., Carlyle, D., Wilson, L., Whitehead, L., Pankhurst, A., O'Brien, A., and Joyce, P. (2012). Feeling out of control: a qualitative analysis of the impact of bipolar disorder. *Journal of Psychiatric and Mental Health Nursing, 19*, 294-302.

Davidson, L. (2003). *Living outside mental illness: Qualitative studies of recovery in schizophrenia*. New York: New York University Press.

Davidson, L., and Strauss, J. S. (1992). Sense of self in recovery from severe mental illness. *British Journal of Medical Psychology, 65*, 131-145. doi:10.1111/j.2044-8341.1992.tb01693.x.

Davidson, L., Tondora, J., Lawless, M. S., O'Connell, M. J., and Rowe, M. (2009). *A practical guide to recovery-oriented practice: Tools for transforming mental health care.* Oxford: Oxford University Press.

Deegan, G. (2003). Discovering recovery. *Psychiatric Rehabilitation Journal, 26*(4), 368-376.

Deegan, P. (1988). Recovery: The lived experience of rehabilitation. *Psychosocial Rehabilitation Journal, 11*, 11-19.

Deegan, P. (1996). Recovery as a journey of the heart. *Psychiatric Rehabilitation Journal, 19*, 91-97.

Deegan, G. (2003). Discovering recovery. *Psychiatric Rehabilitation Journal, 26*, 368-376.

Fink, A. (2005). *Conducting research literature reviews: From the internet to paper (2nd ed.).* Thousand Oaks, CA: Sage.

Forchuk, C., Jewell, J., Tweedell, D., and Steinnagel, L. (2003). Reconnecting: The client experience of recovery from psychosis. *Perspectives in Psychiatric Care, 39*, 141-150.

Frese, F., Stanley, J., Kress, K., and Vogel-Scibilia, S. (2001). Integrating evidence-based practices and the recovery model. *Psychiatric Services, 52*, 1462-1468. doi:10.1176/appi.ps.52.11.1462

Galvez, J., Thommi, S., and Ghaemi, S. (2011). Positive aspects of mental illness: A review in bipolar disorder. *Journal of Affective Disorders, 128*, 185-190. doi:10.1016/j.jad.2010.03.017

Gitlin, M.J., Swendsen J., Heller, T.L., and Hammen, C.(1995). Relapse and impairment in bipolar disorder. *American Journal of Psychiatry, 152,* 1635-1640.

Glover, H. (2005). Recovery based service delivery: Are we ready to transform the words into a paradigm shift? *Australian e-Journal for the Advancement of Mental Health, 4*, 1-4.

Goodwin, F.K. and Jamison, K.R. (1990). *Manic-Depressive Illness: Bipolar disorders and recurrent depression.* Oxford: Oxford University Press.

Harding, C. M., Zubin, J., and Strauss, J. S. (1987). Chronicity in schizophrenia: Fact, partial fact, or artifact? *Hospital and Community Psychiatry, 38*, 477-486.

Harding, C. M., Zubin, J., and Strauss, J. S. (1992). Chronicity in schizophrenia: Revisited. *British Journal of Psychiatry, 16,* 27-37.

Hugo, M. M. (2001). Mental health professionals' attitudes towards people who have experienced a mental health disorder. *Journal of Psychiatric and Mental Health Nursing, 8*, 419-425. doi:10.1046/j.1351-0126.2001.00430.x.

*Inder M., Crowe, M., Joyce, P., Moor, S., Carter, J., and Luty, S. (2010). "I really don't know whether it is still there": Ambivalent acceptance of a diagnosis of bipolar disorder. *The Psychiatric Quarterly*, *81*, 157-165.

*Inder, M., Crowe, M., Moor, S., Luty, S., Carter, J., and Joyce, P. (2008). "I actually don't know who I am": The impact of bipolar disorder on the development of self. *Psychiatry*, *71*, 123-133.

Johnson, S. (2005). Mania and dysregulation in goal pursuit: A review. *Clinical Psychology Review, 25*, 241-262.

*Jönsson, P., Wijk, H., Skärsäter, I., and Danielson, E. (2008). Persons living with bipolar disorder – their view of the illness and the future. *Issues in Mental Health Nursing*, *29*, 1217-1236.

Jorm, A. F., Korten, A. E., Jacomb, P. A., Christensen, H., and Hendersen, S. (1999). Attitudes towards people with a mental disorder: A survey of the Australian public and health professionals. *Australian and New Zealand Journal of Psychiatry*, *33*, 77-83.

Judd, L., Akiskal, H., Schettler, P., Coryell, W., Maser, J., Rice, J., … Keller, M.

(2003). The comparative clinical phenotype and long term longitudinal episode course of bipolar I and II: A clinical spectrum or distinct disorders? *Journal of Affective Disorders, 73*, 19-32.

Judd, L., Akiskal, H., Schettler, P., Endicott, J., Maser, J., Solomon, D., ... Keller, M. (2002). The long-term natural history of the weekly symptomatic status of bipolar I disorder. *Archives of General Psychiatry*, *59*, 530-537.

Kessler, R.C., Berglund., P., Demler, O., Jin, R., Merikangas, K.R., and Walters, E.E. (2005). Lifetime prevalence and age-of-onset distribution of DSM-IV disorders in the National Comorbidity Survey Replication. *Archives of General Psychiatry, 62,* 593-602.

*Lim, L., Nathan, P., O'Brien-Malone, A., and Williams, S. (2004). A qualitative approach to identifying psychosocial issues faced by bipolar patients. *Journal of Nervous and Mental Disease, 192*, 810-817. doi:10.1097/01.nmd.0000146734.39501.57.

*Mansell, W., Powell, S., Pedley, R., Thomas, N., and Jones, S. (2010). The process of recovery from bipolar I disorder: A qualitative analysis of personal accounts in relation to an integrative cognitive model. *British Journal of Clinical Psychology*, *49*, 193-215. doi:10.1348/014466509X45144.

Mays, N., Pope, C; and Popay, J. (2005). Details of approaches to synthesis-a methodological appendix to the paper: Systematically reviewing qualitative and quantitative evidence to inform management and policy making in the health field. Canadian Health Services Research Foundation. NHS Service Delivery and Organisation RandD Programme, Ottawa. Retrieved from: *http://researchonline.lshtm.ac.uk/19432/*

*Mehl-Madrona, L. (2007). Narrative analysis: Alternative constructions of bipolar disorder. *Advances in Mind-Body Medicine, 22*, 12-19.

*Michalak, E.E., Hole, R., Holmes, C., Velyvis, V., Austin, J., and Hou, S. (2012). Implications for psychiatric care of the word 'recovery' in people with bipolar disorder. *Psychiatric Annals, 42,* 173-178. doi: 10.3928/00485713-20120507-04.

*Michalak, E. E., Yatham, L., Kolesar, S., and Lam, R. W. (2006). Bipolar disorder and quality of life: A patient-centered perspective. *Quality of Life Research, 15*, 25-37. doi:10.1007/s11136-005-0376-7.

*Michalak, E. E., Yatham, L., Maxwell, V., Hale, S., and Lam, R. W. (2007). The impact of bipolar disorder upon work functioning: A qualitative analysis. *Bipolar Disorders, 9*, 126-143.

Murray, G., and Johnson, S. L. (2010). The clinical significance of creativity in bipolar disorder. *Clinical Psychology Review, 30*, 721-732. doi:10.1016/j.cpr.2010.05.006.

Murray, C. J., and Lopez, A. D. (1997). Global mortality, disability, and the contribution of risk factors: Global burden of disease study. *The Lancet, 349*, 1436-1442. doi:10.1016/S0140-6736(96)07495-8.

Nordentoft, M., Mortensen, P.B., and Pedersen, C.B. (2011). Absolute risk of suicide after first hospital contact in mental disorder. *Archives of General Psychiatry, 68,* 1058-64.

Oades, L., Deane, F., Crowe, T., Lambert, W., Kavanagh, D., and Lloyd, C. (2005). Collaborative recovery: An integrative model for working with individuals who experience chronic and recurring mental illness. *Australasian Psychiatry, 13*, 279-284. doi:10.1111/j.140-1665.2005.02202.x.

*O'Connor, C., Gordon, O., Graham, M., Kelly, F., and O'Grady-Walshe, A. (2008). Service user perspectives of a psychoeducation group for individuals with a diagnosis of bipolar disorder: A qualitative study. *The Journal of Nervous and Mental Disease*, *196*, 568-571.

Ösby, U., Brandt., L., Correia, N., Ekbom, A., and Sparen, P. (2001). Excess mortality in bipolar and unipolar disorder in Sweden. *Archives of General Psychiatry, 58,* 844-850.

Özer, S., Ulusahin, A., Batur, S., Kabakçi, E., Saka, M. (2002). Outcome measures of inter-episode bipolar patients in a Turkish sample. *Social Psychiatry and Psychiatric Epidemiology, 37*, 31-37.

Pitt, L., Kilbride, M., Nothard, S., Welford, M., and Morrison, A.P. (2007). Researching recovery from psychosis: A user-led project. *Psychiatric Bulletin, 31*, 55-60.

*Pollack, L. E. (1995). Striving for stability with bipolar disorder despite barriers. *Archives of Psychiatric Nursing, 9*, 122-129.

*Pollack, L. E. (1996a). Inpatient self-management of bipolar disorder. *Applied Nursing Research, 9*, 71-79. doi:10.1016/S0897-1897(96)80446-0.

*Pollack, L. E. (1996b). Inpatients with bipolar disorder: Their quest to understand. *Journal of Psychosocial Nursing and Mental Health Services, 34*, 19.

*Pollack, L. E., and Aponte, M. (2001). Patients' perceptions of their bipolar illness in a public hospital setting. *The Psychiatric Quarterly, 72*, 167-179.

*Proudfoot, J. G., Parker, G. B., Benoit, M., Manicavasagar, V., Smith, M., and Gayed, A. (2009). What happens after diagnosis? Understanding the experiences of patients with newly-diagnosed bipolar disorder. *Health Expectations, 12*, 120-129. doi:10.1111/j.1369-7625.2009.00541.x.

Robb, J. C., Cooke, R. G., Devins, G. M., Young, L. T., and Joffe, R. T. (1997). Quality of life and lifestyle disruption in euthymic bipolar disorder. *Journal of Psychiatric Research, 31*, 509-517. doi:10.1016/S0022-3956(97)00030-7.

*Rusner, M., Carlsson, G., Brunt, D., and Nyström, M. (2009). Extra dimensions in all aspects of life – the meaning of life with bipolar disorder. *International Journal of Qualitative Studies on Health and Well-being, 4*, 159-169. doi:10.1080/17482620902864194.

*Russell, S. J., and Browne, J. L. (2005). Staying well with bipolar disorder. *Australian and New Zealand Journal of Psychiatry*, *39*, 187-193.

SAMHSA announces a working definition of recovery from mental disorders and substance use disorders. (2011, December). *SAMHSA News Release*. Retrieved from: *http://www.samhsa.gov/newsroom/advisories/1112223420.aspx.*

Schaffer, A., Cairney, J., Cheung, A., Veldhuizen, S., and Levitt, A. (2006). Community survey of bipolar disorder in Canada: Lifetime prevalence and illness characteristics. *Canadian Journal of Psychiatry, 51*, 9-16.

Slade, M. (2009a). *Personal Recovery and Mental Illness*. Cambridge: Cambridge University Press.

Slade, M. (2009b). The contribution of mental health services to recovery. *Journal of Mental Health, 18*, 367-371.

*Suto, M., Murray, G., Hale, S., Amari, E., and Michalak, E. E. (2010). What works for people with bipolar disorder? Tips from the experts. *Journal of Affective Disorders, 124*, 76-84. doi:10.1016/j.jad.2009.11.004.

*Todd, N.J., Jones, S.H., and Lobban, F.A. (2012). "Recovery" in bipolar disorder: How can service users be supported through a self-management intervention? A qualitative focus group study. *Journal of Mental Health, 21*, 114-126.

Tohen, M., Hennen, J., Zarate, C. M., Baldessarini, R. J., Strakowski, S. M., Stoll, A. L., … Cohen, B. M. (2000). Two-year syndromal and functional recovery in 219 cases of first-episode major affective disorder with psychotic features. *The American Journal of Psychiatry, 157*, 220-228. doi:10.1176/appi.ajp.157.2.220.

Torrey, E.F., and Knable, M.B. (2002). *Surviving manic-depression: A manual on bipolar disorder for patients, families, and providers*. New York: Basic Books.

*Tse, S., and Yeats, M. (2002). What helps people with bipolar affective disorder succeed in employment: A grounded theory approach. *Work, 19*, 47.

*Veseth, M., Binder, P., Borg, M., and Davidson, L. (2012). Toward caring for oneself in a life of intense ups and downs: A reflexive-collaborative exploration of recovery in bipolar disorder. *Qualitative Health Research, 22,* 119-133.

*Wang, G., Tse, S., Michalak, E. E., and Depp, C. (2009). Self-management techniques for bipolar disorder in a sample of New Zealand Chinese. *International Journal of Therapy and Rehabilitation, 16*, 602-608.

Young, A., Green, C., and Estroff, S. (2008). New endeavors, risk taking, and personal growth in the recovery process: findings from the stars study. *Psychiatric Services, 59*, 1430-1436.

In: Bipolar Disorder
Editor: Nickolas B. Moore

ISBN: 978-1-62618-666-8


*Chapter V*

# Computerised Self-Management in Bipolar Disorder: A Useful Treatment Approach?

***Nicholas John Todd***

Psychologist in Clinical Training, Leeds Teaching Hospitals NHS Trust and Leeds University, UK

## Abstract

Bipolar Disorder (BD) is a highly recurrent affective disorder characterised by periods of extreme mood, including depression and mania or hypomania (Goodwin and Jamison, 1990). It has been identified in 2% of the population (Merikangas et al., 2007) and is estimated to cost the UK £5.2 billion per year (Mccrone et al., 2008). There is increasing evidence that people with BD respond well to psychological interventions, evidenced by fewer relapses, improvements in social functioning and reduced hospital admissions (e.g. Morriss et al., 2007). Despite this, few service users receive psychological intervention within routine clinical services (Mind, 2010). Computerised interventions are an innovative way of addressing the accessibility problem by providing highly accessible, around the clock, self-directed support (Kazdin and Blase, 2011). Despite numerous interventions being developed for 'mild to moderate' depression and the majority studies demonstrating clinical effectiveness (Kalthenthaler et al., 2008), the development of this approach in BD is in its infancy. This is somewhat surprising considering there is evidence that self-management is effective in BD (Russell and Browne, 2005), the effective components of self-help and face-to-face psychological therapy can be translated into computerised therapy with a similar treatment effect (e.g. Barak et al., 2008) and the treatment effect in depression has also been observed in 'severely' depressed sample subgroups (e.g. Proudfoot et al., 2004; Purves et al., 2009; De Graaf et al., 2008; Vernmark et al., 2010; Wiersma et al., 2011). Smith et al (2011) have recently published results from a pilot trial failing to find a statistically significant treatment effect, and three other trials (Barnes et al., 2007; Lauder et al., 2008 and Proudfoot et al., 2007) have not yet published on effectiveness outcome. Todd et al (Under Review) however have reported positve findings, demostrating the strongest improvement in psychological and physical domains of quality life, wellbeing and recovery outcomes. Recovery and quality of life outcomes despite being service user priorities (Todd et al., 2012), and recovery focussed approaches being halied as one of the ke prorities for modernising mental health care (New Horrizons, 2009), have not until now been the primary focus of interventions in this area. Interventions have tended to focus on relapse prevention, symptom management and medication compliance (Todd et al., Under Review-a). The content, structure and support provided in these interventions may be an important predictor of outcome and may be related to acceptability (Todd et al., Under Review-b). Statistically powered, hypothesis testing trials are urgently needed to tease these differences apart. Future research needs to focus on the cost effectiveness of such interventions, explore the mechanisms of change and consider the impact of individual components on outcome. The relevance of this approach for people not routinely accessing the internet for self-help would support translation of interventions into practice. This budding research field is starting to demonstrate the promise computerised treatment approaches have to feasibly deliver evidence based psychological intervention to a large number of people with BD. Such approaches are a current government priority to improve access to psychological interventions for people with 'severe' mental health problems (IAPT, 2013).

# Preface

This chapter discusses whether computerised self-management in Bipolar Disorder (BD) is a useful treatment approach. The research into this treatment method and its effectiveness is in its infancy. Todd, Lobban and Jones have developed and evaluated 'Living with Bipolar': a web-based intervention for BD (Todd, Solis-Trapala, Jones, and Lobban, 2012c). The overall aim of this research project was to develop and evaluate the feasibility, acceptability and potential effectiveness of delivering a web-based self-management intervention to people with Bipolar Disorder. This chapter integrates the findings of this research project into the wider literature and discusses the implications for the development of theory and new clinical interventions.

## General Background

Bipolar Disorder (BD) is a highly recurrent affective disorder characterised by periods of extreme mood, including depression and mania or hypomania (Goodwin and Jamison, 2007). It is estimated to affect 2% of the population (Merikangas et al., 2007), cost the UK £5.2 billion per year (McCrone, Dhanasiri, Patel, Knapp, and Lewton-Smith, 2008) and is identified as one of the sixth most debilitating conditions (Murray and Lopez, 1997). However, outcome is highly variable and people can experience long periods of stability (Michalak, Yatham, Kolesar, and Lam, 2006).

Pharmacotherapy is the main treatment of choice, but has limited effectiveness. Relapse rates are high (Geddes, Burgess, Hawton, Jamison, and Goodwin, 2004), psychosocial difficulties between episodes are significant (Judd et al., 2002) and people can find it difficult to manage a medication regime long term; due in part to the side effects and perceived restrictiveness (Adams and Scott, 2000). People with 'severe and enduring' mental health problems such as BD and Psychosis experience problems receiving access to psychological therapy (Bird, 2006), despite the developing evidence for the adjunctive use of such therapies (Miklowitz et al., 2007; Morriss et al., 2007). To date, only "mild to moderate" mental health problems such as depression and anxiety have benefited from receiving psychological support on a large scale, through the improving access to psychological therapies initiative (IAPT), although this is current being extended into 'severe' mental health (IAPT, 2013).

An innovative solution to the accessibility problem has been the use of computerised therapeutic approaches, which are now recommended in the National Institute of Clinical Excellence (NICE) guidelines for 'mild to moderate' anxiety and depression (NICE, 2006b). These approaches are highly accessible (Gournay, 2007), and provide round the clock evidence based self-directed support (Kazdin and Blase, 2011) to many people at a reduced cost to the National Health Service (NHS)(DoH, 2005). There is currently not enough evidence for disorders at the 'severe' end of the spectrum to receive this accessible means of support, but many reasons for the development of this approach. There is evidence that self-management may be effective in these populations (Kennedy, Schepp, and O'Connor, 2000; Rothbaum and Astin, 2000). The internet is one of the top sources of information accessed by people with mental health problems (Powell and Clarke, 2006) but the majority of website provide poor quality information on mental health (Reavley et al., 2012). There are significant advantages for service users and the NHS for the increased use of this treatment modality (Bell, 2007).

## The Theoretical Underpinnings of Computerised Interventions in Bipolar Disorder

A systematic review of the computerised intervention literature indicates that there may be false dichotomy between 'mild to moderate' and 'severe and enduring' mental health problems (Todd, Solis-Trapala, Jones, and Lobban, In Submission-b). These interventions are reported to be clinically effective in depression with all but one intervention reporting positive results (De Graaf et al., 2009, 2011). However, some of these interventions report positive results in 'severely' depressed populations (Meyer et al., 2009; Proudfoot et al., 2004; Purves, Bennett, and Wellman, 2009), and there are some preliminary studies specifically targeting this group (Learmonth and Rai, 2007; Vernmark et al., 2010; Wiersma et al., 2011). In psychosis two interventions were found to be effective on their primary outcomes (Pitkänen et al., 2012; Rotondi et al., 2010). There is evidence that one intervention specifically targeting social rhythms is effective in Bipolar Disorder (BD)(Lieberman, Swayze, and Goodwin, 2011). However, a more general intervention failed to report any notable treatment effects (Smith et al., 2011), but as this result is explained by methodological shortcomings, and suggests further evaluation of psychological outcome.

This evidence provides a useful grounding for the further development of these approaches. The development of accessible evidence based interventions for 'severe' mental illness will contribute to treatment guidelines (NICE, 2006a, 2009) and may form part of the IAPT initiative in 'severe' mental health (IAPT, 2013). When reviewing the content of the interventions for depression it was found that they were primarily focussed on the cognitive behavioural model (Beck, Rush, Shaw, and Emery, 1987), and the interventions for psychosis and BD were focussed on psycho-education (Colom and Vieta, 2006). Interestingly only one intervention (Barnes, Harvey, Mitchell, Smith, and Wilhelm, 2007) contained cognitive behavioural therapy (CBT) for BD despite there being some evidence for this approach in this population (Lam, Hayward, Watkins, Wright, and Sham, 2005; Lam. et al., 2003). There was a clear difference in what material was delivered and how it was supported for people with BD. The material tended to be highly structured (Smith et al., 2011) and supported at a higher level than computerised interventions for depression (Barnes et al., 2007). The interventions for BD are heavily focussed on improving compliance with medication, symptom reduction and relapse prevention with few psychological outcomes assessed (Barnes et al., 2007, Proudfoot et al., 2007; Simpson et al., 2009).

Although there is evidence such approaches may support people to improve their mental health symptoms and reduce relapse (Castle, Berk, Lauder, Berk, and Murray, 2009), they may not be in line with service user priorities. A priority for some service users is 'recovery' which is defined as the process by which people can live fulfilling lives alongside their mental health problems (Anthony, 1993). This is in contrast to clinical recovery which is defined as the absence of symptoms (Mead and Copeland, 2000). In order to develop interventions that are more in line with service user priorities, service users need to be central to this process to ensure they are meaningful to those who use them (DoH, 2003). This is important considering dropout rates can be related to acceptability (Kaltenthaler, Parry, Beverley, and Ferriter, 2008). A qualitative investigation of recovery in BD (Todd, Jones, and Lobban, 2012a) explored service users' concept of recovery and self-management in order to develop a new way of supporting service users which is more compatible with their definition. Supporting recovery without such an investigation is difficult as there is some debate about how it should be supported, when defined both as an individual (Anthony, 1993) and dynamic (Buchanan-Barker and Barker, 2006) process. This study provided further support that recovery is about revaluating service users' condition outside the medical model and living alongside symptoms (Anthony, 1993). Service users provided support for part of recovery being about taking responsibility for their own wellness (Mead and Copeland, 2000) achieved through self-management approaches (Martyn, 2003).

A self-management approach informed by the recovery literature has been suggested as a way to support recovery. This approach aids participants recovery, allows them to take responsibility by learning to self-manage through building on existing techniques (Russell and Browne, 2005) and overcome barriers to recovery by gaining a different perspective on their condition (Young and Ensing, 1999). This approach differs significantly from the current self-management interventions in the literature for BD. There is not a prescriptive focus on treatment and overemphasis on symptom recovery, but instead empowers the service user as an 'expert by experience', integrating recovery into symptom management and outcome being measured through personally defined recovery goals and quality of life. Recovery focussed approaches are one of the key priorities for modernising mental health care (HM Goverment, 2009).

A second qualitative investigation focussed specifically on the content of a recovery informed self-management intervention (Todd, Jones, and Lobban, 2012b). We considered how the cognitive behavioural model of BD (Lam, Jones, and Hayward, 2010) and the individual psycho-education approach (Perry et al., 1999) could be adapted to match service user priorities. Service users described wanting a web-based self-management approach that not only gives them the techniques they need to manage their moods (Lam et al., 2010; Perry, Tarrier, Morriss, McCarthy, and Limb, 1999), but also the techniques to manage their lives alongside the disorder, including; managing stigma (Perlick et al., 2001), increasing self-advocacy (Byrne, 2000), improving relationships (Keller, Levori, Coryell, Endicott, and Mueller, 1993) and managing employment (Michalak, Yatham, Maxwell, Hale, and Lam, 2007). Crucially, participants did not state the absence of symptoms or a cure as their desired outcome (Anthony, 1993), suggesting the need for a focus on promoting a fulfilling life alongside the disorder (Roberts and Wolfson, 2004). Such support included balancing stability but not falling into a false sense of security (Russell and Browne, 2005), and focussing on the positives in their experience(Galvez, Thommi, and Ghaemi, 2011; Lobban, Taylor, Murray, and Jones, 2012). The internet was considered to be a practical solution (Kazdin and Blase, 2011), but a number of recommendations were made to ensure engagement, including the problem with motivation online (Bados, Balaguer, and Saldaña, 2007), the need for reminders (MacGregor, Hayward, Peck, and Wilkes, 2009) and a peer support mechanism (Andersson, Estling, Jakobsson, Cuijpers, and Carlbring, 2011; Spek et al., 2007).

A web-based self-management intervention was developed based on the cognitive behavioural model of mood experience (Lam et al., 2010), individual psycho-education approach (Perry et al., 1999) and the recovery model (Anthony, 1993), drawing on the work from (Todd et al., 2012a; Todd et al., 2012b; Todd et al., In Submission-b). This intervention aimed to support people to: (1) learn more about themselves, their condition and how it effects their lives; (2) increase their self-esteem and self-efficacy; (3) increase their knowledge of self-management techniques to effectively manage their condition and pursue personally meaningful recovery goals, and; (4) increase their knowledge of practical and interpersonal skills to live a fulfilling life alongside their condition. These aims were built into ten interactive audio-visual modules which combined worksheets, case studies and a mood checking tool. A methodological protocol (Todd et al., 2012c) considered the strengths and weaknesses of this treatment modality, and how these could be accounted for in the delivery of the approach.

The main strength of the treatment modality is accessibility, widening access to free evidence based psychological intervention (NICE, 2006), which has been traditionally difficult for people with ‘severe’ mental illness to access (Todd et al., In Submission-b). The challenges to delivering self-management to a ‘severe’ mental illness include symptom severity and service user motivation (Todd et al., 2012b), which have been linked to drop out in previous studies (Kaltenthaler et al., 2008). These were been accounted for through the development of a theoretical underpinning which combined recovery principles with clinical management (Todd et al., 2012a), a flexible interface; allowing the service user to be in control of their recovery, personalised content and access support from their peers and the research team. The flexibility of the interface is not something other interventions in this area have done, with only one allowing participants to be in charge of their own recovery (Proudfoot et al., 2007). Support has been linked to improved engagement in BD (Nicholas et al., 2010) and features in all of the interventions for BD. This intervention had limited professional support with a peer support forum providing the most support.

However, the increased focus on self-management and recovery in services has not always been discussed as a benefit in some of the service user literature. Self-management has been discussed by some service users as being overly restrictive by focussing on maintaining balance and stability (Michalak et al., 2006) and may create ‘hyper-vigilance’ (Mansell, Powell, Pedley, Thomas, and Jones, 2010) in some individuals. Some service users suggest that the term “recovery” has been hijacked by mental health services and become something it was never intended to be. Examples include “recovery” becoming another form of social control (Kalathil, 2011) and the movement being used as a justification for cutting services (Exell, 2007). Although delivering self-management in a recovery framework outside the context of services may be less likely to encounter such criticism, we acknowledge that there are some instances where the recovery approach or the on-line intervention approach may be unhelpful. There are occasions when service users become acutely unwell and do not realise it. In those cases, hospital admission and complex care and treatment teams may be the appropriate treatment, even if it is against the service users wishes.

## Evaluating the Feasibility, Acceptability and Potential Clinical Effectiveness of a Recovery Informed Web-Based Self-Management Intervention for Bipolar Disorder

The systematic review (Todd, et al., In Submission-b) demonstrated that higher quality research trials are needed investigate whether computerised interventions are a useful treatment approach. The current trials have small sample sizes, high drop-out rates and fail to examine the participants who do not respond or drop out of these interventions. A small scale online randomised controlled trial was designed to assess the feasibility, acceptability and potential effectiveness of ‘Living with Bipolar’: a recovery informed web-based self-management intervention for BD. A protocol describes the methodology in detail and considers the strengths and weaknesses of the methodology undertaken (Todd, et al., 2012c). Conducting a randomised controlled trial online, where participants are screened and administered baseline and follow up assessments over the internet can be as rigorous as a traditional RCT and can have significant advantages. These include time and cost efficient evaluation of new interventions through instantaneous data capture and greater reliability, validity and statistical power through national recruitment of a hard to reach clinical group (Formica, Kabbara, Clark, and McAlindon, 2004). However, challenges include the screening for a diagnosis online (Isometsa et al., 2003), demographic differences in internet populations (Robinson, Neustadtl, and Kestenbaum, 2002), social desirability, nonsense responding (Chan, 2009) and adherence to the treatment online (Eysenbach, 2005). A well designed trial can overcome these challenges with evidence suggesting that recruitment, authentication, adherence and retention can be similar to those in a traditional setting (McAlindon, Formica, Kabbara, LaValley, and Lehmer, 2003).

The randomised controlled trial (RCT) (Todd, Jones, Hart, and Lobban, Under Review) compared 122 participants with a diagnosis of BD. Participants were randomised to either treatment as usual (TAU) or TAU plus the Living with Bipolar (LWB) intervention.

Thetrial ran for six months, outcome assessed at three and six months, delivered online with no face to face interaction between the research team and the participants. Participants were contacted primarily through email and the telephone was used for non-responders. Incentives of extended intervention use for the intervention group were offered and a waiting list control group (WLC) was used to incentivise TAU participants. Feasibility was assessed through recruitment, adherence and drop out statistics.

The study over-recruited with 122 of the original target of 100 consenting to take part in the trial, potentially demonstrating a substantial interest in the treatment modality. Retention rates were amongst the highest in the web-based intervention literature (Melville, Casey, and Kavanagh, 2010) and higher than the most recent trial of a web based intervention for BD (Smith et al., 2010). 88% of participants in the intervention group and 92% of participants in the WLC group remained in the trial. This challenges the conventional wisdom that drop outs are "a natural and typical feature" of intervention interventions (Eysenbach, 2005) even amongst participants with a 'severe and enduring' mental health problem.

Acceptability was assessed through website usage statistics and a specifically designed user satisfaction scale. On average, participants engaged with 60% of the programme and the feedback was positive with 92% of participants finding the content positive, and 81% finding the interface positive. Participants engaged with this programme more than any other online approach in the literature in their use of the modules (Smith et al., 2011; Nicholas et al., 2010).

The potential clinical effectiveness, determined by estimating effect sizes was measured through a range of psychological outcome measures delivered at three and six month time points. The primary effectiveness outcome was quality of life and the secondary effectiveness outcomes were symptom severity, social functioning and recovery. The descriptive statistics indicated that participants accessing LWB improved on all the outcomes, apart from 'activation', compared to those receiving TAU. Even after an 'extreme''missing not at random' analyses a number of treatment effects were of a medium effect size on physical and psychological quality of life, wellbeing and recovery; suggesting some robust treatment effects. These effects are not likely to be the consequence of increased medication or service use, as these reduced on average for the treatment group and increased on average for the WLC group. The reason 'activation' failed to improve may be because (hypo)manic symptoms are difficult to address in a self-management intervention or that alternative self-report measures are required to identify change. Interestingly, the only other published web-based BD intervention focusses solely on the chronic depressive features of the disorder so this finding cannot be compared (Smith et al., 2011).

The process measures were cognitive outcome, self-management response, service and medication use. The descriptive statistics of the process measures indicated that a number of psychological mechanisms may be moderating the treatment effect, including illness perceptions, self-efficacy, stigma, coping strategies for mania and depression. It is likely that the online peer support forum interacts with the intervention to improve treatment response. These results are encouraging when compared to a similar trial (Smith et al., 2011) which did not demonstrate an improvement in quality of life outcome. These differences could be explained by both differences with the interventions theoretical orientation and the methodological limitations. Theoretically, the 'Living with Bipolar' (LWB) intervention focussed on improving quality of life rather than improving symptoms, through recovery informed intervention. Participants' access to the intervention was not structured and there was an emphasis on self-directed support. Methodologically, this trial is significantly larger with a higher retention rate and the majority of participants were recruited online with an interest in this approach.

We recognise that self-management interventions are not the answer to everyone's problems, and even with the best support, they may require more intensive intervention. This limitation is dependent on how computerised interventions are delivered. If provided as a choice in a range of intervention, service users will not be in the position of receiving inappropriate levels of intervention. There is understandably ambience in the clinical community about the use and efficacy of computerised and web-based interventions (Perle et al., 2012; Young and Ensing, 1999). Some of these concerns surround around the worry that computers will replace face-to-face interventions (Barak and Grohol, 2011).

However, others consider whether such interventions are without their risks. Although such therapies have been considered "low risk" and "safe" in some studies, this problem has yet to be systematically investigated (Gibbons et al., 2009). Although one of the major advantages of computerised therapies is how easily they can be accessed, there may be unintended effects of providing them to everyone across the spectrum of severity without supervision. People may rely heavily on the intervention; poor outcome may be unmanaged and may affect their engagement in further intervention (Carroll and Rounsaville, 2010). The other side of this argument is whether it is ethical to withhold potentially effective treatments from individuals because of the unknown effects which may not exist.

## The Potential Impact of Intervention Acceptability and Trial Methodology on Participant Engagement and Therapeutic Outcome

Acceptability has been linked to improved engagement and outcome in previous approaches (Nicholas et al., 2010). In-depth qualitative evaluations of service user experience are recommended alongside randomised trials to inform future development of these interventions (Kaltenthaler et al., 2008). These studies are important to investigate reasons for lack of adherence, high dropout rates (Barak, Hen, Boniel-Nissim, and Shapira, 2008) and the mechanisms of change in online interventions (Bendelin et al., 2011). The final qualitative study investigated how participants use an online therapy programme for BD, how acceptable it is and potential change processes (Todd, Jones, and Lobban, In Submission). Participants were purposively sampled providing the views of distinct groups of intervention users to gain valuable insights into the therapeutic process.

In terms of use, participants beliefs about the intervention not being recovery focussed(odd, et al., 2012a), acute symptoms (Nicholas et al., 2010), periods of stability (Proudfoot et al., 2009) and life events taking up time (Todd, et al., 2012b) all impacted on engagement and drop out from the intervention. Participants were motivated by the quality of the content (Proudfoot et al., 2004). However, their use was mood dependent. Participants dipped in and out and accessed modules as and when required (Christensen et al., 2006). Participants decided for themselves which modules were important (Andersson et al., 2011). Support from the peer support forum and prompting emails was related to continued engagement for some participants but a burden for others (Gerhards et al., 2011). Participants used the intervention for one of two things; as a reminder of the techniques learnt in therapy (Bell, 2007) or as a resource for the newly diagnosed (Proudfoot et al., 2007). Acceptability wise, participants found the intervention accessible, practical (Bendelin et al., 2011) and recovery focused, with a flexible interface allowing participants to take responsibility for their wellness (Mead and Copeland, 2000;Todd, et al., 2012b). Participants left the intervention with a less threatening view of their condition (Broadbent, Petrie, Main, and Weinman, 2006; Pollack and Aponte, 2001) and more confidence to take control (Lorig et al., 2001), which meant they used more mood management techniques and changed the way they used services (Leventhal, Leventhal, and Contrada, 1998). Therapeutic gains included improved stability, accessing additional help from friends and family, less reliance on services and more likely to turn to self-management (Lam et al., 2003). These gains were evidenced not just in participants who completed the entire intervention, but also in those who had selected modules important to their needs (Anderrson et al., 2011).

However, some participant's therapeutic gains were to a lesser extent, for instance, seeking more help from services, which may be because they didn't engage well enough in the intervention or their acute symptoms prevented engagement. The peer support forum formed a significant part of the intervention, reducing loneliness, normalising experience and making links with material. This resourse was used significantly more than other similar interventions (Smith et al., 2011). These findings may provide support for the theoretical model underpinning online interventions, which predicts that website use leads to behaviour change via various mechanisms of change and that these behaviour changes result in symptom improvement, maintained through relapse prevention (Ritterband, Thorndike, Cox, Kovatchev, and Gonder-Frederick, 2009; Webb, Joseph, Yardley, and Michie, 2010). Methodological reasons have been cited for lack of engagement with previous approaches (Smith et al., 2011). Trials conducted in 'mild to moderate' depression have reported attrition rates as high as 50% with limited predictors of drop out but theorised to be related to both trial design and the acceptability of the intervention (Christensen, Griffiths, and Farrer, 2009).

This was the first randomised controlled trial (RCT) in 'severe' mental health to be conducted online with other similar trials in 'severe' mental health populations yet to report final results (e.g. Barnes et al., 2007; Proudfoot et al., 2007), one of these trials has reported some problems retaining participants interest in the control arm (Proudfoot et al., 2007). Face to face trials of online interventions in 'severe' mental health (e.g. Pitkänen et al., 2012; Rotondi et al., 2010; Smith et al., 2011)have reported lower attrition rates than in the current online trials, but still below the evidence based medicine cut off (Fewtrell et al., 2008) and Smith et al. (2011) reported problems enrolling participants. It is possible that the trial methodology used in the 'Living with Bipolar' (LWB) trial may have improved the levels of engagement. The mixture of recruitment methods led to significant interest in the project. Methods where the research team could engage with participants were the most useful, such as internet discussion groups (Bull, Lloyd, Rietmeijer, and McFarlane, 2004). The participants were representative of other BD internet treatment trials and other large scale trials in BD (Smith et al., 2011). Participants engaged with the treatment despite no face to face motivation apart from emails and a peer support forum (Bell, 2007). These methods were used more than in similar trials who reported less attention and engagement (Smith et al., 2011). People who engaged with the treatment engaged with the methodology, whereas non engagers in treatment dropped out of the trial. A separate registration and consent procedure may have been equivalent to a 'trial run in period' (Pablos-Méndez, Barr, and Shea, 1998) in maintaining participants with the most interest. We identified 50% of participants dropping out before consent and in other web-based trials 50% drop-out during the trial (Christensen, 2009).

## Contribution of the Current Research to Academic Theory

The current research makes a number of contributions to the current theoretical background around the treatment of Bipolar Disorder (BD) and online interventions in mental health. The research provides a theoretical framework for combining recovery in self-management interventions delivered online, which promotes individual control rather than professional reliance and personal meaningful outcome rather than symptomatic outcome. There is now evidence that self-management can be delivered in a way which is consistent with the individual (Anthony, 1993) and combination between individual and professionals (Buchanan-Barker and Barker, 2006). This may provide a useful framework to delivering the therapeutic techniques from traditional CBT (e.g. Lam et al., 2003) and psycho-education (e.g. Colom and Vieta, 2009; Perry et al., 1999) models in a way which is consistent with the recovery model (Anthony, 1993). The research provides early evidence that the therapeutic gains from an online approach may be similar to those seen in some of the face to face CBT trials; such as improved stability, accessing more help, less reliance on services and using more self-management (Lam et al., 2003). However, one trial of CBT in BD suggests that CBT may only be effective for those with fewer mood episodes (Scott et al., 2006). Additional findings suggest that providing self-management in a recovery framework may prevent hyper-vigilance which has been related to other self-management approaches in BD (Mansell et al., 2011).

The existing model for understanding how and why online interventions provide therapeutic benefit suggests that website use is linked to behaviour change, which results in symptom improvement and relapse prevention (Ritterband et al., 2006). The results in this study provide support and further additions to this model. They suggest that behaviour change may have been promoted through participants developing a less threatening view of their illness, and increased confidence in their ability to cope with their condition (Todd, et al., In Submission). This is consistent with the self-regulation model which suggests service users interpretation of their health predicts the way they decide to cope which is related to outcome (Leventhal et al., 1998; Lorig et al., 2001). At this stage no causal relationships between the variables can be assumed. Crucially however service users did not need to access the entire content of the online intervention to improve (Todd, et al., Under Review). This adds support for the idea that participants may be able to decide for themselves which modules are important to use to produce the maximum benefit for themselves (Anderrson et al., 2011). There is some evidence that participants use these interventions as a reminder of previously learnt techniques (Bell, 2007) or as a resource for the newly diagnosed (Proudfoot et al., 2007). There is also the possibility of non-specific factors in online interventions (Hurling et al., 2006). The most likely in this study was the inclusion of peer support (Todd, et al., Under Review).

The online forum was a significantly utilised addition to website content and improved engagement with the modules (Gerhards et al., 2011). This 'Living with Bipolar' (LWB) project suggests that online interventions may not be completely distinct from face-to-face intervention.

There is further support for the idea that the barriers to the using of online interventions may be similar to face-to-face approaches (Nicholas et al., 2010; Proudfoot et al., 2009). Internet interventions may not always be related to limited engagement and high dropout rates (Eysenbach, 2005). This study provides an additional contribution to methodological theory. Online randomised controlled trials may be a useful way to assess internet interventions in 'severe and enduring' mental health. Motivational research prompts, peer support (Bell, 2007) and a trial 'run in period' (Pablos-Mendez et al., 1998) may be crucial for ensuring high levels of retention and engagement.

## Contribution of the Current Research to Clinical Practice

The 'Living with Bipolar' (LWB) research makes it's most substantial contributions to clinical practice. The most significant is that online self-management may be a feasible, acceptable and clinical effective intervention for people with Bipolar Disorder (BD). Online intervention may be another form of evidence based psychological intervention that can be delivered to a number of people with BD (NICE, 2006). This is a particularly useful finding considering the amount of people needing psychological services will always outstrip demands (Kazdin and Blase, 2011), and there is often limited support for self-management in secondary care mental health services. This finding is particular timely as the improving access to psychological therapies initiative (IAPT) begins trials in 'severe' mental health (IAPT, 2013). This raises questions about how online intervention should be used in 'severe' populations. In 'mild to moderate' depression and anxiety it is delivered as a first step in the treatment pathway (NICE, 2011). This may not be the most useful approach in 'severe' mental health or secondary care mental health services, where people are living alongside their difficulties for many years. Online interventions may instead be one intervention in a series of interventions which service users can move flexibility between, depending on their level of need. This fits with how service users described using the approach in the LWB project. The headline finding has wider implications. It suggests that the traditional challenges to delivering self-management to a 'severe' mental illness population such as engagement, drop out and hyper-vigilance may be averted through delivering therapeutic principles in a recovery framework, on a flexible interface with facilitated peer support. It provides early evidence that recovery focussed CBT and psycho-educational self-management packages may be acceptable and effective form of psychological intervention in BD. This is consistent with recovery focussed approaches being considered a priority for some service users (Mead and Copeland, 2000). In line with this the intervention was most useful for improving non-symptomatic outcomes such as quality of life, recovery and wellbeing. These packages may therefore provide a useful alternative to the symptom focussed approaches currently in the literature. There may not be a need to structure this material heavily (Smith et al., 2011) or support to a higher level (Barnes et al., 2007). This is a useful finding considering that recovery focussed services and approaches are one of the key priorities for the modernisation of mental health (HM Government, 2009).

## Limitations of the Current Research

The systematic review (Todd et al., In Submission-b) is limited in its scope as it only considered published studies which were in English language. No formal statistical analysis of effectiveness or the components which relate to outcome was possible due to the heterogeneity in the studies and the lack of available studies in the Bipolar Disorder (BD) and Psychosis literature. The qualitative phases (Todd et al., 2012a; Todd et al., 2012b, In Submission) share a number of limitations. The qualitative nature of these studies means that valid generalisations cannot be made based on the results. Studies 2 and 3 were a subset analysis based on a series of focus groups and study 6 used purposive sampling method to select intervention users. Ideally separate in-depth qualitative studies would have been performed allowing for greater diversity and depth. All of these studies were not representative of those living with BD in terms of geography and cultural differences. Participants were likely to be interested in the online research approach, had varying levels of knowledge about psychological intervention and there was no formal assessment of diagnosis or current symptoms. These factors could have impacted on the results. There is no way of knowing how far the results generalise to members of the general population not ultilising using the 'Living with Bipolar' intervention.

The randomised controlled trial (RCT) (Todd et al., Under Review) was a feasibly study, not designed for hypothesis testing and requires replication. The trial made no attempt to examine post investigation follow-up or economic impact. The diagnostic screen relied exclusively on self-report and was not independently verified. Participants were randomised before completing the baseline questionnaires which could have impacted how they completed the questionnaires. We cannot be sure that there were no predictors of drop out. Contamination between arms was possible without internet protocol address restriction. There was no measurement of participants' computer literacy which could have affected participants' ability to use the intervention. It is unclear how much effect the personal emails from the researcher and the personalised forum moderation had on outcome. The findings may not be generalisable to those who do not routinely use the internet to access self-help.

The intervention was designed as a low intensity intervention to be useful for a large number of people with BD. However, there are those who need a greater level of input and this approach cannot replace high intensity, structured psychological interventions. There are specific groups of people with BD who may benefit from more specific interventions, for instance, people with a recent vs. established diagnosis and those who rapid cycle. The current intervention was a pilot intervention and lacked the interactivity expected by some participants. The methodology described (Todd, Hart, Jones, and Lobban, In Submission-a) in this paper does not necessarily generalise to recruiting offline or to people who do not use the internet for self-help. The methodological strengths are based on a relatively small sample size. If this trial was to be extended careful consideration of the researcher to participant ratio may be needed to ensure the same high retention and engagement rates. There is currently no ethical consensus on the use of online informed consent which would need to be considered in future trials.

## Future Directions of the Current Research

There are a number of future directions the intervention evaluated and new interventions in the area could take based on the findings of the current research. Although increasing support may be contrary to the self-management approach (Cook, 2004), motivational interviewing may be useful for participants who have problematic beliefs about the intervention and treatment approach (e.g. Andersson and Cuijpers, 2009; Simpson et al., 2009). This research has demonstrated that future interventions focussed on recovery need to give participants choice of different components in order to take responsibility for their own wellness(Davidson, 2005). Completing interventions at participants own pace is a common advantage of the online approach (Bendelin et al., 2011; Gerhards et al., 2011), but not always done in this population, with some interventions giving access to modules in a supervised fashion (e.g. Smith et al., 2011; Barnes et al., 2010). Improvements to the pitch, level and target group of the intervention were suggested (Nicholas et al., 2010). A 'one stop shop' approach to content (Andersson et al., 2005), and from a technical point of view improved interactivity in line with other interventions (e.g. Smith et al., 2011). Taken to its extreme online clinical formulation is possible in web-based interventions (e.g. Copeland and Martin, 2004) and may be a useful direction. Improved interactivity with material has been linked to greater acceptability (Gerhards et al., 2011), and important for therapeutic outcome (Clarke et al., 2005; Hurling, Fairley, and Dias, 2006)

These findings have identified that structured support may be required alongside complex interventions, however, there is currently no consensus confirming either harm or benefit of online communities in mental health (Eysenbach, Powell, Englesakis, Rizo, and Stern, 2004), which would be useful to formally evaluate. The trial design, particularly the use of a waiting list control arm (WLC) instead of treatment as usual (TAU), the comprehensive retention procedure and incentives offered to participants were particularly successful at ensuring participant engagement and retention. The online RCT may provide a feasible way to effectively and efficiently evaluate online interventions in 'severe' mental health. However, it may not be possible to conduct these trials entirely online and the successful outcomes in this trial may be down to a combination of methods recommended for future trials.

A number of recommendations are suggested for the future development of this methodology which could be independently assessed to identify the most important factor. Questionnaires and demands asked of participants may need to be piloted, as there is the danger that too many outcome assessments can distress participants and cause drop out. Participants may need to be pro-actively recruited making use of a trial "run in period" (Eysenbach, 2002). Combining diagnostic screening measures or using a telephone method may improve validity (Revicki et al., 1997) and even engagement (Paul, Seib, and Prescott, 2005). Randomising participants at the same time may facilitate support from the research team. Support from the research team, particularly at the start of the trial, considering the same researcher may foster a therapeutic relationship (Sucala et al., 2012) and improve participants' motivation towards the trial methodology. Fostering this positive, motivation and supportive relationship with participants in both groups with strict guidelines throughput the trial may be important. The availability of an online community and motivational email prompts may be important for improving engagement with the intervention.

In terms of unanswered questions,a statistically powered, hypothesis testing trial is needed to assess the clinical and cost effectiveness of the LWB intervention. This research provides the data needed for this to be conducted. This trial should focus on the evaluation of quality of life and recovery as the primary outcomes over medium to long term. Dropouts are unlikely to be at random and so need careful consideration. Future studies should focus on the mechanisms of change and how important the online community and researcher prompts are to the successfulness of this intervention. The investigation of the generalizability of this approach for people in traditional NHS settings, not routinely accessing the internet for self-help, and the consideration of potential clinical risks would support translation of the intervention into practice.

## Overall Conclusions

This project has contributed to both academic theory and clinical practice. There is now preliminary evidence that the web-based treatment approach in BD is feasible, acceptable and potentially effective. This success may be due to the acceptability with the recovery focussed treatment approach, improvements in the online randomised controlled trial methodology or a combination of both of these factors. Future research needs to focus on the mechanisms of change in this intervention and the impact of the methodology on outcome. These findings have implications for the future development of web-based interventions in Bipolar Disorder and the use of online randomised controlled trials in 'severe and enduring' populations. Web-based interventions could be part of the improving access to psychological therapies (IAPT) initiative which is currently being extended into 'severe' mental health.

# References

Adams, J., and Scott, J. (2000). Predicting medication adherence in severe mental disorders. *Acta. Psychiatrica Scandinavica,* 101, 119-124.

Andersson, G., Bergström, J., Holländare, F., Carlbring, P., Kaldo, V., and Ekselius, L. (2005). Internet-based self-help for depression: randomised controlled trial. *The British Journal of Psychiatry,* 187(5), 456-461.

Andersson, G., and Cuijpers, P. (2009). Internet-based and other computerized psychological treatments for adult depression: a meta-analysis. *Cognitive Behaviour Therapy,* 38(4), 196-205.

Andersson, G., Estling, F., Jakobsson, E., Cuijpers, P., and Carlbring, P. (2011). Can the Patient Decide Which Modules to Endorse? An Open Trial of Tailored Internet Treatment of Anxiety Disorders. *Cognitive Behaviour Therapy,* 40(1), 57-64.

Anthony, W. A. (1993). Recovery from mental illness: the guiding vision of the mental health service system in the 1990s. *Psychosocial Rehabilitation Journal,* (16), 11-23.

Bados, A., Balaguer, G., and Saldaña, C. (2007). The efficacy of cognitive–behavioral therapy and the problem of drop-out. *Journal of Clinical Psychology,* 63(6), 585-592.

Barak, A., and Grohol, J. M. (2011). Current and Future Trends in Internet-Supported Mental Health Interventions. *Journal of Technology in Human Services,* 29(3), 155-196.

Barak, A., Hen, L., Boniel-Nissim, M., and Shapira, N. a. (2008). A Comprehensive Review and a Meta-Analysis of the Effectiveness of Internet-Based Psychotherapeutic Interventions. *Journal of Technology in Human Services,* 26(2-4), 109-160.

Barnes, C., Harvey, R., Mitchell, P., Smith, M., and Wilhelm, K. (2007). Evaluation of an online relapse prevention program for bipolar disorder: an overview of the aims and methodology of a randomized controlled trial. *Disease Management and Health Outcomes,* 15(4), 215-224.

Beck, A. T., Rush, A. J., Shaw, B. F., and Emery, G. (1987). Cognitive therapy of depression: The Guilford Press.

Bell, V. (2007). Online information, extreme communities and internet therapy: Is the internet good for our mental health? *Journal of Mental Health,* 16(4), 445-457.

Bendelin, N., Hesser, H., Dahl, J., Carlbring, P., Nelson, K. Z., and Andersson, G. (2011). Experiences of guided Internet-based cognitive-behavioural treatment for depression: A qualitative study. *BMC Psychiatry,* 11(1), 107.

Bird, A. (2006). We Need to Talk: The case for Psychological Therapy on the NHS. Accessed online: http://www.mind.org.uk/campaigns_and_issues/report_and_resources/899_we_need_to_talk.

Broadbent, E., Petrie, K. J., Main, J., and Weinman, J. (2006). The Brief Illness Perception Questionnaire. *Journal of Psychosomatic Research,* 60(6), 631-637.

Buchanan-Barker, P., and Barker, P. J. (2006). The ten commitments: a value base for mental health recovery. *Journal of Psychosocial Nursing and Mental Health Services,* 44(9), 29.

Bull, S., Lloyd, L., Rietmeijer, C., and McFarlane, M. (2004). Recruitment and retention of an online sample for an HIV prevention intervention targeting men who have sex with men: the smart sex quest project. *AIDS Care,* 16(8), 931-943.

Byrne, P. (2000). Stigma of mental illness and ways of diminishing it. *Adv Psychiatr Treat, 6*(1), 65-72.

Carroll, K. M., and Rounsaville, B. J. (2010). Computer-assisted therapy in psychiatry: be brave—it'sa new world. *Current psychiatry reports,* 12(5), 426-432.

Castle, D. J., Berk, L., Lauder, S., Berk, M., and Murray, G. (2009). Psychosocial interventions for bipolar disorder. *Acta Neuropsychiatrica,* 21(6), 275-284.

Chan, D. (2009). So why ask me? Are self report data really that bad? In Charles E. Lance and Robert J. Vandenberg (Eds.), Statistical and methodological myths and urban legends: Doctrine, verity and fable in the organizational and social sciences (pp309-335). New York, NY: Routledge.

Christensen, H., Griffiths, K. M., and Farrer, L. (2009). Adherence in internet interventions for anxiety and depression. *Journal Of Medical Internet Research,* 11(2), e13.

Clarke, G., Eubanks, D., Reid, C. K., O'Connor, E., DeBar, L. L., Lynch, F., Gullion, C. (2005). Overcoming Depression on the Internet (ODIN)(2): a randomized trial of a self-help depression skills program with reminders. *Journal of Medical Internet Research,* 7(2).

Colom, F., and Vieta, E. (2006). Psychoeducation Manual for Bipolar Disorder. Cambridge: Cambridge University Press.

Cook, J. (2004). Mental illness self-management through wellness recovery action planning. *Mental Health Recovery Newsletter,* 5(3), 6-7.

Copeland, J., and Martin, G. (2004). Web-based interventions for substance use disorders: a qualitative review. *Journal of Substance Abuse Treatment,* 26(2), 109-116.

Davidson, L. (2005). Recovery, self management and the expert patient-Changing the culture of mental health from a UK perspective. *Journal of Mental Health,* 14(1), 25-35.

De Graaf, L., Gerhards, S., Arntz, A., Riper, H., Metsemakers, J., Evers, S., Huibers, M. (2009). Clinical effectiveness of online computerised cognitive–behavioural therapy without support for depression in primary care: randomised trial. *The British Journal of Psychiatry,* 195(1), 73-80.

De Graaf, L., Gerhards, S., Arntz, A., Riper, H., Metsemakers, J., Evers, S., Huibers, M. (2011). One-year follow-up results of unsupported online computerized cognitive behavioural therapy for depression in primary care: A randomized trial. *Journal of behavior therapy and experimental psychiatry,* 42(1), 89-95.

DoH. (2003). Self-help interventions for mental health problems: Expert Briefing. . Accessed online:http://www.dh.gov.uk/en/Publicationsandstatistics/Publications/PublicationsPolicyAndGuidance/DH_4125793. Department of Health.

DoH. (2005). Self care - A real choice: Self care support - A practical option Accessed online: http://www.dh.gov.uk/en/Publicationsandstatistics/Publications/PublicationsPolicyAndGuidance/DH_4100717. Department of Health.

Exell, J. (2007). Recovery: Poem. Accessed online: http://www.voicesforum.org.uk/rec2007.htm.

Eysenbach. (2002). Issues in evaluating health websites in an Internet-based randomized controlled trial. *J. Med. Internet. Res.,* 4(3), e17.

Eysenbach. (2005). The law of attrition. *Journal of medical Internet research,* 7 (11), Eysenbach, Powell, J., Englesakis, M., Rizo, C., and Stern, A. (2004). Health related virtual communities and electronic support groups: systematic review of the effects of online peer to peer interactions. *BMJ,* 328(7449), 1166.

Fewtrell, M. S., Kennedy, K., Singhal, A., Martin, R. M., Ness, A., Hadders-Algra, M., Lucas, A. (2008). How much loss to follow-up is acceptable in long-term randomised trials and prospective studies? *Archives of Disease in Childhood,* 93(6), 458-461.

Formica, M., Kabbara, K., Clark, R., and McAlindon, T. (2004). Can Clinical Trials Requiring Frequent Participant Contact Be Conducted Over the Internet? Results From an Online Randomized Controlled Trial Evaluating a Topical Ointment for Herpes Labialis. *J. Med. Internet. Res.,* 6(1), e6.

Galvez, J. F., Thommi, S., and Ghaemi, S. N. (2011). Positive aspects of mental illness: a review in bipolar disorder. *Journal of Affective Disorders,* 128(3), 185-190.

Geddes, J. R., Burgess, S., Hawton, K., Jamison, K., and Goodwin, G. M. (2004). Long-Term Lithium Therapy for Bipolar Disorder: Systematic Review and Meta-Analysis of Randomized Controlled Trials. *Am. J. Psychiatry.,* 161(2), 217-222.

Gerhards, S. A. H., Abma, T. A., Arntz, A., de Graaf, L. E., Evers, S. M. A. A., Huibers, M. J. H., and Widdershoven, G. A. M. (2011). Improving adherence and effectiveness of computerised cognitive behavioural therapy without support for depression: A qualitative study on patient experiences. *Journal of Affective Disorders,* 129(1-3), 117-125.

Gibbons, M. C., Wilson, R. F., Samal, L., Lehmann, C. U., Dickersin, K., Lehmann, H. P., Ritu, S. (2009). Impact of consumer health informatics applications. Evid Rep Technol Assess (Full Report). (188):1-546.

Goodwin, F., K, and Jamison, K., R. (2007). Bipolar disorder and recurrent depression, 2nd edition. . Oxford University Press: New York.

Gournay. (2007). Review of free to access computerised cognitive behaviour therapy websites. British Association of Behavioural and Cognitive Psychotherapists (BABCP). Accessed online: http://kc.nmhdu.org.uk.

HM Government. (2009). New Horizons: a shared vision for mental health. Accessed online: http://www.dh.gov.uk/en/Publicationsandstatistics/Publications /PublicationsPolicyAndGuidance/DH_109705. Her Majesty's Government.

Hurling, R., Fairley, B. W., and Dias, M. B. (2006). Internet-based exercise intervention systems: Are more interactive designs better? *Psychology and Health,* 21(6), 757-772.

IAPT. (2013). Improving Access to Psychological Therapy in Severe Mental Illness. Accessed online: http://www.iapt.nhs.uk/smi-/ Improving Access to Psychological Therapy.

Isometsa, E., Suominen, K., Mantere, O., Valtonen, H., Leppamaki, S., Pippingskold, M., and Arvilommi, P. (2003). The Mood Disorder Questionnaire improves recognition of bipolar disorder in psychiatric care. *BMC Psychiatry,* 3(1), 8.

Judd, L. L., Akiskal, H. S., Schettler, P. J., Endicott, J., Maser, J., Solomon, D. A., Keller, M. B. (2002). The Long-term Natural History of the Weekly Symptomatic Status of Bipolar I Disorder. *Arch Gen Psychiatry,* 59(6), 530-537.

Kalathil, J. (2011). Recovery and Resilience. Accessed online: http://mentalhealth.org.uk/content/assets/PDF/publications/recovery_and_resilience.pdf.

Kaltenthaler, E., Parry, G., Beverley, C., and Ferriter, M. (2008). Computerised cognitive-behavioural therapy for depression: systematic review. *The British Journal of Psychiatry,* 193(3), 181-184.

Kazdin, A. E., and Blase, S. L. (2011). Rebooting Psychotherapy Research and Practice to Reduce the Burden of Mental Illness. *Perspectives on Psychological Science,* 6(1).

Keller, M. B., Levori, P. W., Coryell, W., Endicott, J., and Mueller, T. (1993). Bipolar I: A Five-Year Prospective Follow-up. *The Journal Of Nervous And Mental Disease,* 181(4), 238-245.

Kennedy, M. G., Schepp, K. G., and O'Connor, F. W. (2000). Symptom self-management and relapse in schizophrenia. *Archives of Psychiatric Nursing,* 14(6), 266-275.

Lam, Hayward, P., Watkins, E. R., Wright, K., and Sham, P. (2005). Relapse Prevention in Patients With Bipolar Disorder: Cognitive Therapy Outcome After 2 Years. *Am. J. Psychiatry,* 162, 324-329.

Lam, Jones, S. H., and Hayward, P. (2010). Cognitive therapy for bipolar disorder: a therapist's guide to concepts, methods and practiceCognitive therapy for bipolar disorder: a therapist's guide to concepts, methods and practice (2nd Edition). Wiley-Blackwell.

Lam., Watkins, E. R., Hayward, P., Bright, J., Wright, K., Kerr, N., Sham, P. (2003). A randomized controlled study of cognitive therapy for relapse prevention for bipolar affective disorder: outcome of the first year. *Archives of General Psychiatry,* 60(2), 145-152.

Learmonth, D., and Rai, S. (2007). Establishing the effectiveness of computerised cognitive behavioural therapy for secondary/tertiary mental healthcare service users with and without physical co-morbidities. *Health Psychology Update,* 16(3), 42.

Leventhal, H., Leventhal, E. A., and Contrada, R. J. (1998). Self-regulation, health, and behavior: A perceptual-cognitive approach. *Psychology and Health,* 13(4), 717-733.

Lieberman, D. Z., Swayze, S., and Goodwin, F. K. (2011). Best Practices: An Automated Internet Application to Help Patients With Bipolar Disorder Track Social Rhythm Stabilization. *Psychiatric Services,* 62(11), 1267-1269.

Lobban, F., Taylor, K., Murray, C., and Jones, S. (2012). Bipolar Disorder is a two-edged sword: a qualitative study to understand the positive edge. *Journal of Affective Disorders.*

Lorig, K. R., Ritter, P., Stewart, A. L., Sobel, D. S., William Brown, B. J., Bandura, A., Holman, H. R. (2001). Chronic Disease Self-Management Program: 2-Year Health Status and Health Care Utilization Outcomes. *Medical Care,* 39(11), 1217-1223.

MacGregor, A. D., Hayward, L., Peck, D. F., and Wilkes, P. (2009). Empirically grounded clinical interventions clients' and referrers' perceptions of computer-guided CBT (FearFighter). *Behavioural and cognitive psychotherapy,* 37(1), 1.

Mansell, W., Powell, S., Pedley, R., Thomas, N., and Jones, S. A. (2010). The process of recovery from bipolar I disorder: A qualitative analysis of personal accounts in relation to an integrative cognitive model. *British Journal of Clinical Psychology,* 49(2), 193-215.

Martyn, D. (2003). Self Management, the experiences and views of self management of people with a diagnosis of Schizophrenia. *London: Rethink.*

McAlindon, T., Formica, M., Kabbara, K., LaValley, M., and Lehmer, M. (2003). Conducting clinical trials over the internet: feasibility study. *BMJ,* 327(7413), 484-487.

McCrone, P., Dhanasiri, S., Patel, A., Knapp, M., and Lewton-Smith, S. (2008). Paying the Price, King's Fund. Accessed online: www.kingsfund.org.uk/publications.

Mead, S., and Copeland, M. E. (2000). What Recovery Means to Us: Consumers' Perspectives. *Community Mental Health Journal,* 36(3), 315-328.

Melville, K. M., Casey, L. M., and Kavanagh, D. J. (2010). Dropout from Internet-based treatment for psychological disorders. *British Journal of Clinical Psychology,* 49(4), 455-471.

Merikangas, K. R., Akiskal, H. S., Angst, J., Greenberg, P. E., Hirschfeld, R. M. A., Petukhova, M., and Kessler, R. C. (2007). Lifetime and 12-Month Prevalence of Bipolar Spectrum Disorder in the National Comorbidity Survey Replication. *Arch. Gen. Psychiatry,* 64(5), 543-552.

Meyer, B., Berger, T., Caspar, F., Beevers, C. G., Andersson, G., and Weiss, M. (2009). Effectiveness of a novel integrative online treatment for depression (Deprexis): randomized controlled trial. *Journal of Medical Internet Research,* 11(2).

Michalak, Yatham, L., Kolesar, S., and Lam, R. (2006). Bipolar Disorder and Quality of Life: A Patient-Centered Perspective. *Quality of Life Research,* 15(1), 25-37.

Michalak, Yatham, L., Maxwell, V., Hale, S., and Lam, R. (2007). The impact of bipolar disorder upon work functioning: a qualitative analysis. *Bipolar Disorders,* 9(1-2), 126-143.

Miklowitz, D. J., Otto, M. W., Frank, E., Reilly-Harrington, N. A., Wisniewski, S. R., Kogan, J. N., Sachs, G. S. (2007). Psychosocial treatments for bipolar depression: A 1-year randomized trial from the Systematic Treatment Enhancement Program. *Archives of General Psychiatry,* 64(4), 419-427.

Morriss, R., Faizal Mohammad, A., Jones Ashley, P., Williamson Paula, R., Bolton Catherine, A., and McCarthy James, P. (2007). Interventions for helping people recognise early signs of recurrence in bipolar disorder. Cochrane Database of Systematic Reviews,(1). Retrieved from http://www.mrw.interscience.wiley.com/cochrane/clsysrev/articles/CD004854/frame.html

Murray, C. J. L., and Lopez, A. D. (1997). Global mortality, disability, and the contribution of risk factors: Global Burden of Disease Study. *The Lancet,* 349(9063), 1436-1442.

NICE. (2006a). Bipolar Disorder: The management of bipolar disorder in adults, children and adolescents, in primary and secondary care. Accessed online: http://guidance.nice.org.uk/index.jsp?action=byIdando=10989andhistory=t. National Institute of Clinical Excellence.

NICE. (2006b). Depression and anxiety - computerised cognitive behavioural therapy (CCBT). Accessed online: http://guidance.nice.org.uk/TA97. National Institute of Clinical Excellence.

NICE. (2009). Depression in adults: The treatment and management of depression in adults. Accessed online: http://publications.nice.org.uk/depression-in-adults-cg90. National Insitute of Clinical Excellence.

NICE. (2011). Generalised anxiety disorder and panic disorder (with or without agoraphobia) in adults: Management in primary, secondary and community care Accessed online: http://publications.nice.org.uk/generalised-anxiety-disorder-and-panic-disorder-with-or-without-agoraphobia-in-adults-cg113. National Institute of Clinical Excellence.

Nicholas, J., Proudfoot, J., Parker, G., Gillis, I., Burckhardt, R., Manicavasagar, V., and Smith, M. (2010). The ins and outs of an online bipolar education program: a study of program attrition. *Journal of Medical Internet Research,* 12(5), e57-e57.

Pablos-Méndez, A., Barr, R. G., and Shea, S. (1998). Run-in periods in randomized trials. *JAMA: The Journal of the American Medical Association,* 279(3), 222-225.

Paul, J., Seib, R., and Prescott, T. (2005). The Internet and Clinical Trials: Background, Online Resources, Examples and Issues. *J. Med. Internet. Res.,* 7(1), e5.

Perle, J. G., Langsam, L. C., Randel, A., Lutchman, S., Levine, A. B., Odland, A. P., Marker, C. D. (2012). Attitudes Toward Psychological Telehealth: Current and Future Clinical Psychologists' Opinions of Internet Based Interventions. *Journal of Clinical Psychology,* 69(1):100-13.

Perlick, D. A., Rosenheck, R. A., Clarkin, J. F., Sirey, J. A., Salahi, J., Struening, E. L., and Link, B. G. (2001). Stigma as a Barrier to Recovery: Adverse Effects of Perceived Stigma on Social Adaptation of Persons Diagnosed With Bipolar Affective Disorder. *Psychiatr. Serv.,* 52(12), 1627-1632.

Perry, A., Tarrier, N., Morriss, R., McCarthy, E., and Limb, K. (1999). Randomised controlled trial of efficacy of teaching patients with bipolar disorder to identify early symptoms of relapse and obtain treatment. [Article]. *British Medical Journal,* 318(7177), 149-153.

Pitkänen, A., Välimäki, M., Kuosmanen, L., Katajisto, J., Koivunen, M., Hätönen, H., Knapp, M. (2012). Patient education methods to support quality of life and functional ability among patients with schizophrenia: a randomised clinical trial. *Quality of Life Research,* 21(2), 247-256.

Pollack, L. E., and Aponte, M. (2001). Patients' perceptions of their bipolar illness in a public hospital setting. *Psychiatric Quarterly,* 72(2), 167-179.

Powell, J., and Clarke, A. (2006). Internet information-seeking in mental health. *The British Journal of Psychiatry,* 189(3), 273-277.

Proudfoot, Parker, G., Hyett, M., Manicavasagar, V., Smith, M., Grdovic, S., and Greenfield, L. (2007). Next generation of self-management education: Web-based bipolar disorder program. *Australian and New Zealand Journal of Psychiatry,* 41(11), 903-909.

Proudfoot, Parker, G. B., Benoit, M., Manicavasagar, V., Smith, M., and Gayed, A. (2009). What happens after diagnosis? Understanding the experiences of patients with newlydiagnosed bipolar disorder. *Health Expectations,* 12(2), 120-129.

Proudfoot, Ryden, C., Everitt, B., Shapiro, D. A., Goldberg, D., Mann, A., Gray, J. A. (2004). Clinical efficacy of computerised cognitive–behavioural therapy for anxiety and depression in primary care: randomised controlled trial. *The British Journal of Psychiatry,* 185(1), 46-54.

Purves, D. G., Bennett, M., and Wellman, N. (2009). An Open Trial in the NHS of Blues Begone (R): A New Home Based Computerized CBT Program. *Behavioural and Cognitive Psychotherapy, 37*(5), 541.

Reavley, N. J., Mackinnon, A. J., Morgan, A. J., Alvarez-Jimenez, M., Hetrick, S. E., Killackey, E., Jorm, A. F. (2012). Quality of information sources about mental disorders: a comparison of Wikipedia with centrally controlled web and printed sources. *Psychological Medicine,* 42(08), 1753-1762.

Revicki, D. A., Tohen, M., Gyulai, L., Thompson, C., Pike, S., Davis-Vogel, A., and Zarate, C. (1997). Telephone versus In-Person Clinical and Health Status Assessment Interviews in Patients with Bipolar Disorder. *Harvard Review of Psychiatry,* 5(2), 75-81.

Ritterband, L. M., Thorndike, F. P., Cox, D. J., Kovatchev, B. P., and Gonder-Frederick, L. A. (2009). A behavior change model for internet interventions. *Annals of Behavioral Medicine,* 38(1), 18-27.

Roberts, G., and Wolfson, P. (2004). The rediscovery of recovery: open to all. *Adv Psychiatr Treat,* 10(1), 37-48.

Robinson, J. P., Neustadtl, A., and Kestenbaum, M. (2002). Why public opinion polls are inherently biased: Public opinion differences among Internet users and non-users. Paper presented at the annual meeting of the American Association for Public Opinion Research, St. Petersburg Beach, Florida.

Rothbaum, B. O., and Astin, M. C. (2000). Integration of pharmacotherapy and psychotherapy for bipolar disorder. *Journal of Clinical Psychiatry,* 61, 68-75.

Rotondi, A. J., Anderson, C. M., Haas, G. L., Eack, S. M., Spring, M. B., Ganguli, R., Rosenstock, J. (2010). Web-Based Psychoeducational Intervention for Persons With Schizophrenia and Their Supporters: One-Year Outcomes. *Psychiatric Services,* 61(11).

Russell, S. J., and Browne, J. L. (2005). Staying well with bipolar disorder. *Australian and New Zealand Journal of Psychiatry,* 39(3), 187-193.

Scott, J., Paykel, E., Morriss, R., Bentall, R., Kinderman, P., Johnson, T., Hayhurst, H. (2006). Cognitive-behavioural therapy for severe and recurrent bipolar disorders: Randomised controlled trial. *The British Journal of Psychiatry,* 188(4), 313-320.

Simpson, S., Barnes, E., Griffiths, E., Hood, K., Cohen, D., Craddock, N., Smith, D. (2009). The Bipolar Interactive Psychoeducation (BIPED) study: trial design and protocol. *BMC Psychiatry,* 9(1), 50.

Smith, D. J., Griffiths, E., Poole, R., di Florio, A., Barnes, E., Kelly, M. J., Simpson, S. (2011). Beating Bipolar: exploratory trial of a novel internet-based psychoeducational treatment for bipolar disorder. *Bipolar Disorders,* 13(5-6), 571-577.

Spek, V., Cuijpers, P., Cek, I., Riper, H., Keyzer, J., and Pop, V. (2007). Internet-based cognitive behaviour therapy for symptoms of depression and anxiety: a meta-analysis. *Psychological Medicine,* 37(03), 319-328.

Sucala, M., Schnur, J. B., Constantino, M. J., Miller, S. J., Brackman, E. H., and Montgomery, G. H. (2012). The Therapeutic Relationship in E-Therapy for Mental Health: A Systematic Review. *Journal of medical Internet research,* 14(4).

Todd, N. J., Hart, A., Jones, S., and Lobban, F. (In Submission-a). Conducting a randomised controlled trial online in a severe mental health population: feasibility and recommendations for practice.

Todd, N. J., Jones, S. H., Hart, A., and Lobban, F. A. (Under Review). A web-based self-management intervention for Bipolar Disorder 'Living with Bipolar': a feasibility randomised controlled trial.

Todd, N. J., Jones, S. H., and Lobban, F. A. (2012a). "Recovery" in bipolar disorder: how can service users be supported through a self-management intervention? A qualitative focus group study. *Journal of Mental Health,* 21(2), 114-126.

Todd, N. J., Jones, S. H., and Lobban, F. A. (2012b). What Do Service Users with Bipolar Disorder Want from a Web-Based Self-Management Intervention? A Qualitative Focus Group Study. Clinical Psychology and Psychotherapy.

Todd, N. J., Jones, S. H., and Lobban, F. A. (In Submission ). The use, acceptability and change in 'Living with Bipolar' a web-based self-management intervention for Bipolar Disorder: a qualitative interview study.

Todd, N. J., Solis-Trapala, I., Jones, S. H., and Lobban, F. A. (2012c). An online randomised controlled trial to assess the feasibility, acceptability and potential effectiveness of 'Living with Bipolar': A web-based self-management intervention for Bipolar Disorder: Trial design and protocol. *Contemporary Clinical Trials,* 33(4), 679-688.

Todd, N. J., Solis-Trapala, I., Jones, S. H., and Lobban, F. A. (In Submission-b). Effectiveness and essential components of computerised psychosocial interventions for Mood and Psychotic Disorders: a Systematic Review.

Vernmark, K., Lenndin, J., Bjärehed, J., Carlsson, M., Karlsson, J., Öberg, J., Andersson, G. (2010). Internet administered guided self-help versus individualized e-mail therapy: A randomized trial of two versions of CBT for major depression. *Behaviour Research and Therapy,* 48(5), 368.

Webb, T. L., Joseph, J., Yardley, L., and Michie, S. (2010). Using the internet to promote health behavior change: a systematic review and meta-analysis of the impact of theoretical basis, use of behavior change techniques, and mode of delivery on efficacy. *Journal of Medical Internet Research,* 12(1).

Wiersma, J. E., Titov, N., Van Schaik, D. J., Van Oppen, P., Beekman, A. T., Cuijpers, P., and Andrews, G. A. (2011). Treating chronic symptoms of depression in the virtual clinic: findings on chronicity of depression in patients treated with internet-based computerized cognitive behaviour therapy for depression. *Psychotherapy and Psychosomatics,* 80(5), 313-315.

Young, S. L., and Ensing, D. S. (1999). Exploring recovery from the perspective of people with psychiatric disabilities. *Psychiatric Rehabilitation Journal,* 22(3), 219-231.

In: Bipolar Disorder
Editor: Nickolas B. Moore
ISBN: 978-1-62618-666-8


*Chapter VI*

# Memantine in the Long-Term Prophylaxis of Treatment-Resistant Bipolar Mood Disorders

***Giulia Serra*[2]*, Paolo Stefano D'Aquila*[1]*,***
***Francesca Demontis*[1]*, Lavinia De Chiara*[2]*,***
***Alexia Emilia Koukopoulos*[2]*, Adriana Galistu*[1]*,***
***Athansios Koukopoulos*[3] *and Gino Serra*[1*]**

[1]Department of Biomedical Sciences, University of Sassari, Italy
[2]NeSMOS Department, School of Medicine and Psychology,
Sapienza University, UOC Psichiatry, Sant'Andrea Hospital, Rome, Italy
[3]Centro Lucio Bini, Rome, Italy

## Abstract

Memantine is a non-competitve NMDA receptor antagonist with a low affinity for the receptor and a voltage/use dependent action. Interestingly, it has been recently demonstrated that the drug by selectively blocking the extrasynaptic (excitotoxic) receptor but preserving the normal synaptic function has a neuroprotective action.

It is currently used in the treatment of moderate to severe Alzheimer's Disease (AD). Although its efficacy on the AD patient's quality of life has proven to be moderate, several studies have demonstrated the excellent safety and tolerability profile of the drug.

Moreover, Memantine has been used off-label in a number of neurological and psychiatric conditions, including depression, with conflicting and inconclusive results.

We have recently suggested the use of memantine as an antimanic and mood-stabilizing agent in treatment-resistant bipolar disorder. This use is absolutely at variance

* Corresponding Author: Prof. Gino Serra M. D. Full Professor of Pharmacology, Psychiatrist, Dipartimento di Scienze Biomediche, Università di Sassari, Viale San Pietro 43/b, 07100 SASSARI. Email: dsfserra@uniss.it. +39-3290092278.

with the prevalent hypotheses which take NMDA receptor antagonists to be potential antidepressant drugs (mainly on the basis of their effect on the forced swimming test).

In keeping with our hypothesis, based on experimental pharmacological evidence obtained in an animal model of bipolar disorder, we have observed a clinically relevant antimanic and sustained mood-stabilizing effect of memantine, as augmenting agent, in treatment-resistant bipolar disorders.

## Introduction

Bipolar Disorders (BD) comprise: BD I (which presents with an alternation of episodes of major depression and recurrent episodes of mania); BD II (which is made up of episodes of major depression and recurrent hypomanias); Cyclothymic Disorder (for at least two years several hypomanic and depressive episodes which must not be major). Further, a Mixed Episode is when symptoms of major depression and mania are present in the same episode.

The depression that manifests in BD is also commonly defined as Bipolar Depression, while that of Major Depressive Disorder is often called Unipolar Depression (or Unipolar Depressive Disorder).

Since affective disorders are often highly recurrent, prophylaxis is of primary importance. Many cases, however, do not respond to current mood stabilizing treatments.

Cole et al. (1993) identified four different patterns of treatment-resistant Bipolar Disorder: rapid cycling (37%), other form of cycling (32%), chronic depression (26%) and mixed states (6%). They identified some risk factors for treatment resistant Bipolar Disorder, including female gender (for rapid cycling), high prevalence of family history of affective disorders (72%) and electroencephalografic abnormalities (54% of recordings).

Particularly resistant to prophylactic treatments are the patients with the rapid cycling course.

Dunner and Fieve (1974) defined as Rapid Cyclers those patients that showed a course with four or more affective episodes in the 12 previous months, and this course specifier was adopted by DSM-IV.

Today, most clinicians waive the duration criterion of episodes and intervals because in many cases the episodes become progressively shorter and we see ultra-rapid (within the course of weeks or days) and ultradian cyclers (mood shifts within 24 hours). Some patients indeed show an alternation of phase within a few hours.

The general impression of clinicians today is that the course of recurrences of manic-depressive illness has substantially changed in the last 40 years. The recurrences of many patients have become more frequent. One sees more manias and hypomanias and therefore more bipolar cases than before, more rapid cyclers, and more chronic depressions (Koukopoulos et al 1983; Ghaemi, 2008). This phenomenon is called today mood destabilization.

In his monograph on *la folie a double forme,* Ritti (1883) presented only 17 cases with a rapid course; he collected them from various French and German authors. Kraepelin (1913) illustrated one case with a rapid cycling course in his graphs of type of course. This was case C, and he commented, "I had to seek for a long time in my cases until I finally found at least one course of the type that case C represents.' In a meta-analysis of 8 studies including 2054 bipolar patients, Kupka et al. (2003) found a percentage of 16.3% of rapid cyclers. Women and bipolar II patients were slightly but significantly more prevalent. Maj et. al (1994) found a prevalence of 19.5% of rapid cyclers among BPI patients.

Among the first 500 BP patients of the STEP-BD study 20% were rapid cyclers while in 2008 among 1,742 BD patients the percentage at entry was 32% (Schneck et al., 2008).

Among women, rapid cycling is more frequent than among men and the age of onset of the bipolar disorder is earlier than among non-rapid cycling patients (Yildiz et al., 2004).

Particularly frequent is rapid cycling among prepubertal and early adolescent bipolar patients. Geller at al. (1998) found a proportion of 83.3% rapid, ultra-rapid or ultradian cyclers among such young patients.

Rapid-cycling is more frequent among BPII than among BPI and in patients with hyperthymic and cyclothymic temperament. They are very energetic, very emotional and reactive (Kukopoulos et al., 1983). One could posit the hypothesis that they are equally reactive to chemical stimulations. Because of this temperament they are diagnosed often as borderline personality disorders and in the past as hysterics. In patients with cyclothymic temperament the rapid-cycling course could be viewed as the accentuation of longstanding subclinical mood oscillations.

Patients that more likely remain rapid-cyclers for many years are those with a DMI (depression-mania-interval) or DmI (depression-hypomania-interval) cycle patterns, those with a switch process and/or agitated depression in their course and those who have not been stabilized after the first year of an adequate treatment.

The investigation of the course of manic-depressive illness is a difficult task in itself, and the investigation of possible factors that influence this course is extremely difficult due to the variability of the spontaneous course. Yet the above-mentioned changes and the general increase of bipolar cases today make this investigation necessary. Of all the possible factors that unfavourably influence the course of the disease, the treatments themselves are in the most urgent need to be investigated, firstly because they certainly influence the disease, and secondly, because treatments are given by the doctor and therefore can be easily modified. This is certainly not the case of other factors like menopause, old age, life situations, and so forth.

The increase of substance abuse, including alcohol and cannabis among young people, certainly plays an important role in the worsening of the course of affective disorder.

Antidepressant treatments should also be reconsidered. They have been largely employed in the treatment of affective disorders during the last five decades, although many authors observed an increase of the frequency of episodes compared to the course of the disease before the introduction of antidepressants (Arnold and Kryspin Exner, 1965; Freyhan, 1960; Heinz and Grunze, 2008; Hoheisel, 1966; Lauber, 1964; Till, 1970).

Particularly associated to the use of antidepressants is the rapid cycling course (Kukopulos et al., 1983). The stabilization of rapid cyclers is often very difficult. It requires prolonged effort: it is necessary to know the life of the patient, his premorbid temperament and personality, the history of his illness and its course, the treatments used in the past, and the events and treatments associated with the onset of rapid cycling.

Patients with rapid cycling course are usually of cyclothymic or hyperthymic temperament, therefore particularly excitable and emotional persons. It is important to advise them to avoid coffee, tea, alcohol and all psychostimulant substances, intense physical exercise and also to avoid, as much as possible, stressful situations and events. Sleep is particularly important and they should go to sleep early and try to sleep as long as possible.

The resistance of rapid cyclers to all mood-stabilizing treatments is well established. None of these treatments (carbamazepine, lithium, lamotrigine, topiramate and valproate) showed a clear advantage over the others (Baldessarini et al., 2000; Tondo et al., 2003). Also the efficacy of atypical antipsychotics as mood stabilazers in maintenance therapy has not been demonstrated, and current data do not support their use as maintenance agents (Zupancic, 2011, Goodwin et al., 2011). The authors, however, agree with Muzina (2009) about the fundamental importance of lithium in the treatment of rapid cyclers.

We apply the following strategy. Given that most cases of rapid cycling are induced by antidepressants, it is of primary importance to suspend the antidepressants and to continue the treatment with mood stabilizing agents. In most cases without antidepressants the depressive phase will last longer but the following mania/hypomania will be less intense. The anti-manic action of mood stabilizers will be more effective in the absence of antidepressants. Gradually, both the excitatory and the depressive phase will be attenuated and stabilization will eventually be achieved, over a variable period of time. This therapeutic strategy is based on the idea that the suppression of the excitatory phase prevents or attenuates the following depression (Koukopoulos and Ghaemi, 2009). Indeed, all mood stabilizers like lithium, anticonvulsants, calcium antagonists, old or new antipsychotics (Koukopoulos and Ghaemi, 2009), and also memantine (Koukopoulos et al., 2010) are essentially anti-excitatory agents.

In the presence of suicide risk, electroconvulsive therapy (ECT) could be used to end the depressive phase and immediately afterwards mood stabilizing treatment should be administered.

A study from Sainte-Anne hospital in Paris shows that maintenance ECT is effective against the RC course, with full or partial remission for 100% of RC patients (Vanelle et al., 1994).

Other authors have shown that maintenance ECT is effective against rapid cycling course: Minnai et al. (2011) found a percentage of remission of 58% of patients, and other similar results were obtained by Fazzari (2009, *personal comunication*). Continuous treatment was more effective against mania/hypomania than against depression, yet in all persisting rapid cycler cases the mania/hypomania remitted only partially.

## Memantine and Currently Used Mood Stabilizers

Memantine is a non-competitve NMDA receptor antagonist, but, at variance with the most potent NMDA receptor blockers, such as Ketamine, Phencyclidine and MK-801, has a low affinity for the receptor and its action is voltage/use dependent (Gillin et al., 2009; Johnson and Kotermanski, 2006; Rammes et al., 2008). Moreover it has been recently demonstrated that this compound selectively blocks the extrasynaptic (excitotoxic) receptor but preserves the normal synaptic function (La Spada, 2009).

These peculiar pharmacological properties explain the lack of psychotomimetic/ psychedelic effect and of interference with the normal physiological functions [memory and learning, synaptic plasticity, etc. etc. (Van Dongen, Editor, 2009)].

The drug has been on the market in Germany as Akatinol Memantine since 1982 for the treatment of Parkinsonism, cerebral and peripheral spasticity, and organic brain syndrome, without apparent cause for concern before its approval in 2002 and 2004 by EMEA and FDA for the treatment of moderate to severe Alzheimer's Disease.

A recent review (Jones, 2010) of most recent safety/tolerability data for memantine (derived from meta-analyses, pooled analyses, European SPCs, and EMEA publications) confirmed that memantine has a favorable tolerability profile when used in monotherapy or in combination with other agents. Moreover, results of studies of a total treatment period of up to two years show that memantine is safe and tolerated, with an adverse event profile almost indistinguable from that of placebo. Side effects are usually mild to moderate in severity, and are commonly represented by dizziness, constipation, headache, hypertension and somnolence.

The incidence of serious adverse events (SAEs) was slightly lower for memantine than for placebo.

Warnings and precautions are few: caution is recommended in epileptic patients or with a former history of convulsions or predisposing factors for epilepsy. Close supervision is recommended in patients with myocardial infarction, uncompensated congestive heart failure or uncontrolled hypertension.

There are no contraindications for the use of memantine, apart from the sensitivity to tablets excipients. However, due to the lack of clinical experience, the drug should be avoided in patients with severe hepatic impairment. Drug-drug interactions: memantine should not be administered alongside other compounds acting at NMDA receptors such as amantadine, ketamine and dextromethorphan, due to the risk of psychotic symptoms. Moreover memantine might enhance the effects of antiparkinson drugs such as levodopa, dopamine agonists and anticholinergic compounds. On the contrary, the effects of neuroleptics and barbiturates might be reduced. Finally, memantine may also influence the effect of baclofen and dantrolene (antispamodic agents). Although its actual efficacy on the AD patient's quality of life has proven to be moderate (Emre et al., 2008; Kaduszkiewicz and Hoffmann, 2008), several pre-marketing and post-marketing studies have demonstrated the excellent safety and tolerability profile of the drug (Farlow and Phillips, 2008; Jones, 2010).

Moreover, the drug has been used off-label in a number of neurological and psychiatric conditions, including depression, with conflicting and inconclusive results (Zdanis and Tampi, 2008, Sani et al., 2012 ).

We have recently suggested, on the basis of preclinical experimental evidence obtained in our laboratory (Serra 2009, 2010) the use of memantine, as having an antimanic and mood-stabilizing effect, in treatment-resistant bipolar disorder. This use is absolutely at variance with the prevalent hypotheses which take NMDA receptor antagonists to be potential antidepressant drugs [mainly on the basis of their effect on the forced swimming test (Rogoz et al., 2002, Reus et al., 2010), a widely used animal model of depression].

In keeping with our experimental pharmacological evidence, we have observed in bipolar patients a significant clinical antimanic and sustained mood-stabilizing effect of memantine, both as augmenting agent and as a monotherapy (Serra et al. 2013a, 2013b) in treatment-resistant bipolar disorders.

Lithium is the drug of choice for the treatment of mania and the prophylaxis (as a mood stabilizer) of manic and/or depressive recurrences of Bipolar Disorders (BD) and Unipolar Depression (Goodwin, 2002). In cases of severe mania with a strong component of psychomotor agitation and/or psychotic symptoms, antipsychotic drugs are generally combined.

Anticonvulsants (carbamazepine, valproic acid, lamotrigine) are used [in mania and/or as mood stabilizers (Rapoport, 2009)] in combination with lithium when the latter does not produce a satisfactory response or in monotherapy in patients for whom lithium is contraindicated. The effectiveness of these drugs, both as antimanics and mood stabilizers, is however modest, and therefore patients who do not respond adequately to lithium (Koukopoulos et al. 1995, Tohen et al., 2005) today constitute the real problem of long-term treatment of mood disorders.

The use of antipsychotics as mood stabilizers is not advisable both because of their dubious efficacy (Culpepper and Ghaemi, 2011, Goodwin et al., 2011) and their long-term safety and/or tolerability.

Traditional antipsychotics, as well as having undesirable effects of a psychiatric type (emotional blunting, etc.), may, if administered for a long time, provoke sometimes debilitating and irreversible neurological damage (Serra and Gessa, 1990). The so-called atypical antipsychotics, on which the jury is still out on whether they do not cause long-term neurological damage (Gardener et al., 2005), have the drawback (except for some) of being able to cause what is called "metabolic syndrome" (Gardner et al., 2005), which constitutes a serious cardiovascular risk factor and thus risk of early death (which is aggravated by the fact that BD patients *per se* have an increased cardiovascular risk). Finally, it should be stressed that most antipsychotics, whether traditional or atypical, may cause, albeit rarely, death by sudden cardiac arrest (Ray et al., 2009) or by neuroleptic malignant syndrome (Serra and Gessa, 1990).

Concern has also been raised by a recent alarm (FDA Alert, 2008) over the possibility that anti-epileptics may bring a two-fold increase in suicide risk compared to placebo.

Along with the approved old anticonvulsants, a plethora of "new" antiepileptics [Gabapentin, Oxcarbazepine, Clonazepam, Pregabaline, Tiagabine, Topiramate, etc. (Kaufman, 2011)] are usually used off-label in combination with lithium, anticonvulsants and antipsychotics, when these associations fail to produce a satisfactory clinical response. Thus, the overwhelming majority of bipolar patients, today, receive a combination of 4 or 5 drugs or even more, often with questionable pharmacological rationale and little additional relevant clinical benefit.

The problem of the therapy and prophylaxis of mood disorders in patients who do not respond to lithium, whose numbers appear to be continually rising, therefore remains unsolved (Koukopoulos et al., 1995; Ghaemi, 2008).

Indeed, while the acute phases of the manic/hypomanic and depressive episodes of the illness appear to be relatively easy to control, the failure on the stabilization of treatment-resistant bipolar disorders is becoming an emergengy of psychiatry today and represents an increased risk of suicide.

Unfortunately, the currently available lithium-alternative mood-stabilizers not only are of limited efficacy, but have a number of acute troublesome and sometimes long-term severe side effects along with clinically relevant drug-drug interaction (Mc Namara, 2011).

Hence, the need for new more effective and safe mood-stabilizing drugs.

# The Possible Mechanism of Antimanic and Mood-Stabilizing Action of Memantine

The first evidence-based hypothesis of the neurobiology of mood disorders was proposed by Schildkraut in 1965 (Schildkraut, 1965). Mainly on the basis of the supposed mechanism of therapeutic effect of tricyclic antidepressants and MAO inhibitors (blockade of serotonin and noradrenaline reuptake or inhibition of MAO, respectively) he suggested that depression may be associated with a decreased function of serotonin and noradrenaline transmission. Further support for this hypothesis is provided by the observation that reserpine, which induces depression in humans, causes a depletion of the neurotransmitters in monoaminergic neurons.

As a consequence of this hypothesis the role of dopamine (DA) in the pathophysiology of mood disorders has long been neglected although reserpine also depletes dopaminergic neurons.

In 1979 (Serra et al., 1979) we first reported that antidepressant drugs act not only on serotonin and noradrenaline, but also activate dopaminergic transmission. In fact we found that chronic treatment with antidepressants, potentiate dopaminergic transmission in rats, and suggested that this effect may play an important role both in the therapeutic action and in the ability of antidepressants to induce mania/hypomania.

Since then, in the last three decades, an amount of preclinical and clinical evidence has been accumulated strongly suggesting a key role of dopamine in the pathophysiology of bipolar disorders (Berk et al., 2007; Cousins and Butts, 2009; Dihel and Gershon, 1992).

A detailed description of this clinical and preclinical evidence supporting a key role of dopamine in the pathophysiology of bipolar disorders is beyond the aim of this chapter: the reader may find such a description in a number of excellent recent reviews (Berk et al., 2007; Cousins and Butts, 2009; Dihel and Gershon, 1992; Dunlop and Nemeroff, 2007).

In our first report (Serra et al., 1979) we observed that chronic treatment with antidepressants reduces the sedative effect of apomorphine and potentiates its stimulatory action on locomotor activity, thus potentiating dopamine transmission. We interpreted these effects as a consequence of a development of sedative dopamine autoreceptor subsensitivity, and suggested that the potentiation of dopamine transmission may play an important role both in the antidepressant action and in the ability to induce switching from depression to mania/hypomania of antidepressant drugs.

Subsequent studies in the following 30 years have produced conflicting results (Chiodo and Antelman, 1980a, 1980b; Diggory and Buckett, 1984; Dziedzicka-Wasylewska, 1997; Holcomb et al., 1982; Muscat et al., 1988; Serra et al., 1980, 1981a, 1981b; Spyraki and Fibiger, 1981) on the ability of ADs to induce subsensitivity in DA autoreceptors.

However numerous studies have confirmed that virtually all AD treatments (including electroconvulsivechock, REM-sleep deprivation ), increase the motor-stimulant effect of DA receptor agonists (Collu et al., 1997a; D'Aquila et al., 2000a; Gershon et al., 2007; Spyraki and Fibiger, 1981; Serra et al., 1990, 1991, 1992; Willner, 1997). In particular, Spyraki and Fibiger in 1981 (Spyraki and Fibiger, 1981) observed that chronic Desipramine treatment potentiated dopaminergic transmission by inducing a supersensitivity of postsynaptic dopamine receptors in the mesolimbic system.

Strong evidence now exists suggesting a key role of mesolimbic DA in the mechanism of action of antidepressants (Collu et al., 1997b; D'Aquila et al., 2000a; Fibiger and Philips, 1981; Gershon et al., 2007; Spyraki and Fibiger, 1981; Serra et al., 1990, 1992; Willner, 1997).

Gershon et al. (2007) recently published an elegant review on the experimental and clinical evidence indicating the role of dopamine D2 receptors in the mechanism of action of antidepressants.

In 1990 we re-evaluated the effect of chronic antidepressant treatments on pre- and post-synaptic dopamine receptor sensitivity (Serra et al., 1990). We found that chronic antidepressant treatment does not induce a subsensitivity of dopamine autoreceptors, but, confirming the results of Spiraki and Fibiger (1981), we observed that such a treatment sensitizes dopamine D2, but not D1, receptors selectively in the mesolimbic system. The key role of mesolimbic DA D2 receptor sensitization in the mechanism of action of antidepressants is now widely accepted (Collu et al., 1997a; D'Aquila et al., 2000a; Fibiger and Philips, 1981; Gershon et al., 2007; Spyraki and Fibiger, 1981; Serra et al., 1990, 1991, 1992; Willner, 1997).

In keeping with these observations, it may be suggested that the increased dopaminergic transmission in the mesolimbic system (the reward system) due to D2 receptor sensitization, induced by antidepressants, may contribute to their therapeutic effect, and in particular for symptoms such as anhedonia, loss of motivation, decreased libido and psychomotor retardation (Collu, 1997b; D'Aquila, 2000a; Serra et al. 1990, 1992).

Moreover, the sensitization of mesolimbic dopamine D2 receptors induced by antidepressants may be responsible, in "vulnerable subjects" (bipolar disorder, the presence of previous mixed states, early age at onset, a cyclothymic or hyperthymic temperament, genetic factors?), for the switches from depression to mania/hypomania (Collu et al., 1997b; D'Aquila e al., 2000a; Gessa et al., 1995; Serra et al., 1990, 1992, Serra and D'Aquila, 2008; Serra, 2009, 2010) which, in turn, trigger a rapid-cycling course (Serra et al., 2008; Serra, 2009, 2010).

Koukopoulos et al. (1980) suggested that *"The intensification of an underlying hypomanic process by antidepressants would precipitate another depression and establish continuous circularity"*.

Consistent with this hypothesis we recently found that chronic treatment with imipramine induced a 'bipolar-like behaviour' (i.e. a cycle of mania-depression (D'Aquila et al., 2003; D'Aquila et al., 2004). In fact, as expected, imipramine induces a sensitization of dopamine D2 receptors (mania/hypomania ), which is followed after imipramine withdrawal by a progressive desensitization of dopamine D2 receptors (depression) (D'Aquila et al., 2003) associated with a depressive-like behaviour as assessed in the forced swimming test animal model of depression in rats (D'Aquila et al., 2004).

This observation provides strong experimental support for the hypothesis that antidepressant-induced mania/hypomania is the trigger phenomenon of rapid-cycling course (Collu et al., 1997b; Serra and D'Aquila, 2008; Serra, 2009, 2010) and that the prevention of both spontaneous or antidepressant-induced mania/hypomania (Koukopoulos and Reginaldi, 1973; Koukopoulos and Ghaemi, 2009) (in neurobiological terms, dopamine D2 receptor sensitization) is essential to avoid the development of a rapid-cycling bipolar disorder.

The prevention of mania, whether induced by antidepressants or spontaneous, is the essential element in the therapy and prophylaxis of bipolar disorders (Koukopoulos and

Reginaldi, 1973; Koukopoulos and Ghaemi, 2009). When, in fact, treatments currently in use do not achieve this aim, the course of the disorder becomes 'malign', i.e refractory to treatment, as in the rapid-cycling course.

According with the clinical observations that demonstrate the ineffectiveness of currently used mood stabilizers in preventing antidepressant-induced switch from depression to mania (Leverich et al., 2006; Tondo et al., 1981, 2010), we found that the concomitant administration of lithium (D'Aquila et al., 2000b), carbamazepine (D'Aquila et al., 2001), valproate (D'Aquila et al 2006) and lamotrigine (unpublished results) with imipramine fails to prevent the development of dopamine D2 receptor sensitization. Actually, carbamazepine seems to be effective, but its effect is due to the reduction of imipramine plasma levels due to the induction of the drug metabolism.

These observations led us to further investigate the mechanism by which antidepressants induce dopamine receptor sensitization. In fact, this mechanism may represent a possible target to develop drugs effective in preventing this phenomenon as potential new antimanic and mood stabilizing agents.

There is ample experimental evidence showing that the NMDA glutamate receptor plays an essential role in the phenomenon of sensitization. Its stimulation is, in fact, necessary for the sensitization to amphetamine (Battisti et al., 2000; Groning et al., 2004; Ohmori et al., 1994; Pacchioni et al., 2002; Vezina and Quen, 2000; Wolf et al., 1994), methylphenidate (Gaytan et al., 2000), cocaine ( Heusner and Palmiter 2005; Li et al., 2000; Kim et al., 1996; Rompré and Bauco 2006), apomorphine (Acerbo et al., 2004; Pacchioni et al., 2002; Voikar et al., 1999) and other dopamine mimetics (Kalivas, 1995; Rockhold, 1998), nicotine (Kelsey et al., 2002), morphine (Jeziorski et al., 1994; Trujillo, 2002) and ethanol (Broadbent and Weiemier, 1999; Camarini et al., 2000; Kotlinska et al., 2006), as well as several types of stress such as, for instance, 'restraint stress' (Pacchioni et al., 2002) and 'social defeat stress' (Yap et al., 2005).

The stimulation of NMDA receptors is required for the development of dopamine receptor sensitization induced by antidepressants. Indeed, we found that the administration of MK-801, a selective non-competitive NMDA receptor blocker, completely prevents the dopamine receptor sensitization induced by imipramine (D'Aquila et al., 1992) and by electroconvulsive shock (D'Aquila et al., 1997).

These observations strongly suggest that the non-competitive blockade of NMDA receptors should result in an anti-manic and mood stabilizing action, and that it should also be effective in the treatment of the disorders resistant to currently used antimanic and mood stabilizers.

Consistently with this hypothesis, we have recently found that memantine prevents both the up-regulation induced by chronic imipramine and the down-regulation of dopamine D2 receptors associated with a depressive-like behaviour observed after imipramine withdrawal (Demontis et al. 2012).

These observations provide strong experimental evidence supporting the hypothesis of the antimanic and prophylactic effect of memantine in bipolar disorders resistant to conventional treatments.

Moreover, an antimanic-like activity of memantine has been observed in other animal models of mania by Gao et al.( 2011).

These observations prompted us to suggest the use of memantine, the only safe and well-tolerated non-competitive NMDA antagonist that may be proposed for long-term clinical use, as antimanic and mood-stabilizer in treatment-resistant bipolar disorder (Serra, 2009, 2010).

In addition, it may be interesting to recall that memantine, like the "gold standard" antimanic and mood-stabilizer, lithium, seems to posses a powerful neuroprotective activity (La Spada, 2009), an effect that may contribute to its mood-stabilizing properties. Indeed, in accordance with the neurotrophic hypothesis of mood-disorders (Dumas, 2004; Serra and Fratta, 2007), an excessive glutamatergic stimulation of NMDA receptors [that seems to be associated with mania (Ongur et al., 2009)] could result in a neurodegeneration that appears to be associated with depression (Dumas, 2004, Macqueen, 2003, Videbech and Ravnkilde, 2004 ) and can be reversed by an effective antidepressant treatment (Sheline et al., 2003; Malberg, 2004, Malberg and Blendy, 2005; Paizanis et al., 2007).

Thus, it may be suggested that memantine, by blocking NMDA receptors, prevents both the up (mania) and down (depression) regulation of dopamine D2 receptors, and the neurodegeneration that results from the excessive glutamatergic neurotransmission during mania, which might underlie the following depressive phase.

## Antimanic and Mood Stabilizing Effect of Memantine in Treatment-Resistant Bipolar Patients

In order to evaluate the antimanic and mood stabilizing effects of memantine we have recently carried out seven naturalistic clinical studies.

In the first study (Koukopoulos et al., 2010) we administered memantine (10-30 mg/day), as augmenting agent, to 18 treatment-resistant bipolar patients monitored for 24 weeks. The severity of the patients' condition before memantine and the change after memantine augmentation was evaluated on the Clinical Global Impression-Bipolar (Spearing et al., 1997 ) Overall Bipolar Illness scale.

The patients had been ill for an average of 21 years and had been resistant to very intense standard treatments (lithium, anticonvulsants, typical and atypical antipsychotics, electroconvulsive therapy, and antidepressants). Of these 18 patients, 13 were bipolar I and 5 bipolar II, 10 were rapid cyclers, Thirteen patients exhibited psychotic symptoms. The 10 rapid cyclers had a mean duration of rapid cycling course of 11 years.

The average of CGI-BP score before memantine was 6.6, which indicates a very severe condition. After 24 weeks of memantine addition 72.2% of patients were very much or much improved. Among the rapid cyclers 60% reached stability. The mean time to improvement was 55 days.

The second study (Koukopoulos et al., 2012) encompassed 40 treatment-resistant bipolar patients monitored for 12 months. Of these 40 patients 21 were bipolar I and 19 bipolar II, 19 were rapid cyclers. Nineteen exhibited psychotic symptoms. All patients had been resistant for many years to very intense long-term standard treament. The mean duration of illness was 22 years, while the average duration of rapid cycling course of rapid cyclers was 8.6 years.

The average of CGI-BP Overall Bipolar Illness score before the memantine addition was 6.7, indicating a very severe condition.

After 6 months of memantine augmentation (10-30 mg/day added to ongoing treatment which was left unmodified) 72.5% of patients were very much or much improved and remained stabilized for 12 months. Among the rapid cyclers 68.5% reached stability after 6 months and remained free of recurrences for 12 months.

In order to evaluate the long-term effect of memantine, we studied the action of the drug on 22 treatment-resistant bipolar patients with a follow-up of 36 (Serra, 2012). Sixteen were BPI and 6 BPII, 10 were rapid cyclers. The average of CGI-BP score was 6.6 before the addition of memantine. The mean duration of illness was 22.4 years, and the duration of rapid cycling course 11 years. Patients very much (scored 1) or much (scored 2) improved were 77.3%, 81.8%, 68.2%, 72.7%, 72.7% and 72.7%, at 6, 12, 18, 24, 30 and 36 months, respectively.

More recently we found that memantine has antimanic and mood stabilizing effect also when used as a monotherapy, both in BP I (Serra et al., 2013a) and BP II (Serra et al., 2013b).

Moreover, we observed that memantine is able to prevent the severe affective reccurrences occurring after lithium discontinuation (in peparation).

Finally we recently confirmed that memantine has a clinically relevant and substained mood stabilizing effect in rapid cycling bipolar disorders (in preparation). The side effects observed during our studies are the already described dizziness (one patient), constipation (one patient) and drowsiness (one patient), thus confirming the excellent safety and tolerability profile of the drug, also when used in combination with other drugs currently used in the treatment of bipolar disorders.

Our results strongly suggest that memantine, both as augmenting agent and as a monotherapy, was associated with clinically substantial antimanic and sustained mood-stabilizing effects in treatment-resistant bipolar disorder patients with excellent safety and tolerability.

As in all naturalistic studies, the limitation of our clinical observations is the lack of a placebo control. Hovewer, the prior history of treatment resistance of the study patients and the long-lasting effect of the drug argues against a placebo effect contributing in any substantial way to what we observed. Nevertheless, we are going to start an RCT to confirm our naturalistic observations.

Consistent with our results is the observation by Keck et al (2009) of an antimanic effect of memantine monotherapy in bipolar disorder patients.

In addition, our results are consistent with a recent analysis on the effect of memantine on the management of behavioural disorders in AD patients (Gauthier et al., 2010) which suggest an antimanic and mood-stabilizing effect of memantine.

In fact, the analysis demonstrates that memantine reduces “manic” symptoms such as agitation, aggression, irritability, lability, and even delusions and hallucinations in AD patients. Moreover, suggestive of a prophylactic/ mood-stabilizing effect, the observation that patients who do not exhibit such symptoms at baseline, showed a reduction of their emergence.

Taken together these clinical observations and considering the safety/tolerability and the drug-drug interaction of the drug, we are tempted to suggest, pending the results of our controlled clinical trial, the use of memantine, as augmenting agent, in treatment-resistant bipolar disorders, which have no therapeutic alternative.

## Conclusion

Memantine is a non competitive NMDA receptor antagonist, with peculiar pharmacological properties, which explain its excellent safety and tolerability profile, at variance with the most potent NMDA receptor blockers such as Ketamine, Phencyclidine and MK-801. The drug, has been used in Germany since 1982, and approved by EMEA in 2002 and by FDA in 2004 for the treatment of moderate to severe Alzheimer's Disease. Moreover it has been recently used off-label in a number of neurological and psychiatric disorders, including depression, with conflicting and inconclusive results.

At variance with the hypothesis that, mainly on the basis of the effect of these compounds in the forced swimming animal model of depression, suggests that NMDA receptors antagonists might have an antidepressant activity, we have recently demonstrated that MK-801 and Memantine show an antimanic and mood-stabilizing-like effects in an animal model of bipolar disorder resistant to standard treatments.

Thus, we have suggested (Serra, 2009, 2010) the use of Memantine as antimanic and mood-stabilizing agent in the treatment of resistant bipolar disorders. This hypothesis prompted us to carry out naturalistic trials to test memantine in the management of treatment resistant bipolar disorders.

The results of our studies strongly suggest that memantine has a clinically relevant antimanic effect and a long-term prophylactic action in treatment of resistant and very severe bipolar patients, with very good safety and tolerability.

Although our naturalistic observations lack of placebo control and need to be confirmed by a RCT (wihch we are going to start), we believe that they provide enough information to suggest the safe use of memantine augmentation in severely ill bipolar patients, who are resistant to conventional treatments and have not therapeuthic alternative.

## Acknowledgments

The authors would like to thank Denis Greenan for his precious contribution to the drafting of the paper.

## References

Acerbo, M.J., Lee, J.M., Delius, J.D. (2004). Sensitization to apomorphine, effects of dizocilpine NMDA receptor blockades. *Behav. Brain Res.* May 5; 151(1-2):201-208.

Arnold, O.H., Kryspin-Exner, K. (1965). Zur Frage der Beeinflussung des Venlaufes des manish-depressiven Krankheitsgeschehens durch Antidepressiva. *Wiener Medizinische Wochenschrift* 45/46:929-934,1965.

Baldessarini, R.J., Tondo, L., Floris, G., Hennen, J. (2000). Effects of rapid cycling on response to Lithium maintenance treatment in 360 bipolar I and 11 disorder patients. *J. Affect. Disord.* 61, 13—22.

Baldessarini, R.J. in Goodman and Gilman's. *The Pharmacological Basis of Therapeutics 11 Edition 2005*; 429-500.

Battisti, J.J., Shreffler, C.B., Uretsky, N.J., Wallace, L.J. (2000). NMDA antagonists block expression of sensitization of amphetamine- and apomorphine-induced stereotypy. *Pharmacol. Biochem. Behav.* Oct; 67(2):241-246.

Berk, M., Dodd, S., Kauer-Sant'anna, M., Malhi, G.S., Bourin, M., Kapczinski, F., Norman, T. (2007). Dopamine dysregulation syndrome: implications for a dopamine hypothesis of bipolar disorder. *Acta Psychiatr Scand. Suppl.* (434):41-49.

Broadbent, J., Weitemier, A.Z. (1999). Dizocilpine (MK-801) prevents the development of sensitization to ethanol in DBA/2J mice. *Alcohol Alcohol.* May-Jun; 34(3):283-288.

Camarini, R., Frussa-Filho, R., Monteiro, M.G., Calil, H.M. (2000). MK-801 blocks the development of behavioral sensitization to the ethanol. *Alcohol Clin. Exp. Res.* 24(3):285-290.

Chiodo, L.A., Antelman, S.M. (1980). Electroconvulsive shock: progressive dopamine autoreceptor subsensitivity independent of repeated treatment. *Science.*14; 210(4471):799-801.

Chiodo, L.A., Antelman, S.M. (1980). Repeated tricyclics induce a progressive dopamine autoreceptor subsensitivity independent of daily drug treatment. *Nature*; 287(5781):451-454.

Chiodo, L.A., Antelman, S.M. (1980). Tricyclic antidepressants induce subsensitivity of presynaptic dopamine autoreceptors. *Eur. J. Pharmacol.* Jun 13;64(2-3):203-204.

Cole AJ, Scott J, Ferrier IN, Eccleston D. (1993). Patterns of treatment resistance in bipolar affective disorder. *Acta Psychiatr Scand.* 1993 Aug;88(2):121-3.

Collu, M., Poggiu, A.S., Devoto, P., Serra, G. (1997a). Behavioural sensitization of D2 mesolimbic dopamine receptors in chronic fluoxetine treated rats. *Eur. J. Pharm.* 322, 123-127.

Collu, M., D'Aquila, P., Gessa, G.L., Serra, G. (1997b). Do antidepressant treatments induce mania by activating dopaminergic trasmission? *Second International Conference on Bipolar Disorders,* Pittsburg, USA, June 19-21.

Culpepper, L., Ghaemi, N. (2011) Are antipsychotics overprescribed? *Medscape Psychiatric and Mental Illness.* Posted: 02/18/2011.

Cuosins, D.A., Butts, K. (2009). Young AH The role of dopamine in bipolar disorders. *Bipolar Disord,* 11: 787-806.

D'Aquila, P..S., Sias, A., Gessa, G.L., Serra, G. (1992). The NMDA receptor antagonist MK-801 prevents imipramine-induced supersensitivity to quinpirole. *Eur. J. Pharmacol.* 224: 199-202.

D'Aquila, P.S., Collu, M., Gessa, G.L., Serra, G. (1997). Dizolcipine prevents the enhanced locomotor response to quinpirole induced by repeated electroconvulsive shock. *Eur. J. Pharm.* 330, 11-14.

D'Aquila PS, Collu M, Gessa GL, Serra G. The role of dopamine in the mechanism of action of antidepressant drugs. *Eur. J. Pharmacol.* 2000a; 405(1-3):365-73.

D'Aquila P.S., Collu M., Devoto P., Serra G (2000b): Chronic lithium chloride fails to prevent imipramine-induced sensitization to the dopamine-D2- like receptor-agonist quinpirole. *Eur. Journ Pharmacol*, 395: 157-160.

D'Aquila, P.S., Peana, A.T., Tanda, O., Serra, G. (2001): Carbamazepine prevents imipramine-induced behavioural sensitization to the D2-like dopamine receptor agonist quinpirole. *Eur. Journ Pharmacol* 416: 107-111.

D'Aquila, P.S., Peana, A.T., Panin, F., Grixoni, C., Cossu, M., Serra, G. (2003). Reversal of antidepressant-induced dopaminergic behavioural supersensitivity after long-term chronic imipramine withdrawal. *Eur. Journ Pharmacol.* 458, 129-134.

D'Aquila, P.S., Panin, F., Serra, G. (2004). Long-term imipramine withdrawal induces a depressive-like behaviour in the forced swimming test. *Eur. Journ Pharmacol.* 492, 61-63.

D'Aquila, P.S., Panin, F., Serra, G. (2006). Chronic valproate fails to prevent imipramine-induced behavioural sensitization to the dopamine D2-like receptor agonist quinpirole. *Eur. Journ Pharmacol.* 535, 208-212.

Demontis F., Cubeddu A., Serra G.(2012): Memantine prevents the "bipolar-like behaviour" induced by chronic treatment with imipramine in rats. IRBD, Nice 21-23 May, 2012.

Diehl, D.J., Gershon, S. (1992). The role of dopamine in mood disorders. *Compr Psychiatry*; 33(2):115-120.

Diggory, G.L., Buckett, W.R. (1984). Chronic antidepressant administration fails to attenuate apomorphine-induced decreases in rat striatal dopamine metabolites. *Eur. J. Pharmacol.*; 105(3-4):257-263.

DSM-IV-TR: American Psychiatric Association. 2000.

Dumas, R.S. (2004). Role of Neurotrophic factors in the etiology and treatment of mood disorders. *Neuromolecular Medicine.* 5: 11-25.

Dunlop, B.W., Nemeroff, C.B. (2007). The role of dopamine in the pathophysiology of depression. *Arch. Gen. Psychiatry.* Mar;64(3):327-337.

Dunner, D.L., Fieve, R.R. (1974). Clinical factors in lithium carbonate prophylaxis failure. *Arch. Gen. Psychiatry* 30: 229 233.

Dziedzicka-Wasylewska, M. (1997). The effect of imipramine on the amount of mRNA coding for rat dopamine D2 autoreceptors. *Eur. J. Pharmacol.* ;337(2-3):291-294.

Emre, M., Mecocci, P., Stender, K. (2008). Pooled analyses on cognitive effects of memantine in patients with moderate to severe Alzheimer's disease. *J. Alzheimers Dis*;14(2):193-197.

Farlow, M.R., Graham, S.M., Alva, G. (2008). Memantine for the treatment of Alzheimer's disease: tolerability and safety data from clinical trials. *Drug Saf.* 31(7): 577-585.

Fibiger, H.C., Phillips, A.G. (1981). Increased intracranial self stimulation in rats after long-term administration of desipramine. *Science.*; 214(4521):683-685.

Fibiger, H.C. (1995). Neurobiology of depression: focus on dopamine. In: *Depression and Mania: From neurobiology to treatment.(Gessa G.L., Fratta W., Pani L., Serra G. (eds), Adv. Biochem. Psychopharmacol. 49, Raven Press) pp 1-17,*

Freyhan, F.A. (1960). Zur modernen psychiatrischen Behandlung der Depressionen.

Gao Y, Payne RS, Schurr A, Hougland T, Lord J, Herman L, Lei Z, Banerjee P, El-Mallakh RS. Memantine reduces mania-like symptoms in animal models. *Psychiatry Res.* 2011; 188(3):366-371.

Gardner, D.M., Baldessarini, R.J., Waraich, P. Modern antipsychotics drugs: a critical overview. *CMAJ.;* 2005; 172 (13).

Gauthier S, Cummings J, Ballard C, Brodaty H, Grossberg G, Robert P, Lyketsos C. Management of behavioral problems in Alzheimer's disease. *Int Psychogeriatr. 2010 ;22(3):346-372.*

Gaytan, O., Nason, R., Alagugurusamy, R., Swann, A., Dafny, N. (2000). MK-801 blocks the development of sensitization to the locomotor effects of methylphenidate. *Brain Res. Bull.* 51(6):485-492.

Geller, B., Williams, M., Zimerman, B., Frazier, J., Beringer, L., Warner, K.L. (1998) Prepubertal and early adolescent bipolarity. *J. Affect Disord.* 1998 ; 51 (2): 81-91.

Gershon, A.A., Vishne, T., Grunhaus, L. (2007). Dopamine D2-like receptors and the antidepressant response. *Biol Psychiatry.*; 61(2):145-153.

Gessa, G.L., Pani, L., Serra, G., Fratta, W. (1995). Animal models of Mania. In: *Depression and Mania: From neurobiology to treatment. (Gessa G.L., Fratta W., Pani L., Serra G. (eds), Adv. Biochem. Psychopharmacol. 49, Raven Press)pp 43-66.*

Ghaemi, S.N. (2008). Treatment of Rapid-Cycling Bipolar Disorder: Are Antidepressants Mood Destabilizers? *Am. J. Psychiatry* 165(3): 300-302.

Gilling, K.E., Jatzke, C., Hechenberger, M., Parsons, C.G. (2009). Potency, voltage-dependency, agonist concentration-dependency, blocking kinetics and partial untrapping of the uncompetitive N-methyl-D-aspartate (NMDA) channel blocker memantine at human NMDA (GluN1/GluN2A) receptors. *Neuropharmacology. 2009*;56(5):866-875.

Goodwin, F.K. (2002). Rationale for long-term treatment of bipolar disorder and evidence for long-term lithium treatment. *J. Clin. Psychiatry.* 2002;63 (10):5-12.

Goodwin FK, Whitham EA, Ghaemi SN. Maintenance treatment study designs in bipolar disorder: do they demonstrate that atypical neuroleptics (antipsychotics) are mood stabilizers? CNS Drugs. 2011; 25(10):819-827.

Grönig, M., Atalla, A., Kuschinsky, K. (2004). Effects of dizocilpine [(+)-MK-801] on the expression of associative and non-associative sensitization to D-amphetamine. *Naunyn Schmiedebergs Arch. Pharmacol.*; 369(2):228-231.

Heusner, C.L., Palmiter, R.D. (2005). *Expression of mutantNervenarzt* 31:112—118, 1960.

NMDA receptors in dopamine D1 receptor-containing cells prevents cocaine sensitization and decreases cocaine preference. *J. Neurosci.* Jul 13; 25(28): 6651-6657.

Hoheisel, H.P. (1966) Zur Frage der Veirzung von Intervallzeiten psychophar makologisch behandelter phasischer Psychosen. *Nervenarzt* 37:259—263.

Heinz, C.R., Grunze, M.D. (2008). Switching, Induction of Rapid Cycling, and Increased Suicidality With Antidepressants in Bipolar Patients: Fact or Overinterpretation? *CNS Spectr.* 13(9):790-795.

Holcomb, H.H., Bannon, M.J., Roth, R.H. (1982). Striatal dopamine autoreceptors uninfluenced by chronic administration of antidepressants. *Eur. J. Pharmacol.* 27;82(3-4):173-178.

Jeziorski, M., White, F.J., Wolf, M.E. (1994). MK-801 prevents the development of behavioral sensitization during repeated morphine administration. *Synapse.*; 16(2): 137-147.

Johnson, J.W., Kotermanski, S.E. (2006). Mechanism of action of memantine. *Curr. Opin. Pharmacol.;* 6(1):61-67.

Jones, R.W. (2010). A review comparing the safety and tolerability of memantine with the acetylcholinesterase inhibitors. *Int. J. Geriatr Psychiatry.* 24: 547–553.

Lauber, H. (1964) Studie zur Frage der Krankheitsdauer unter Behandlung mit Psychopharmaka. *Nervenarzt* 35:488 – 491.

Li, Y., White, F.J., Wolf, M.E. (2000). Pharmacological reversal of behavioral and cellular indices of cocaine sensitization in the rat. *Psychopharmacology (Berl)*; 151(2-3):175-183.

Kaduszkiewicz,, H., Hoffmann, F. (2008). Review: cholinesterase inhibitors and memantine consistently but marginally improve symptoms of dementia. *Evid. Based Ment Health.* Nov; 11(4): 113-120.

Kalivas, P.W. (1995). Interactions between dopamine and excitatory amino acids in behavioral sensitization to psychostimulants. *Drug Alcohol Depend.* Feb; 37(2): 95-100.

Kaufman, K.R. (2010) Antiepileptic drugs in the treatment of psychiatric disorders. *Epilepsy Behav.* 2011 May;21(1):1-11.

Keck, P.E., Jr Hsu H.A., Papadakis, K., Russo, J. Jr. (2009). Memantine efficacy and safety in patients with acute mania associated with bipolar I disorder: a pilot evaluation. *Clin. Neuropharmacol.*;32(4):199-204.

Kelsey, J.E., Beer, T., Lee, E., Wagner, A. (2002). Low doses of dizocilpine block the development and subsequent expression of locomotor sensitization to nicotine in rats. *Psychopharmacology (Berl).*; 161(4):370-378.

Kim, H.S., Park, W.K., Jang, C.G., Oh, S. (1996). Inhibition by MK-801 of cocaine-induced sensitization, conditioned place preference, and dopamine receptor supersensitivity in mice. *Brain Res. Bull.* 40(3): 201-207.

Kotlinska, J., Bochenski, M., Danysz, W. (2006). N-methyl-D-aspartate and group I metabotropic glutamate receptors involved in the expression of ethanol-induced sensitization in mice. *Behav. Pharmacol.* Feb; 17(1):1-8.

Koukopoulos, A., Reginaldi, D. (1973). Does lithium prevent depression by suppressing mania? *Int. Pharmacopsychiatry* 8 (3): 152-158.

Kukopulos, A.(variant of Koukopoulos), Reginaldi, D., Laddomada, P., Floris, G., Serra, G., Tondo, L. (1980). Course of the manic-depressive cycle and changes caused by treatments. *Pharmakopsychiatry* 13: 156—167.

Kukopulos, A. (variant of Koukopoulos), Caliari, B., Tundo, A., Floris. G., Reginaldi, D., Tondo, L. (1983) Rapid cyclers temperament and antidepressants. *Compr. Psychiatry* 24, 249-258.

Koukopoulos A., Reginaldi D., Minnai G., Serra G., Pani L., Johnson F.N. (1995). The long-term prophylaxis of affective disorders. In: Depression and Mania: From neurobiology to treatment; (Gessa G.L., Fratta W., Pani L., Serra G. (eds.), *Adv. Bichem. Psychopharmacol.* 49 Raven Press), pp. 127-147.

Koukopoulos, A., Ghaemi, S.N. (2009). The primacy of mania: a reconsideration of mood disorders. *Eur. Psychiatry* ;24(2):125-134.

Koukopoulos A, Reginaldi D, Serra G, Koukopoulos AE, Sani G, Serra G. (2010). Antimanic and mood stabilizing effect of memantine as an augmenting agent in treatment resistant bipolar disorder. *Bipolar Disorders.* 12: 348-349.

Koukopoulos, A., Serra, G., Koukopoulos, A.E., Reginaldi, D., Serra, G. (2012) The sustained mood stabilizing effect of memantine in the manegement of treatment resistant bipolar disorders: findings from a 12-month naturalistic trial. J. Affective Disorders 2012; 136: 163-166.

Kraepelin, E., 1913. Psychiatry, 8th Edition. Barth. Leipzig.

Kupka, R.W., Luckenbaugh, D.A., Post, R.M., Leverich, G.S., Nolen, W.A. (2003) Rapid and non-rapid cycling bipolar disorder: a meta-analysis of clinical studies. *J. Clin. Psychiatry* ; 64 (12): 1483-94.

La Spada, A.R. (2009). Memantine strikes the perfect balance. *Nat. Med.* Dec;15(12):1355-1356.

Leverich, G.S., Altshuler, L.L., Frye, M.A., Suppes, T., McElroy, S.L., Keck, PE. Jr, et al. (2006). Risk of switch in mood polarity to hypomania or mania in patients with bipolar depression during acute and continuation trials of venlafaxine, sertraline, and bupropion as adjuncts to mood stabilizers. *Am. J. Psychiatry.* ; 163(2):232-239.

Macqueen, G.M., Campbell, S., Mcewen, B.S., Macdonald, K., Amano, S., Joffe, R.T., Nahmias, C., Young, L.T. (2003) Course of illness, hippocampal function, and hippocampal volume in major depression. *PNAS.* 100(3):1387-1392.

Malberg, J.E. (2004) Implication of adult hippocampal neurogenesis in antidepressant action. *J. Psychiatry Neurosci*, 29(3):196-205.

Malberg, J.E., Blendy, J.A. (2005). Antidepressant action: to the nucleus and beyond. *Trends Pharmacol. Sci.*; 26(12):631-638.

Maj, M., Magliano, L., Pirozzi, R., Marasco, C., Guameri, M. (1994). Validity of rapid cycling as a course specifier for bipolar disorder. *Am. J. Psychiatry* 151, 1015-1019.

Mc Namara J.O.2001 Pharmacotherapy of the Epilepsies. In Goodman and Gilman's, 12 Edition pp: 583-607.

Minnai G.P., Salis P.G., Oppo R, Loche A.P., Scano F. Tondo L. (2011) Effectiveness of maintenance electroconvulsive therapy (m-ECT) in rapid cycling bipolar disorder. *J. ECT*; 27(2):123-6.

Muscat, R., Towell, A., Willner, P. (1988). Changes in dopamine autoreceptor sensitivity in an animal model of depression. *Psychopharmacology* (Berl); 94(4):545-550.

Muzina, D.J. (2009). Pharmacologic treatment of rapid cycling and mixed states in bipolar disorder: an argument for the use of lithium. Bipolar Disord. 2009 Jun;11 (2):84-91.

Ohmori, T., Abekawa, T., Muraki, A., Koyama, T. (1994). Competitive and noncompetitive NMDA antagonists block sensitization to methamphetamine. *Pharmacol. Biochem. Behav.*; 48(3):587-591.

Ongur, D., Jensen, E., Prescot, A.P., Stork, C., Lundy, M., Cohen, B.M. (2008). Renshaw PF. Abnormal glutamatergic neurotransmission and neuronal-glial interaction in acute mania. *Biol. Psychiatry.* 64: 718-726.

Pacchioni AM, Gioino G, Assis A, Cancela LM. A single exposure to restraint stress induces behavioral and neurochemical sensitization to stimulating effects of amphetamine: involvement of NMDA receptors. Ann N Y Acad Sci. 2002 ; 965:233-46.

Paizanis, E., Hamon, M., Lanfumey, L. (2007). Hippocampal neurogenesis, depressive disorders, and antidepressant therapy. *Neural Plast.* 2007: 1-7.

Peet, M.(1994). Induction of mania with selective serotonin reuptake inhibitors and tricyclic antidepressants. *Br. J. Psychiatry;* 164:549–550.

Rammes, G., Danysz, W., Parsons, C.G. (2008) Pharmacodynamics of memantine: an update. *Curr. Neuropharmacol.*;6(1):55-78.

Rapoport, S.I., Basselin, M., Kim, H.W., Rao, J.S. (2009) Bipolar disorder and mechanisms of action of mood stabilizers. *Brain Res. Rev.* Oct;61(2):185-209.

Ray, W.A., Chung, C.P., Murray, K.T., Hall, K., Stein, C.M. (2009) Atypical antipsychotic drugs and the risk of sudden cardiac death. N Engl J Med. 2009; 360(3):225-35. *N. Engl. J. Med.* 2009 ;361(18):1814.

Réus, G.Z., Stringari, R.B., Kirsch, T.R., Fries, G.R., Kapczinski, F., Roesler, R., Quevedo, J. (2010). Neurochemical and behavioural effects of acute and chronic memantine administration in rats: Further support for NMDA as a new pharmacological target for the treatment of depression? *Brain Res. Bull.*; 81(6):585-9.

Ritti, A. (1883) Traité Clinique de la Folie à Double Forme. Paris, Octave Doin, Rockhold RW. Glutamatergic involvement in psychomotor stimulant action. *Prog Drug Res.* 1998;50:155-92.

Rogóz, Z., Skuza, G., Maj, J., Danysz, W. (2002) Synergistic effect of uncompetitive NMDA receptor antagonists and antidepressant drugs in the forced swimming test in rats. *Neuropharmacology.* Jun;42(8):1024-30.

Rompré, P.P., Bauco, P. (2006). Neurotensin receptor activation sensitizes to the locomotor stimulant effect of cocaine: a role for NMDA receptors. *Brain Res.*;1085(1):77-86.

Sani G, Serra G, Kotzalidis GD, Romano S, Tamorri SM, Manfredi G, Caloro M, Telesforo CL, Caltagirone SS, Panaccione I, Simonetti A, Demontis F, Serra G, Girardi P. The role of memantine in the treatment of psychiatric disorders other than the dementias: a review of current preclinical and clinical evidence. *CNS Drugs*. 2012; 26(8):663-690.

Schildkraut, J.J. (1965) The catecholamine hypothesis of affective disorders: a review of supporting evidence. *Am. J. Psychiatry.* Nov;122(5):509-522.

Schneck, C. D., Miklowitz, D. J., Miyahara, S., Araga, M., Wisniewski, S., Gyulai, L., Allen, M.H., Thase, M.E., Sachs, G.S. (2008). The Prospective Course of Rapid-Cycling Bipolar Disorder: Findings From the STEP-BD, *Am. J. Psychiatry* 165:3, 370-377.

Serra, G., Argiolas, A., Klimek, V., Fadda, F., Gessa, G.L. (1979). Chronic treatment with antidepressants prevents the inhibitory effect of small doses of apomorphine on dopamine synthesis and motor activity. *Life Sci.* 25: 415-424.

Serra, G., Argiolas, A., Fadda, F., Gessa G.L. (1980). Hyposensitivity of dopamine autoreceptore induced by chronic administration of tricyclic antidepressants. *Pharmacol. Res. Comm.* 12: 619-624.

Serra, G., Argiolas, A., Fadda F., Melis, M.R., Gessa, G.L. (1981). Repeated electroconvulsive shock prevents the sedative effect of small doses of apomorphine. *Psychopharmacology* 73: 194-196.

Serra, G., Melis, M.R., Argiolas, A., Fadda, F., Gessa, G.L. (1981). REM sleep deprivation induces subsensitivity of dopamine receptors mediating sedation in rats. *Eur. J. Pharmacol.* 72: 131-135.

Serra, G., Gessa, G.L. (1990) Manuale di Psicofarmacologia. Masson Editore, Milano.

Serra, G., Collu, M., D'Aquila, P.S., De Montis, G.M., Gessa G.L (1990). Possible role of dopamine D1 receptor in the behavioural supersensitivity to dopamine agonists induced by chronic treatment with antidepressant. *Brain Res.* 527: 234-243.

Serra, G., Collu, M., D'Aquila, P., De Montis, G.M., Gessa, G.L (1991). Chronic imipramine "reverses" B-HT 920-induced hypomotility in rats. *J. Neural Transm.* 84: 237-240.

Serra, G., Collu, M., D'Aquila, P.S., Gessa, G.L. (1992). Role of the mesolimbic dopamine system in the mechanism of action of antidepressants. *Pharmacol Toxicol.* 71 (1):72-85.

Serra, G., Fratta, W. (2007). A possible role for the endocannabinoid system in the neurobiology of depression. *Clinical Practice and Epidemiology in Mental Healt*; 3: 25.

Serra, G., D`Aquila, P.S. (2008). Do antidepressants induce mania and rapid cycling by increasing dopaminergic transmission? *TDM 2008 International Meeting-Bologna Ottobre* 2008. pp. 54-55.

Serra, G. (Patent, 2009) Uso della memantina per il trattamento dei disturbi dell'umore. N° MI2009A000174. 11/02/2009.

Serra, G. (EP Patent, 2010) Memantine for treating bipolar mood disorders resistant to conventional treatments. EP 2 218 450 A1. Priority: 11.02.2009 IT MI20090174. 18.08.2010 Bulletin 2010/33.

Serra, G. (2012) A 3 years open label naturalistic study of adjuntive memantine in treatment resistant bipolar disorder. IRBD, Nice 21-23 May, 2012.

Serra G., Koukopoulos A., Serra G.(2013): Antimanic and long-lasting mood stabilizing effect of Memantine in Bipolar I Mood Disorder: two case reports. *J. Clinic. Psychopharmacol.* (in press).

Serra G., De Chiara L., Reginaldi D., Koukopoulos A., Serra G. (2013): Efficacy of memantine in the treatment and prophylaxis of bipolar type II mood disorder: two case reports. *Clin. Neuropharmacol.* (submitted).

Sheline, Y.I., Gado Mokhtar, H., Kroemer, H.C. (2003) Untreated depression and hippocampal volume loss. *Am. J. Psychiatry.* 160:1516-1518.

Spearing, M.K., Post, R.M., Leverich, G.S., Brandt, D., Nolen, W. (1997) Modification of the Clinical Global Impressions (CGI) Scale for use in bipolar illness (BP): the CGI-BP. *Psychiatry Res.* Dec 5;73(3):159-71.

Spyraki, C., Fibiger, H.C. (1981). Behavioural evidence for supersensitivity of postsynaptic dopamine receptors in the mesolimbic system after chronic administration of desipramine. *Eur. J. Pharmacol.* 11;74(2-3):195-206.

Till, E., Vuckovic, S. (1970). Ueber den Einfluss der thymoleptischen Behandlung auf den Verlauf endogener Depressionen. *Im Pharmacopsychiatry* 4:210—2 19.

Tohen, M., Greil, W., Calabrese, J.R., Sachs, G.S., Yatham, L.N., Oerlinghausen, B.M., Koukopoulos, A., Cassano, G.B., Grunze, H., Licht, R.W., Dell'Osso, L., Evans, A.R., Risser, R., Baker, R.W., Crane, H., Dossenbach, M.R., Bowden, C.L. (2005). Olanzapine versus lithium in the maintenance treatment of Biolar Disorders: a 12-month, randomized, double-blind, controlled clinical trial. *Am. J. Psychiatry.*; 162(7):1281-90.

Tondo L., Laddomada P., Serra G., Minnai G., Kukopulos A (1981). Rapid cyclers and antidepressants. *Int. Pharmacopsychiat.* 16: 119-123.

Tondo, L., Hennen, J., Baldessarini, R.J. (2003). Rapid-cycling bipolar disorder: effects of long-term treatments. *Acta Psychiatr Scand.*;108(1):4-14.

Tondo, L., Vázquez, G., Baldessarini, R.J. (2010). Mania associated with antidepressant treatment: comprehensive meta-analytic review. *Acta Psychiatr Scand.* 121(6):404-414.

Trujillo, K.A. (2002). The neurobiology of opiate tolerance, dependence and sensitization: mechanisms of NMDA receptor-dependent synaptic plasticity. *Neurotox Res.*; 4(4): 373-391.

Van Dongen, A.M. Editor. (2009). Biology of NMDA receptor. Frontiers in Neuroscience.

Vanelle JM, Loo H, Galinowski A, de Carvalho W, Bourdel MC, Brochier P, Bouvet O, Brochier T, Olie JP. (1994). Maintenance ECT in intractable manicdepressive disorders. *Convulsive Therapy*. Sep; 10 (3): 195-205.

Vezina P, Queen AL (2000). Induction of locomotor sensitization by amphetamine requires the activation of NMDA receptors in the rat ventral tegmental area. *Psychopharmacology*. 151(2-3): 184-191.

Videbech, P., Ravnkilde, B. (2004) Hippocampal volume and depression. A meta-analysis of MRI studies. *Am. J. Psychiatry*, 161(11):1957-1966.

Võikar V, Soosaar A, Volke V, Kõks S, Bourin M, Männistö PT, Vasar E (1999). Apomorphine-induced behavioural sensitization in rats: individual differences, role of dopamine and NMDA receptors. *Eur. Neuropsychopharmacol.;* 9(6): 507-514.

Warnings About Suicidality Risk With Antiepileptic Drugs FDA, Alert 2008, Dec 16.

Wehr, TA, Goodwin, FK. (1979). Rapid cycling in manic-depressives induced by tricyclic antidepressants. *Arch. Gen. Psychiatry*. May; 36(5): 555-559.

Westfall TC, Westfall DP. In Goodman and Gilman's The Pharmacological Basis of Therapeutics 11 Edition 237-295.

Willner, P. (1997). The mesolimbic dopamine system as a target for rapid antidepressant action. *Int. Clin. Psychopharmacol.*;12 (3):S7-14.

Wolf ME, White FJ, Hu XT.(1994): MK-801 prevents alterations in the mesoaccumbens dopamine system associated with behavioral sensitization to amphetamine. *J. Neurosci.*; 14(3):1735-1745.

Yap JJ, Covington HE 3rd, Gale MC, Datta R, Miczek KA (2005). Behavioral sensitization due to social defeat stress in mice: antagonism at mGluR5 and NMDA receptors. *Psychopharmacology* (Berl).; 179(1):230-239.

Yildiz A, Sachs GS., Characteristics of rapid cycling bipolar I patients in a bipolar speciality clinic. *J. Affect Disord*. 2004 Apr; 79 (1-3):247-51

Zdanys, K., Tampi, R.R. (2008). A systematic review of off-label uses of memantine for psychiatric disorders. *Prog Neuropsychopharmacol Biol Psychiatry.*;32(6):1362-74.

Zupancic, M.L. (2011). Role of atypical antipsychotics in rapid cycling bipolar disorder: a review of the literature. *Ann Clin Psychiatry*. 2011;23(2): 141-149.

In: Bipolar Disorder
Editor: Nickolas B. Moore

ISBN: 978-1-62618-666-8


*Chapter VII*

# Potential Biomarkers for Bipolar Disorder: P11 Expression and PET

***Lei Zhang, Cheng-Ta Li,[1] Tung-Ping Su,[1] Xian-zhang Hu, Stanley Smerin, He Li, Xiaoxia Li and Robert Usano***

Center for the Study of Traumatic Stress, Department of Psychiatry, Uniformed Services University of the Health Sciences, Bethesda, MD, US

[1]Division of Psychiatry, Faculty of Medicine, National Yang-Ming University, Taipei, Taiwan

## Abstract

Bipolar disorder (BD) is a complex, chronic psychiatric condition characterized by recurring episodes of depression and mania or hypomania. It is subdivided into BD-I and BD-II, based on the nature and severity of the mood episodes experienced. Substantial evidence demonstratesthat p11 (S100A10) and positron emission tomography (PET) are potential biomarkers for BD. For example, peripheral blood mononuclear cell (PBMC) p11 mRNA was over-expressed in BD compared with non-BD controls. Comparing BD patients to healthy controls (HCs), normalized glucose metabolism (NGM) was higher in the hippocampus, parahippocampus, and amygdala, but lower in the anterior cingulate cortex (aCC), medial prefrontal cortex (mPFC), dorsolateral prefrontal cortex (dlPFC), insula and thalamus. Compared to BD-II, BD-I had hypometabolism of glucose in the aCC, bilateral middle and inferior temporal gyrus, insula and striatum, and hypermetabolism of glucose in the left parahippocampus. In addition, PBMC p11 mRNA levels were significantly positively correlated with NGM in the mPFC, aCC, left insula, bilateral orbitofrontal cortex (OFC), and left middle, inferior and superior temporal gyri, and withthe number of depressive episodes in BD patients, especially in BD-I patients. These data demonstrate that PBMC p11 mRNA expression is associated with neural activation in the brain of BD patients and warrants a larger translational study to determine its clinical utility. In this chapter, we will discuss the background information of p11 as a potential biomarker for BD. In addition, we develop the concept of combining blood p11 levels with PET as biomarkers for BD diagnosis. We will also discuss the current status of this research, including methods, such as blood sample collection, mRNA purification, real time PCR and PET data analysis for BD biomarker identification. Specifically, we will discuss the strategies for developing a blood test and PET for BD diagnosis from bench to bedside and/or from bedside to bench, a two-way approach.

## Introduction

BD is a complex, chronic psychiatric condition characterized by recurring episodes of depression and mania or hypomania [1]. According to the Diagnostic and Statistical Manual of Mental Disorders, BD is subdivided into BD-I and BD-II, based on the nature and severity of the mood episodes experienced. Patients with BD-I must have one or more manic episodes, while a depressive or hypomanic episode is not required. Patients with BD-II must have one or more major depressive episode and no manic episodes, but may have one or more hypomanic episodes. BD-II is sometimes difficult to distinguish from BD-I clinically since the hypomanic episodes may simply appear as a period of high productivity, and 'social or occupational impairment' is hard to define under certain circumstances. Currently, the diagnosis of BD is based on a subjective description by the patient and observation by the psychiatrist. Although there have been efforts to develop a clinical strategy to diagnose BD, there is still no objective biological assay for the diagnosis of BD or for the differentiation of BD-I from BD-II. The lack of quantitative objective measures of BD is one reason why the causative factors of BD remain obscure. To examine the role of genetic factors and variability in neuronal activity in the development of BD [2], the relationship between PBMC p11 mRNA levels and neuronal activity was examined using qPCR and PET in a group of BD patients in remission. The results demonstrate that the blood p11 levels and PET might serve as biomarkers for identifying BD.

P11 may be a valuable candidate for identifying several psychiatric disorders, including BD and post-traumatic stress disorder (PTSD) [3].P11 (annexin II light chain),a member of the S100 protein family [4] was first described by Gerkeand Weber [5]. The p11 gene islocated on chromosome 1q21 in humans and expresses in many types of cells and tissues, such as in the lung, intestine, kidney and brain in many species [6]. Its protein may regulate exocytosis and endocytosis. In cells, p11 can form a p11/annexin A2 complex, which has heterotetrameric and symmetric entities. The p11 half-life is dramatically increased when it complexesto annexin A2, indicating that in the presence of annexin A2 the p11 protein is more stable [7-9]. In the p11 promoter there are a number of binding sites for specific transcription factors [10] including glucocorticoid receptor response elements (GERs). Structurally, unlike other S100, p11 has crucial amino acid substitutions in the two EF-hand loops that render both $Ca^{2+}$-binding sites inactive [5]. It is locked in the equivalent of a $Ca^{2+}$-loaded structure and is in a permanently activated state [11]. In the absence of $Ca^{2+}$, p11 binds to the target protein in cellular hydrophobic surfaces [11].

Many studies demonstrate the interaction of P11 with annexins, phospholipid-binding proteins, which are structurally highly conserved and have been implicated in a wide range of cellular activities [12]. For example, the p11 dimer contains two identical annexin A2-binding sites [13]. The p11- binding site resides exclusively in the N-terminal residues [14] that form an amphiphatic α-helix [15]. The hydrophobic face of this helix interacts with a hydrophobic surface on the p11 dimer that primarily encompasses residues in the C-terminal region

[6,16,17]. Therefore, p11 is able to interact with additional binding partners. The complex of p11/annexin A2 regulates the distribution of proteins in cellular membranes and/or stabilizes membrane lipids and proteins. Membrane binding of the p11/annexin A2 complex and its specificity is mediated through the annexin A2 sub-unit, which has a preference for negatively charged phospholipids found on the cytosolic leaflets of cellular membranes. However, membrane-bound annexin A2 is also predominantly associated with the plasma membrane and the membrane of early endosomes [15].p11/annexin A2 directly binds to phosphatidylinositol (4,5) bisphosphate (PI(4,5)P2) [18,19]. Hence, p11/annexin A2 is recruited to PI(4,5)P2 and cholesterol-rich membrane domains [19]. Increasing evidence suggests that p11/annexin A2 plays an important role in linking thismicro-domain formation to actin rearrangementsas well [20].p11/annexin A2 binds to the apical PI(4,5)P2 and in turn recruits GTP binding protein (Cdc42)which initiates the formation of an actin belt and subsequent full morphological polarization [8]. Cdc42 interacts with the annexin A2 chain in the p11/annexin A2 complex and competes for p11 binding. Since Cdc42 is a Rho-GTPase that transduces extracellular signals from G-coupled protein receptors (GPCR), in this example, through the p11-induced inhibition ofCdc42 recruitment to annexin A2-decorated membrane sites, p11 regulates cell signaling of integrins and growth factor receptors.

Much evidence demonstrates that p11 plays an important role in regulation of certain channels and receptors. For example, cells expressing p11 with the sodium channel Nav 1.8 complementary deoxyribonucleic acid showed channel membrane translocation and increase of sodium currents. Anti-sense-mediated down regulation of endogenous p11 resulted in lowerNav1.8 activity in sensory neurons [21]. P11 is also an interaction partner for the background TWIK-related acidsensitive $K^+$ (TASK) channel [22] and regulates TASK'splasma membrane activity [23]. In addition, p11 is an interaction factor involved in the functional expression of the transient receptor potential (TRP) channels TRPV5 and TRPV6 at the cell surface. TRPV5 and TRPV6, are calcium selective ion channels and are known to be expressed in calcium-transporting epithelial tissues. Downregulation of annexin A2 lead to a reduction in p11 levels and interfered with TRPV5 and TRPV6 currents in cells ectopically expressing the channels [24]. It is found that p11 also binds to and regulates the activity of the acid-sensing ion channel ASIC1a [25] and the serotonin 5-hydroxytryptamine receptor 1B (5-HT1B receptor) [26]. ASIC1a expresses in the brain, especially in the basolateral amygdala (BLA) [27], where it is involved in the fear [28]. In an animal study, disrupting the ASIC1a protein produced an antidepressant-like effect in mice [29]. The 5-HT1B receptor expresses in the brain, where it induces presynaptic inhibition. Knockout ofthe 5-HT1B gene in miceresulted in an increase of aggression and a higher preference for alcohol [30]. Data also demonstrated that the p11/annexin A2 complex can interact with neuroblast differentiation-associated protein AHNAK (AHNAK) [31,32], which is essential for pseudopod protrusion and cell migration [33].p11/Annexin A2by binding to specific membrane phosphoinositidesstabilizes their local accumulation and recruits other factors to the sites of channels and receptors.

At protein levels, p11 increases the dimerization of ANXA2/p36.p36 (also termed annexin II) is a 39 kDa $Ca^{2+}$/phospholipid-binding, membrane-associated protein that is a protein-tyrosine kinase substrate [34,35]. Thus, p11regulatsprotein phosphorylation. Extracellular p11, probably locates in a complex with annexin A2, is a receptor for tissue-type plasminogen activator (tPA) [36-38]. The interaction of the carboxyl-terminal lysine residues of the p11 subunit of AIIt with the lysine-binding kringle domains of plasminogen is believed to play a key role in plasminogen binding and stimulation of the tPA-catalyzed cleavage of plasminogen to plasmin [39].

Evidences show that p11 may play an important role in depressive disorders. Svenningsson et al. provided compelling data supporting the association of p11 down-regulation in cortical tissue of patients with depression [40]. The possible role of p11 in depression has been further supported by the finding that p11 knockout mice exhibited a depression-like phenotype and had reduced responsiveness to 5 HT1B receptor agonists [40]. Furthermore, p11 over-expression increased localization of 5-HT1B receptors at the cell surface and enhanced 5-HT1B receptor function [40]. Previously, we found that p11 mRNA was over-expressed in the PBMCs of patients with BD compared to normal controls and that BD patients have abnormal neural activity in the limbic-thalamic-cortical circuit [41]. Comparing BD patients to healthy controls (HCs)s, normalized glucose metabolism (NGM) was higher in the hippocampus, parahippocampus, and amygdala, but lower in the anterior cingulate cortex (aCC), medial prefrontal cortex (mPFC), dorsolateral prefrontal cortex (dlPFC), insula and thalamus. Compared to BD-II, BD-I had hypometabolism of glucose in the aCC, bilateral middle and inferior gyrus, insula and striatum, and hypermetabolism of glucose in the left parahippocampus. In addition, PBMC p11 mRNA levels significantly positively correlated with NGM in the mPFC, aCC, left insula, bilateral orbitofrontal cortex (OFC), and left middle, inferior and superior temporal gyri, and with the number of depressive episodes in BD patients, especially in BD-I patients. These data demonstrate that PBMC p11 mRNA expression is associated with neural activation in the brain of BD patients and warrants a translational study to determine its clinical utility [41].

Glucose metabolism is abnormalin the patients with BD. For example, medication-free depressed outpatients with bipolar disorder had decreased metabolism in prefrontal, anterior cingulate, insula, and ventral striatal areas [42]. BD patients in remission have increased neuronal activity in several limbic areas, such as hippocampus, parahippocampus and amygdala [41]. Visualization of resting glucose metabolism in part of the prefrontal cortex (PFC), ACC, insula, and striatum can be used to distinguish subtypes of mood disorders [41]. Although PET provides direct evidence of changes in glucose metabolism, which may be used as a biomarker for BD diagnosis, the expense and radiation exposure limits its utility. Therefore, a blood biomarker for BD-I and BD-II, such as PBMC p11, may complement the PET strategy in routine clinical practice since analysis for mRNA markers in PBMCs is much less expensive than PET, and carries no risk of radiation exposure. PBMC p11 mRNA levels can serve as an adjunctive biomarker for BD and are correlated with neuronal activity, possibly indicating a role for p11 in the pathophysiology of BD. We found that comparing BD patients to HCs, NGM was higher in the hippocampus, parahippocampus, and amygdala, but lower in the anterior cingulate cortex (ACC), medial prefrontal cortex (mPFC), dorsolateral prefrontal cortex (DLPFC), insula and thalamus (Figure 1). Compared to BD-II patients, BD-I patients had hypometabolism of glucose in the aCC, bilateral middle and inferior temporal gyrus, insula and striatum, and hypermetabolism of glucose in the left parahippocampus (Figure 1). PBMC p11 mRNA was over-expressed in both BD-I and BD-II, although there was no significant difference in its expression levels between BD-I and B-II patients (Figure 1). Further, there were significant positive correlations between PBMC p11 mRNA and NGM in the mPFC, aCC, left insula, bilateral orbitofrontal cortex (OFC), and left middle, inferior and superior temporal gyri. Also, PBMC p11 mRNA was positively correlated to the number of depressive episodes in BD patients, especially in BD-I patients (Table 1) [41].

The PBMC p11 mRNA over-expression might serve as a compensatory mechanism for the decreased neuronal activity in the brain of BD patients [41]. p11 protein is linked with the transport of 5-HT1B receptors from the cytosol to the membrane [26], which has been implicated in the regulation of mood and stress through the HPA axis and is involved in the pathophysiology of BD. It is possible that the over-expression of PBMC p11 mRNA in remission patients with BD is caused by the dysregulation of certain brain regions, particularly the hippocampus and amygdala, in response to stress. There are two specific glucocorticoid receptor response elements (GRE) in the p11 promoter region [10].

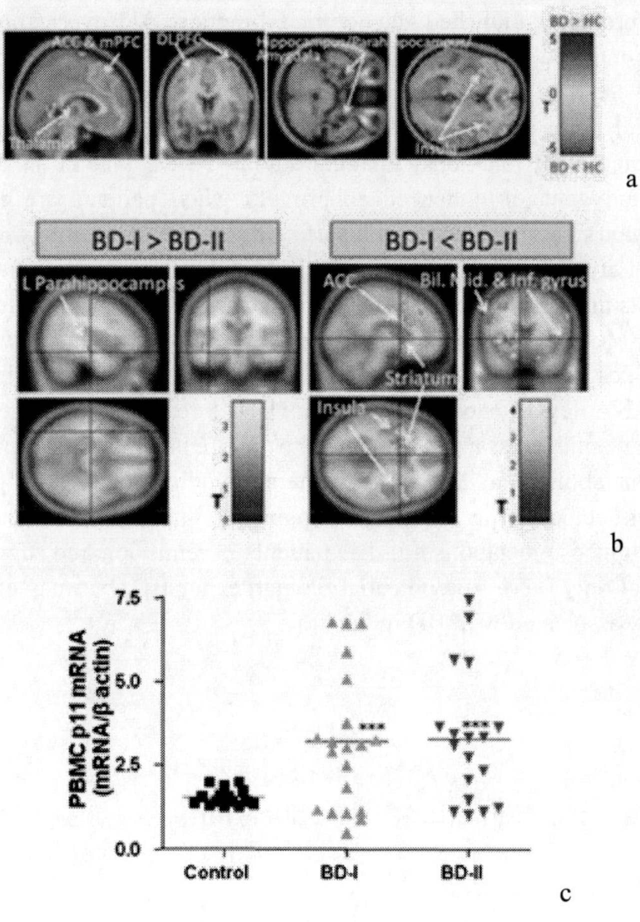


Figure 1. Normalized glucose metabolism in patients with BD-I and BD-II and in HCs under a corrected $p<.05$, after controlling for age and sex. a) glucose metabolism in hippocampus and amygdala was significantly higher in BD patients as compared to controls; and significantly lower in aCC, mPFC, dlPFC, insula and thalami of BD patients compared to HCs. b) There were significant differences in glucose metabolism between BD-I and BD-II patients. BD-I patients had lower glucose metabolism in PFC, aCC, striatum and bilateral insula (left panel), while BD-II patients demonstrated hypermetabolism of glucose in left parahippocampus/fusiform gyrus (right panel). c) PBMC p11 mRNA levels in BD-I and BD-II patients compared to HCs. Quantitative real-time PCR analysis revealed that p11 mRNA levels are significantly elevated in PBMCs of both BD-I and BD-II patients compared to HCs. There is no significant difference in PBMC p11 mRNA levels between BD-I and BD-II patients. ***$p <.001$.

**Table 1. Linear regressive analysis of number of depressive episodes and p11 expression level**

| | B | r | t | P value |
|---|---|---|---|---|
| All (N=40) | 2.58 | 0.38 | 2.45 | 0.02 |
| BD-I (N=20) | 1.22 | 0.51 | 2.34 | 0.03 |
| BD-II (N=20) | 2.81 | 0.24 | 1.03 | 0.31 |

Stress-induced glucocorticoids activate glucocorticoid receptors (GR), which translocate from the cytosol to the nuclear membrane. In the nuclei, GR binds to the GRE in the p11 promoter and regulates p11 expression. Treatment with a GR antagonist or mutation of the GRE in the p11 promoter abolished glucocorticoid-induced p11 over-expression [10].

Thus, stress-induced p11 expression is mediated by GR and GRE in the p11 promoter, and this circuit may be involved in stress-related diseases such as PTSD and affective disorders. Several brain regions in which p11 is expressed [10] are involved in the stress response. Evidence from functional imaging studies reveal that in anxiety disorders, brain activity in the amygdala is enhanced abnormally when patients are exposed to stressful situations. Elevated neural activity was also found in the hippocampus., These data indicate an increased activity along the HPA axis, which has been implicated in the etiology of BD. Even BD patients in remission present abnormal activity in these stress-related brain regions. In addition, PBMC p11 mRNA levels were positively correlated with the number of depressive episodes of BD-I but not BD-II, . There is no data indicating that the differences of PBMC p11 mRNA levels between BD-I and BD-II resulted from the differences of the administration of antidepressants. Compared to BD-II patients, BD-I patients in remission exhibited hypometabolism in the ACC, bilateral middle and inferior gyrus, striatum and insula and hypermetabolism in the hippocampus [41]. Ourresults are consistent with studies showing altered glucose metabolism in BD patients in remission and suggest that PBMC p11 mRNA levels not only serve as a potential biomarker for BD, but may also reflect the status of neural activity associated with BD in the brain.

# Notes

## Blood Sample Collection and RNA Purification

### *Materialsfor RNA Purification*

There are several protocols for blood RNA isolation on the market. Two protocols have been used and validated in the lab. The protocols use the PAXgene Blood RNA System and GodenRNA Tube system to isolate blood RNA. The difference between PAXgene and GodenRNA tube is that the GodenRAN tube can be used for blood RNAcollection and stored at RT for a week. This tube can also be used for DNA sample collection. There are two kinds of PAXgene tubes, one for RNA and one for DNA.

1 GodenRNA Tube or PAXgene Blood RNA Tube
2 PAXgene RNA spin columns

3 PAXgene Shredder spin columns
4 Proteinase K
5 Buffers BR1 to BR5
6 The RNase-Free DNase Set, which contains DNase I, Buffer RDD, and RNase-free water.

### *RNA Purification*

The purification process is designed to provide high quality RNA from samples that have been stabilized in the reagent of the PAXgene Blood RNA Tube. This system consists of several steps: whole blood collection, nucleic acid stabilization, and RNA purification. By minimizing the irregularity associated with RNA processing, the system provides enhanced accuracy of intracellular RNA analysis. PAXgene tubes contain a proprietary reagent that immediately stabilizes intracellular RNA for 3 days at room temperature (18-25°C) and 5 days at 2-8°C. This system has a specific isolation kit for RNA isolation from collected blood samples. The following method is adopted from the manufacture's protocol (Invitrogen, Inc).

1 Centrifuge blood sample tubes for 10 minutes at 3000–5000 x g.
2 Remove the supernatant and add 4 ml RNase-free water to the pellet.
3 Vortex and centrifuge for 10 minutes at 3000–5000 x g. Remove the entire supernatant. Small debris remaining in the supernatant after vortexing but before centrifugation will not affect the procedure.
4 Add 350 μl Buffer BR1, and vortex.
5 Transfer the sample into a 1.5 ml micro-centrifuge tube containing 300 μl Buffer BR2 and 40 μl proteinase K. Mix by vortexing for 5 seconds, and incubate for 10 minutes at 55°C using a shaker–incubator at 400–1400 rpm. After incubation, set the temperature of the shaker–incubator to 65°C (for step 20).
6 Transfer the lysate into a PAXgene Shredder spin column (lilac) placed in a 2 ml processing tube, and centrifuge for 3 minutes at maximum speed (but not to exceed 20,000 x g).
7 Transfer the supernatant of the flow-through fraction to a fresh 1.5 ml tube without disturbing the pellet in the processing tube.
8 Add 350 μl ethanol (96–100%). Mix by vortexing, and then centrifuge briefly (1–2 seconds at 500–1000 x g) to remove drops from the inside of the tube lid.
9 Transfer 700 μl sample into the PAXgene RNA spin column (red) placed in a 2 ml processing tube, and centrifuge for 1 minute at 8000–20,000 x g. Place the spin column in a new 2 ml processing tube, and discard the old processing tube containing flow-through.
10 Transfer the remaining sample into the PAXgene RNA spin column, and centrifuge for 1 minute at 8000–20,000 x g. Place the spin column in a new 2 ml processing tube, and discard the old processing tube containing flow-through.
11 Transfer 350 μl Buffer BR3 into the PAXgene RNA spin column. Centrifuge for 1 minute at 8000–20,000 x g. Place the spin column in a new 2 ml processing tube, and discard the old processing tube containing flow-through.
12 Add 10 μlDNase I stock solution to 70 μl Buffer RDD in a 1.5 ml tube. Mix by gently flicking the tube, and then centrifuge briefly to collect residual liquid from the

sides of the tube. If processing, for example, 10 samples, add 100 µlDNase I stock solution to 700 µl Buffer RDD. Use the 1.5 ml tubes supplied with the kit.

13 Transfer the DNase I incubation mix (80 µl) directly onto the PAXgene RNA spin column membrane, and place on the benchtop (20–30°C) for 15 minutes.

14 Transfer 350 µl Buffer BR3 into the PAXgene RNA spin column, and centrifuge for 1 minute at 8000–20,000 x g. Place the spin column in a new 2 ml processing tube, and discard the old processing tube containing flow-through.

15 Transfer 500 µl Buffer BR4 to the PAXgene RNA spin column, and centrifuge for 1 minute at 8000–20,000 x g. Place the spin column in a new 2 ml processing tube, and discard the old processing tube containing flow-through.

16 Add another 500 µl Buffer BR4 to the PAXgene RNA spin column. Centrifuge for 3 minutes at 8000–20,000 x g.

17 Discard the tube containing the flow-through, and place the PAXgene RNA spin column in a new 2 ml processing tube. Centrifuge for 1 minute at 8000–20,000 x g.

18 Discard the tube containing the flow-through. Place the PAXgene RNA spin column in a 1.5 ml microcentrifuge tube, and add 40 µl Buffer BR5 directly onto the PAXgene RNA spin column membrane. Centrifuge for 1 minute at 8000–20,000 x g to elute the RNA.

19 Repeat the elution step (step 18) as described, using 40 µl Buffer BR5 and the same tube.

20 Incubate the eluate for 5 minutes at 65°C in the shaker–incubator (from step 5) without shaking. After incubation, immediately chill on ice.

21 If the RNA samples will not be used immediately, store at –20°C or –70°C. Since the RNA remains denatured after repeated freezing and thawing, it is not necessary to repeat the incubation at 65°C.

## PBMC p11 mRNA Assay

PBMCs are separated by centrifugation on a Ficoll-Hypaque (Invitrogen) density gradient. The blood samples were stored at -80 $^{0}$C. RNA is extracted from blood lysates using a PAXgen blood RNA validationKit (PreAnalytiX, Qiagen, Valencia, CA). cDNAwas generatedfrom 3 µg of total RNA using Superscript III RT (reverse transcriptase)and oligo (dT) primers (Invitrogen). Real-time PCR is performed on the generated cDNA product in the IQ5 sequence detection system using SYBR Green (Bio-Rad). The following sequences are used for human p11 mRNA analyses: forward 5'AAATTCGCTGGGGATAAAGG-3' and reverse 5'AGCCCACTTTG CCATCTCTA-3'primers.

β-actin mRNA levels are used as an internal control for normalizing p11 mRNA levels in control and experimental samples. The sequences for b-actin primers are 5'-ACCTGTACGCCAACACAGTG-3'and 5'-ACACGGAGTACTTGCGCTCA-3' (Applied Biosystems). Dilution curves confirm the linear dependence of the threshold cycle number on the concentration of template RNAs.

Relative quantitation of p11 mRNA in control and experimental samples is obtained using the standard curve method.

### PET Study: Imaging Acquisition and Analysis

Patients fasted for at least 4 h before the PET examination. PET scans of glucose utilization are acquired on a PET/CT scanner with a 3D brain mode. PET images are acquired in 45 min after an intravenous injection of 370 MBq FDG. In the combined PET/CT imaging, the standard PET transmission scan is replaced by a low-dose CT scan. Then a CT-based attenuation correction is given. PET images are scanned in the resting state with eyes covered with a mask. The brain acquisition time is 15 min.

The system produces 47 consecutive slices over an axial length of 15.7 cm with a slice thickness of 3.75 mm and a transaxialFOV of 70 cm. PET images arereconstructed in a 128 X 128 matrix using CT for attenuation correction with an ordered-subset expectation maximization iterative reconstruction algorithm. Then the axial images are realigned to yield sagittal and coronal images.

### Statistical Analysis

PET data are analyzed using the Statistical Parametric Mapping, version 2 (SPM2; Wellcome Department of Cognitive Neurology, Institute of Neurology, University College London, London, England) implemented in Matlab 7.0 (The MathworksInc., Sherborn, MA, US). First, an 18F-FDG template is created for all subjects including all BD patients and HCs [43,44]. Then, each subject's images are normalized to the 18FFDG template and smoothed with a 3D Gaussian kernel. The overall grand mean from PET scans is centered and normalized to 100, and global variance across scans is removed by analysis of covariance (ANCOVA) [45]. To assess potential group differences of normalized brain glucose uptake, an ANCOVA with age, gender [46]and global gray matter values as covariates of no interest is used for between-group comparisons (BD-I vs. BD-II). The significance thresholds are set at $p < .05$ uncorrected at the voxel level, followed by a cluster-level analysis with a corrected $p < .05$. In addition, voxel-based partial correlations are performed for investigating the association between 18F-FDG uptake and PBMC p11 mRNA levels after accounting for age, gender andtotal gray matter counts. Since the brain regions selected forstudy are those known to be involved in the neural system underlying BD-PFC, thalamus, aCC, insula, and striatum-the identified brain regions within a priori areas are further examined by Small Volume Correction (SVC) with an anatomically defined regional mask in the relevant gray matter area [47]. Those brain regions passing through a SVCcorrectedp-value <.05 are considered significant.

## References

[1] Michalak, E.E., Murray, G., Young, A.H., and Lam, R.W. Burden of bipolar depression: impact of disorder and medications on quality of life. *CNS drugs* 22, 389-406 (2008).

[2] Saus, E., et al. Comprehensive copy number variant (CNV) analysis of neuronal pathways genes in psychiatric disorders identifies rare variants within patients. *Journal of psychiatric research* 44, 971-978 (2010).

[3] Su, T.P., et al. Levels of the potential biomarker p11 in peripheral blood cells distinguish patients with PTSD from those with other major psychiatric disorders. *Journal of psychiatric research* 43, 1078-1085 (2009).

[4] Grabarek, Z. Structural basis for diversity of the EF-hand calcium-binding proteins. *Journal of molecular biology* 359, 509-525 (2006).

[5] Gerke, V. and Weber, K. The regulatory chain in the p36-kd substrate complex of viral tyrosine-specific protein kinases is related in sequence to the S-100 protein of glial cells. *The EMBO journal* 4, 2917-2920 (1985).

[6] Johnsson, N., Gerke, V. and Weber, K. P36, member of the CA2+/lipid binding proteins (annexins, calpactins, lipocortins) and its complex with P11; molecular aspects. *Progress in clinical and biological research* 349, 123-133 (1990).

[7] Rescher, U., Ruhe, D., Ludwig, C., Zobiack, N. and Gerke, V. Annexin 2 is a phosphatidylinositol (4,5)-bisphosphate binding protein recruited to actin assembly sites at cellular membranes. *Journal of cell science* 117, 3473-3480 (2004).

[8] Hayes, M.J., et al. Annexin 2 binding to phosphatidylinositol 4,5-bisphosphate on endocytic vesicles is regulated by the stress response pathway. *The Journal of biological chemistry* 279, 14157-14164 (2004).

[9] Solito, E., et al. Dexamethasone induces rapid serine-phosphorylation and membrane translocation of annexin 1 in a human folliculostellate cell line via a novel nongenomic mechanism involving the glucocorticoid receptor, protein kinase C, phosphatidylinositol 3-kinase, and mitogen-activated protein kinase. *Endocrinology* 144, 1164-1174 (2003).

[10] Zhang, L., et al. p11 is up-regulated in the forebrain of stressed rats by glucocorticoid acting via two specific glucocorticoid response elements in the p11 promoter. *Neuroscience* 153, 1126-1134 (2008).

[11] Mischke, D., Korge, B.P., Marenholz, I., Volz, A., and Ziegler, A. Genes encoding structural proteins of epidermal cornification and S100 calcium-binding proteins form a gene complex ("epidermal differentiation complex") on human chromosome 1q21. *The Journal of investigative dermatology* 106, 989-992 (1996).

[12] Moss, S.E. and Morgan, R.O. The annexins. *Genome biology* 5, 219 (2004).

[13] Bianchi, R., Pula, G., Ceccarelli, P., Giambanco, I., and Donato, R. S-100 protein binds to annexin II and p11, the heavy and light chains of calpactin I. *Biochimica et biophysica acta* 1160, 67-75 (1992).

[14] Harder, T., Kube, E. and Gerke, V. Cloning and characterization of the human gene encoding p11: structural similarity to other members of the S-100 gene family. *Gene* 113, 269-274 (1992).

[15] Becker, T., Weber, K. and Johnsson, N. Protein-protein recognition via short amphiphilic helices; a mutational analysis of the binding site of annexin II for p11. *The EMBO journal* 9, 4207-4213 (1990).

[16] Rety, S., et al. The crystal structure of a complex of p11 with the annexin II N-terminal peptide. *Nature structural biology* 6, 89-95 (1999).

[17] Kube, E., Becker, T., Weber, K., and Gerke, V. Protein-protein interaction studied by site-directed mutagenesis. Characterization of the annexin II-binding site on p11, a

member of the S100 protein family. *The Journal of biological chemistry* 267, 14175-14182 (1992).

[18] Lambert, O., Gerke, V., Bader, M.F., Porte, F., and Brisson, A. Structural analysis of junctions formed between lipid membranes and several annexins by cryo-electron microscopy. *Journal of molecular biology* 272, 42-55 (1997).

[19] Menke, M., Ross, M., Gerke, V., and Steinem, C. The molecular arrangement of membrane-bound annexin A2-S100A10 tetramer as revealed by scanning force microscopy. *Chembiochem: a European journal of chemical biology* 5, 1003-1006 (2004).

[20] Rescher, U. and Gerke, V. Annexins--unique membrane binding proteins with diverse functions. *Journal of cell science* 117, 2631-2639 (2004).

[21] Hayes, M.J., Rescher, U., Gerke, V., and Moss, S.E. Annexin-actin interactions. *Traffic* 5, 571-576 (2004).

[22] Girard, C., et al. p11, an annexin II subunit, an auxiliary protein associated with the background K+ channel, TASK-1. *The EMBO journal* 21, 4439-4448 (2002).

[23] Mathie, A., Rees, K.A., El Hachmane, M.F., and Veale, E.L. Trafficking of neuronal two pore domain potassium channels. *Current neuropharmacology* 8, 276-286 (2010).

[24] Van de Graaf, S.F., et al. Functional expression of the epithelial Ca(2+) channels (TRPV5 and TRPV6) requires association of the S100A10-annexin 2 complex. *The EMBO journal* 22, 1478-1487 (2003).

[25] Foulkes, T., et al. Deletion of annexin 2 light chain p11 in nociceptors causes deficits in somatosensory coding and pain behavior. *The Journal of neuroscience: the official journal of the Society for Neuroscience* 26, 10499-10507 (2006).

[26] Svenningsson, P. and Greengard, P. p11 (S100A10)--an inducible adaptor protein that modulates neuronal functions. *Current opinion in pharmacology* 7, 27-32 (2007).

[27] Wemmie, J.A., et al. Acid-sensing ion channel 1 is localized in brain regions with high synaptic density and contributes to fear conditioning. *The Journal of neuroscience: the official journal of the Society for Neuroscience* 23, 5496-5502 (2003).

[28] Kim, M., Campeau, S., Falls, W.A., and Davis, M. Infusion of the non-NMDA receptor antagonist CNQX into the amygdala blocks the expression of fear-potentiated startle. *Behavioral and neural biology* 59, 5-8 (1993).

[29] Coryell, M.W., et al. Acid-sensing ion channel-1a in the amygdala, a novel therapeutic target in depression-related behavior. *The Journal of neuroscience: the official journal of the Society for Neuroscience* 29, 5381-5388 (2009).

[30] Hoyer, D., Hannon, J.P. and Martin, G.R. Molecular, pharmacological and functional diversity of 5-HT receptors. *Pharmacology, biochemistry, and behavior* 71, 533-554 (2002).

[31] De Seranno, S., et al. Identification of an AHNAK binding motif specific for the Annexin2/S100A10 tetramer. *The Journal of biological chemistry* 281, 35030-35038 (2006).

[32] Benaud, C., et al. AHNAK interaction with the annexin 2/S100A10 complex regulates cell membrane cytoarchitecture. *The Journal of cell biology* 164, 133-144 (2004).

[33] Shankar, J., et al. Pseudopodial actin dynamics control epithelial-mesenchymal transition in metastatic cancer cells. *Cancer research* 70, 3780-3790 (2010).

[34] MacLeod, T.J., Kwon, M., Filipenko, N.R., and Waisman, D.M. Phospholipid-associated annexin A2-S100A10 heterotetramer and its subunits: characterization of the

interaction with tissue plasminogen activator, plasminogen, and plasmin. *The Journal of biological chemistry* 278, 25577-25584 (2003).

[35] Ayala-Sanmartin, J., Gouache, P. and Henry, J.P. N-Terminal domain of annexin 2 regulates Ca(2+)-dependent membrane aggregation by the core domain: a site directed mutagenesis study. *Biochemistry* 39, 15190-15198 (2000).

[36] Lobov, S., Croucher, D.R., Saunders, D.N., and Ranson, M. Plasminogen activator inhibitor type 2 inhibits cell surface associated tissue plasminogen activator in vitro: potential receptor interactions. *Thrombosis and haemostasis* 100, 319-329 (2008).

[37] Tsai, S.J. The P11, tPA/plasminogen system and brain-derived neurotrophic factor: Implications for the pathogenesis of major depression and the therapeutic mechanism of antidepressants. *Medical hypotheses* 68, 180-183 (2007).

[38] Roda, O., et al. New insights into the tPA-annexin A2 interaction. Is annexin A2 CYS8 the sole requirement for this association? *The Journal of biological chemistry* 278, 5702-5709 (2003).

[39] Fogg, D.K., et al. The p11 subunit of annexin II heterotetramer is regulated by basic carboxypeptidase. *Biochemistry* 41, 4953-4961 (2002).

[40] Svenningsson, P., et al. Alterations in 5-HT1B receptor function by p11 in depression-like states. *Science* 311, 77-80 (2006).

[41] Zhang, L., et al. P11 expression and PET in bipolar disorders. *Journal of psychiatric research* 45, 1426-1431 (2011).

[42] Brooks, J.O., 3rd et al. Decreased prefrontal, anterior cingulate, insula, and ventral striatal metabolism in medication-free depressed outpatients with bipolar disorder. *Journal of psychiatric research* 43, 181-188 (2009).

[43] Gispert, J.D., et al. Influence of the normalization template on the outcome of statistical parametric mapping of PET scans. *NeuroImage* 19, 601-612 (2003).

[44] Gispert, J.D., Pascau, J., Reig, S., Garcia-Barreno, P., and Desco, M. [Statistical parametric mapping (SPM) in nuclear medicine]. *Revista espanola de medicina nuclear* 22, 43-53 (2003).

[45] Friston, K.J., et al. The relationship between global and local changes in PET scans. *Journal of cerebral blood flow and metabolism: official journal of the International Society of Cerebral Blood Flow and Metabolism* 10, 458-466 (1990).

[46] Willis, M.W., et al. Age, sex and laterality effects on cerebral glucose metabolism in healthy adults. *Psychiatry research* 114, 23-37 (2002).

[47] Friston, K.J., Stephan, K.M. and Frackowiak, R.S. Transient phase-locking and dynamic correlations: Are they the same thing? *Human brain mapping* 5, 48-57 (1997).

In: Bipolar Disorder
Editor: Nickolas B. Moore
ISBN: 978-1-62618-666-8


*Chapter VIII*

# Neurocognitive Impairment in Bipolar Disorder

***Lokesh Shahani****
Southern Illinois University, Springfield, IL, US

## Abstract

Bipolar disorder was once thought to be an episodic affective disease with complete inter-episodic remission. However research in the area of neurocognition has demonstrated varying degree of impairment even in the period of remission.

Cognitive deficits within bipolar disorders have been studied and overall pattern of impairment in tests of attention, executive function, and verbal memory has become evident. Increased cognitive dysfunction often is associated with greater symptom severity as well as greater likelihood of poor social and vocational outcomes. The further effect of psychotropic medication on cognitive slowing remains a challenging issue.

Consensus is lacking with respect to the use of mood stabilizers and antipsychotics towards their effect on cognitive impairment or therapeutic effects on neurocognition. Use of non-pharmacological options such as social skills training, cognitive-behavioral therapy and cognitive remediation needs to be further studied. Neuroimaging techniques have identified endophenotypic markers whose identification would help to identify at-risk individuals and facilitate early intervention.

## Introduction

Bipolar disorder is estimated to affect around 2% of the US population and known to be among the leading cause of disability and suicide worldwide [1]. Mood disturbance has been the hallmark of bipolar disorder, however psychosis and psychosocial dysfunction is commonly seen and is often a marker for the severity of the disease. The similarity and

* Email – lokesh83@hotmail.com.

differences in symptoms between bipolar disorder and schizophrenia has a topic of controversy since the start of the era of modern psychiatry. Emil Kraepelin distinguished between the two with the notion that Bipolar disorder usually fully remits between episodes of acute mood disturbance [1].

## Neuropsychological Deficits

Standardized neuropsychological testing has been utilized to evaluate the cognitive impairment seen among chronically mentally ill patients. Studies among patient with bipolar disorder which will be discussed later in this chapter have consistently demonstrated impairment in tests of attention, executive function, and verbal memory in the both the phases of acute mood impairment as well as in euthymic phase.

A recent review of literature by Malhi et al. indicated that deficits in executive function, verbal fluency, attention, and memory were most commonly reported [2]. The severity of the cognitive impairment that persists during euthymia is medium-to-large in magnitude compared to healthy individuals across several recent meta-analyses [3, 4, 5]. Martinez in a meta-analytic review of 39 studies comparing cognitive functioning in 948 euthymic bipolar disorder patients and 1,128 healthy controls, matched for age, sex, education, and estimated IQ, found significant impairments in attention and processing speed, episodic memory, and executive functioning [6]. Another meta-analysis by Robinson et al. also found substantial deficits in measures of executive functions, verbal learning and memory, abstraction, sustained attention, and psychomotor speed in euthymic bipolar disorder patients compared to matched healthy controls [5]. The most recent meta-analyses from Bora and colleagues [3], which included 1,423 euthymic bipolar disorder subjects as well as their unaffected first-degree relatives found results consistent with the prior work, implicating attention, verbal learning, and executive functioning as core deficits in remitted bipolar patients.

Research into cognitive functions in bipolar patients has indicated a relationship between the degree of cognitive dysfunction and patient's disease severity/chronicity. For example, bipolar patients who are more symptomatic, psychotic, chronically ill, and elderly tend to have greater and more diffuse cognitive impairment [7]. Tham et al [8] reported that the number of hospitalizations was negatively correlated with intelligence in bipolar disorder, and van Gorp et al [9] noted that number of mood episodes (mania or depression) was negatively correlated with cognition. It also has been observed that severity of prior course of illness in bipolar disorder, along with higher numbers of affective episodes, was associated with lower cognitive performance which relates to the negative neurochemical cascade during affective episodes [10, 11].

With the existence of Bipolar II disorder and traditionally it being considered a less severe form of Bipolar I, the degree of cognitive impairment in these patients has been investigated. Cognitive deficits in the area of working memory and some measures of executive function as well as some impairment in verbal memory have been reported. Studies have detected mild differences in the two sub-types and these differences could be helpful in differentiating between them at times [24].

With increasing prevalence of Bipolar disorder among youths and adolescents there has been increasing interest in the cognitive profiles of pediatric patients with bipolar disorder.

Meta-analysis of the existing literature comparing individuals with BD to healthy controls indicated that the largest differences are observed for measures of verbal memory. Moderate differences were found in the areas of attention, executive functioning, working memory, visual memory, visual perceptual skills, and verbal fluency. Small differences were found for measures of reading, motor speed, and full-scale intelligence quotient [25]. These findings are consistent with previous meta-analyses of the adult BD neurocognitive literature, suggesting that many of the deficits observed in adults are present earlier in the course of the illness [25].

Similarly with increasing life span among bipolar patient, the cognitive impairment in geriatric bipolar patients gets challenging. A study among bipolar geriatric patients found impairments on measures of memory and executive dysfunction among these patients as compared to the controls. The cognitive dysfunction among the geriatric bipolar patients is consistent with those with symptomatic young bipolar patients [26]. These additional cognitive impairments predispose the geriatric bipolar patients towards further functional compromise.

## Functional Impairment

Neurocognitive impairment has been found to limit creativity, work performance, quality of life, selfesteem, and psychosocial functioning substantially in patients with other severe mental illnesses, especially schizophrenia [12]. In bipolar disorder, there has been increasing recognition of more functional impairment particularly with regard to independent living, personal relationships, and vocational success [12]. In one recent review, only 19%–23% of adult bipolar patients were married (versus 60% of adults in the general population); 19%–58% were not living independently and usually resided with family members; 57%–65% were unemployed (versus 6% of the general population); and up to 80% were considered to have at least partial vocational disability [13]. It is highly likely that sustained neurocognitive deficits critically contribute to major occupational, social, and other dysfunctions commonly observed in bipolar patients [13, 14]. The McLean-Harvard First Episode Mania study found that within two years of initial hospitalization for DSM-IV mania or mixed manic-depressive state, only 43% of the patients achieved functional recovery, defined as regaining their own individual premorbid occupational and residential status, whereas 98% no longer met DSM syndromal criteria, and 72% had achieved symptomatic recovery, based on low scores on standard mania and depression ratings [15]. Another study of midcourse bipolar patients found that only 24% achieved similarly defined functional recovery within a year of an index hospitalization for mania or a mixed state. These findings indicate that 57%– 75% of bipolar patients failed to attain functional recovery within 1–2 years after psychiatric hospitalization, even early in the illness course [16]. A significant correlation between impaired neurocognitive performance and lower psychosocial functioning was found in euthymic bipolar patients as well as those in uncertain mood states, usually after adjusting for relevant demographic and clinical variables [12]. These results are consistent with observations that bipolar disorder is often associated with disability, even early in the course of the illness, and suggest that current treatments are of limited value in facilitating functional recovery.

Studies of performance-based assessment in bipolar patient have also shown bipolar patients performed less well on subtests measuring comprehension and planning, financial skills, communication, transportation skills, and household management. For example a recent study of elderly bipolar patients demonstrated that these patients made more errors in medication management, such as taking fewer pills than prescribed [17].

Decreased cognitive functioning and impairment in performing activities of daily living is a well understood concept in patients with schizophrenia. A study by Masuback et al. [18] compared ambulatory patients with schizophrenia (n = 116) to patients with bipolar illness (n = 89) on their performance on a performance based skill assessment scale and neuropsychological assessments. They then related the results of these performance-based assessments to real-world functional milestones, including independence in residential status and employment as well as informant ratings of the ability to perform real-world functional activities in domains of social, residential, and vocational outcomes. They found that bipolar patients were less impaired than people with schizophrenia on the performance based skill assessment scale, had better overall real-world outcomes, and were rated by informants as less impaired in the three functional domains. Dysthymic symptoms were correlated with poorer work and vocational outcomes in the real world. This finding provides direct evidence that residual depression in bipolar disorder may lead to reductions in real-world success in a manner relatively independent of influences on the ability to perform these critical everyday living skills.

In a follow up study [19], an expanded version of this same sample of subjects was used to develop confirmatory path models of the relationships between affective and psychotic symptoms, cognitive impairments, performace based skill assessment scale score, and real-world functional outcomes. In the model predicting real world community activities rated by informants, it was found that performace based skill assessment scale scores were the single best predictor of everyday activities in the real world in both samples. Further, clinical symptoms in both samples were also negatively related to real-world functional outcomes, with amotivation and mania predicting worse functioning in bipolar patients and amotivation and depression predicting worse functioning in schizophrenia.

An important review published by Green at al. [20] reviewed 37 studies examining relationships between various neurocognitive measures and indications of functional status in schizophrenic patients. They found that verbal learning and memory, executive functioning, attention, concentration, or mental tracking, and immediate memory were particularly strongly or consistently associated with functional outcomes. Functioning was assessed as independent living, medication management, social competence, social problem solving, and occupational functioning. Using the similar concept and identifying neuropsychological traits which could help identify deficits leading to functional impairment in bipolar patients will be of immense importance.

## Biological Evidence

Scientific evidence suggests progressive degeneration of the neurons and the glial cells in the central nervous system as the pathological etiology for development of bipolar disorder. Postmortem study in these patients has suggested mitochondrial dysfunction, inflammation, oxidative stress and enzymatic disturbance to further accelerate this degeneration. Radiological studies have described reduction in brain volume and function and abnormalities in specific brain regions which impact the cognitive and affective functioning [21].

Executive dysfunction has been recognized in patient with bipolar disorder as mentioned above. Executive function includes working memory and attention. Working memory tasks such as the digit-sorting task have been shown to reliably increase dorsolateral prefrontal cortex (DLPFC) activity, whereas attentional tasks, including the Stroop interference task and continuous performance task, have implicated DLPFC, dorsal regions of the anterior cingulate gyrus, and ventral prefrontal cortex (VPFC) in healthy controls [22]. Functional studies using an auditory discrimination continuous performance task (CPT) found that depressed bipolar disorder patients had absolute decreased prefrontal cortex and increased, normalized, subcortical (ventral striatum, thalamus, right amygdala) metabolism compared with healthy controls. Degree of depression correlated negatively with prefrontal and positively with anterior paralimbic subcortical metabolism [23].

## Co-Morbidities Contributing to Cognitive Loss

Patients with bipolar disorder are known to be at a higher risk for several medical disorders including diabetes mellitus, hyperlipidemia and other cardiovascular and cerebrovacular diseases. This is in part because of the pharmacotherapy use to treat bipolar disorder and poor life style among these patients. These medical co-morbidities have been known to be associated with a higher risk of cognitive impairment. A study specifically looked for association of diabetes mellitus and cognitive impairment among bipolar patient and found a positive association [27].

Substance use has a high prevalence among patients with bipolar disorder. Co morbid alcohol dependence was a risk factor for patients to develop cognitive dysfunction in an outpatient setting [9]. Further these patients were more impaired in measures of visual memory, verbal recall and executive functioning [28].

Lithium is a mood stabilizer and has been considered a first-line treatment of bipolar disorder. Controversies on the negative impact of lithium on cognition have existed. Conclusions from studies in normal subjects indicate that acute lithium does not affect short-term memory; subchronic administration spares basic short-term memory of ongoing events but higher task demands (as in neuropsychological testing) occasionally reveal mild deficits.

A similar picture emerges with respect to lithium's effects on human long-term recall. In animal studies, subchronic and chronic lithium with clinically relevant serum levels does not affect spatial reference or object recognition memory and actually enhances working memory under certain conditions. This is consistent with recent clinical MRI findings noting improved immediate verbal memory after a 4-year period of lithium treatment, along with MRI evidence of increased hippocampal volume over the same period [31].

A recent meta-analysis assessing the effects of lithium on cognition, demonstrated small impairments in immediate verbal learning and memory and creativity among patients taking lithium. No significant differences were found in delayed verbal memory, visual memory, attentions, executive functioning, processing speed, and psychomotor performance. Healthy subjects gave no indication of altered cognition with short term exposure and affective patients showed adverse effects on immediate verbal learning and memory, creativity and psychomotor performance on long term exposure. Neither short term nor long term lithium treatment was associated with altered delayed verbal memory, visual memory, attention, executive functioning or processing speed [32].

## Cognitive Endophenotype

Endophenotypes are subclinical quantitative traits that are assumed to be located along the pathway between the genotype and the phenotypic disease. Endophenotypes are conceived as subcomponents of the illness, providing an opportunity for a less complex genetic analysis than the diagnostic phenotype.

Endophenotypes should meet certain criteria: they should be associated with illness, they should be heritable, and co-segregate within families with illness. Furthermore, they should be state-independent traits present in illness as well as in remission, and they should be more frequent in unaffected relatives of patients than in general population [29]. Meta-analysis of family studies of bipolar disorder suggests the existence of cognitive endophenotypes for this disorder.

Strong evidence supports executive function and processing speed as endophenotypes marking the vulnerability to bipolar disorder. In bipolar patients, comparisons with healthy controls yielded large effect sizes for executive functions (working memory, executive control, and fluency) and verbal memory.

Medium effect sizes were reported for other tests of executive function (concept shifting, executive control), mental speed, visual memory, and sustained attention. In first-degree relatives, size effects were small, but significantly different from healthy controls for executive function and verbal memory in particular. The authors concluded that executive function and verbal memory are candidate bipolar endophenotypes given large deficits in these domains in bipolar patients and smaller impairments in first-degree relatives [30].

## Rehabilitation Treatment

Pharmacological therapy for cognitive enhancement in Bipolar disorder has been studied; however the evidence supporting the same is not promising. A lot more studies studying pharmacological therapy has been conducted among patients with schizophrenia. Most of these studies have yielded little evidence of superiority [33].

Cognitive rehabilitation has been well studied among patients with schizophrenia with promising results. Cognitive remediation typically consists of computerized cognitive training or non-computerized drill and practice exercises, varying in frequency and duration. A recent meta-analysis found cognitive remediation to be associated with significant, though modest, improvements in cognitive performance and psychosocial functioning, as well as measurable general symptomatic improvement [34]. Specific improvements in attention, processing speed, verbal learning and memory, visual memory, reasoning, and problem solving and psychosocial functioning were demonstrated. In these trials, improved psychosocial functioning included obtaining work or taking on more competitive jobs, reporting higher quality of and satisfaction with interpersonal relationships, and better ability to solve interpersonal problems. Furthermore, as reviewed in the meta-analysis, improved performance in cognitive abilities was maintained at a similar magnitude during follow-up, averaging eight months in at least six longitudinal studies.

Since cognitive remediation improved both cognitive performance and functional outcomes in schizophrenia patients, it may also have analogous benefits in bipolar patients. In schizophrenia treatment research, multiple interventions have been delivered to improve vocational outcomes. The most common of these is referred to as supported employment, which is an intervention aimed at obtaining and sustaining employment. Methods in this intervention include job interview practice, intensive interviewing, job coach assistance, and individualized programs of support. This intervention has obtained the status of an evidence-based intervention in people with schizophrenia, leading to consistent but moderate gains in employment success.

One study which directly compared bipolar and schizophrenia patients on the employment outcomes and total service costs over a 10-year follow-up period, found that people with bipolar disorder were significantly more likely to have achieved steady work over the period, with significantly lower total service costs as well [35]. These data suggest that supported employment programs might provide a substantial benefit to people with bipolar disorder [33].

## Conclusion

Much greater development in the field of neurocognition is expected in the next decade; however the current existing knowledge should influence patient care. The evidence of neurocognitive deficits warrants routine neuropsychological testing in evaluation of patient with bipolar disorder.

This testing could help us better assess the prognosis and the outcome for the patient and also decide the level of support needed in the community. Neurocognitive deficits could be a factor influencing poor adherence to recommended care and understanding these deficits could guide us deliver better care to these patients. Therapy addressing cognitive rehabilitation should have been shown to be beneficial in patient with chronic schizophrenia and needs to be included in treatment plans to improve psychosocial and vocational training [1].

## References


[1] Manove E, Levy B. Cognitive impairment in bipolar disorder: an overview. *Postgrad. Med.* 2010; 122(4):7-16.

[2] Malhi GS, Ivanovski B, Szekeres V, et al. Bipolar disorder: it's all in your mind? The neuropsychological profile of a biological disorder. *Can. J. Psychiatry* 2004; 49:813–9.

[3] Bora E, Yucel M, Pantelis C. Cognitive endophenotypes of bipolar disorder: a meta-analysis of neuropsychological deficits in euthymic patients and their first-degree relatives. *J. Affect. Disord.* 2009; 113: 1–20.

[4] Arts B, Jabben N, Krabbendam L, van Os J. Metaanalyses of cognitive functioning in euthymic bipolar patients and their first-degree relatives. *Psychol. Med.* 2008; 38: 771–785.

[5] Robinson LJ, Thompson JM, Gallagher P et al. A metaanalysis of cognitive deficits in euthymic patients with bipolar disorder. *J. Affect. Disord.* 2006; 93: 105–115.

[6] Martı´nez-Ara´n A, Vieta E, Reinares M et al. Cognitive function across manic or hypomanic, depressed, and euthymic states in bipolar disorder. *Am. J. Psychiatry* 2004; 161: 262–270.

[7] Bearden CE, Hoffman KM, Cannon TD. The neuropsychology and neuroanatomy of bipolar affective disorder: a critical review. *Bipolar Disord.* 2001; 3:106–50.

[8] Tham A, Engelbrektson K, Mathe AA, et al. Impaired neuropsychological performance in euthymic patients with recurring mood disorders. *J. Clin. Psychiatry* 1997; 58:26–9.

[9] van Gorp WG, Altshuler L, Theberge DC, et al. Cognitive impairment in euthymic bipolar patients with and without prior alcohol dependence. A preliminary study. *Arch. Gen. Psychiatry* 1998; 55:41–6.

[10] Denicoff KD, Ali SO, Mirsky AF, et al. Relationship between prior course of illness and neuropsychological functioning in patients with bipolar disorder. *J. Affect. Disord.* 1999; 56: 67–73.

[11] Altshuler LL. Bipolar disorder: are repeated episodes associated with neuroanatomic and cognitive changes? Biol Psychiatry 1993; 33:563–5.

[12] Wingo AP, Harvey PD, Baldessarini RJ. Neurocognitive impairment in bipolar disorder patients: functional implications. *Bipolar Disord.* 2009; 11(2):113-25.

[13] Huxley N, Baldessarini RJ. Disability and its treatment in bipolar disorder patients. *Bipolar Disord.* 2007; 9: 183–196.

[14] Altshuler L, Tekell J, Biswas K et al. Executive function and employment status among veterans with bipolar disorder. *Psychiatric Serv.* 2007; 58: 1441–1447.

[15] Tohen M, Zarate CA Jr, Hennen J et al. McLean- Harvard First-Episode Mania Study: prediction of recovery and first recurrence. *Am. J. Psychiatry* 2003; 160: 2099–2107.

[16] Keck PE Jr, McElroy SL, Strakowski SM et al. Twelvemonth outcome of patients with bipolar disorder following hospitalization for a manic or mixed episode. *Am. J. Psychiatry* 1998; 155: 646–652.

[17] Gildengers AG, Butters MA, Chisholm D et al. Cognitive functioning and instrumental activities of daily living in late-life bipolar disorder. *Am. J. Geriatr. Psychiatry* 2007; 15: 174–179.

[18] Mausbach BT, Harvey PD, Pulver AE et al. Relationship of the Brief UCSD Performance-based Skills Assessment (UPSA-B) to multiple indicators of functioning in people with schizophrenia and bipolar disorder. *Bipolar Disord.* 2010; 12: 45–55.

[19] Bowie CR, Depp CA, McGrath JA et al. Prediction of real world functional impairments in community-dwelling schizophrenia and bipolar disorder patients. *Am. J. Psychiatry*. 2010; 167(9):1116-24.

[20] Green MF, Kern RS, Braff DL, Mintz J. Neurocognitive deficits and functional outcome in schizophrenia: are we measuring the ''right stuff''? *Schizophr. Bull.* 2000; 26: 119– 136.

[21] Kucyi A, Alsuwaidan MT, Liauw SS, McIntyre RS. Aerobic physical exercise as a possible treatment for neurocognitive dysfunction in bipolar disorder. *Postgrad. Med.* 2010; 122(6):107-16.

[22] Keener MT, Phillips ML. Neuroimaging in bipolar disorder: a critical review of current findings. *Curr. Psychiatry Rep.* 200;9(6):512-20.

[23] Ketter TA, Kimbrell TA, George MS, et al. Effects of mood and subtype on cerebral glucose metabolism in treatment-resistant bipolar disorder. *Biol. Psychiatry* 2001; 49:97–109.

[24] Solé B, Martínez-Arán A, Torrent C, Bonnin CM, Reinares M, Popovic D, Sánchez-Moreno J, Vieta E. Are bipolar II patients cognitively impaired? A systematic review. *Psychol. Med.* 2011; 41(9):1791-803.

[25] Joseph MF, Frazier TW, Youngstrom EA, Soares JC. A quantitative and qualitative review of neurocognitive performance in pediatric bipolar disorder. *J. Child Adolesc. Psychopharmacol.* 2008; 18(6): 595-605.

[26] Young RC, Murphy CF, Heo M, Schulberg HC, Alexopoulos GS. Cognitive impairment in bipolar disorder in old age: literature review and findings in manic patients. *J. Affect. Disord.* 2006; 92(1):125-31.

[27] Tsai SY, Lee HC, Chen CC, Huang YL. Cognitive impairment in later life in patients with early-onset bipolar disorder. *Bipolar Disord.* 2007 Dec; 9(8):868-75.

[28] Levy B, Monzani BA, Stephansky MR, Weiss RD. Neurocognitive impairment in patients with co-occurring bipolar disorder and alcohol dependence upon discharge from inpatient care. *Psychiatry Res*. 2008 Oct 30; 161(1):28-35.

[29] Latalova K, Prasko J, Diveky T, Velartova H. Cognitive impairment in bipolar disorder. *Biomed. Pap. Med. Fac. Univ. Palacky Olomouc. Czech. Repub.* 2011 Mar; 155(1):19-26.

[30] Arts B, Jabben N, Krabbendam L, van OJ. Meta-analyses of cognitive functioning in euthymic bipolar patients and their first-degree relatives. *Psychol. Med.* 2008; 38(6):771-785.

[31] Tsaltas E, Kontis D, Boulougouris V, Papadimitriou GN. Lithium and cognitive enhancement: leave it or take it? *Psychopharmacology* (Berl). 2009 Jan; 202(1-3):457-76.

[32] Wingo AP, Wingo TS, Harvey PD, Baldessarini RJ. Effects of lithium on cognitive performance: a meta-analysis. *J. Clin. Psychiatry*. 2009 Nov; 70(11):1588-97.

[33] Harvey PD, Wingo AP, Burdick KE, Baldessarini RJ. Cognition and disability in bipolar disorder: lessons from schizophrenia research. *Bipolar Disord.* 2010; 12(4):364-75.

[34] McGurk SR, Twamley EW, Sitzer DI, McHugo GJ, Mueser KT. Meta-analysis of cognitive remediation in schizophrenia. *Am. J. Psychiatry* 2007; 164: 1791–1802.

[35] Bush PW, Drake RE, Xie H, McHugo GJ, Haslett WR. The long-term impact of employment on mental health service use and costs for persons with severe mental illness. *Psychiatr. Serv.* 2009; 60: 1024–1031.

# Index

## A

## G



## H

## I



## J



## K



## L

## M

## Q



## R

## S